Living with Lymphoma

Living with Lymphoma

Lymphoma

A Patient's Guide

Elizabeth M. Adler, Ph.D.

Introduction by
Michael R. Bishop, M.D.

THE JOHNS HOPKINS UNIVERSITY PRESS
Baltimore

Note to the reader. This book is not meant to substitute for medical care of people with lymphoma, and treatment should not be based solely on its contents. If you have lymphoma, you need to be under a physician's care. Lymphoma is a complex group of diseases, and the best treatment for any one person may be entirely different from the best treatment for someone else. Treatment must be developed in a dialogue between the individual and his or her physician. This book has been written to help with that dialogue.

Drug dosage. The author and publisher have made reasonable efforts to determine that the selection and dosage of drugs discussed in this text conform to the practices of the general medical community. The medications described do not necessarily have specific approval by the U.S. Food and Drug Administration for use in the diseases and dosages for which they are recommended. In view of ongoing research, changes in governmental regulations, and the constant flow of information relating to drug therapy and drug reactions, the reader is urged to check the package insert of each drug for any change in indications and dosage and for warnings and precautions. This is particularly important when the recommended agent is a new and/or infrequently used drug.

© 2005 The Johns Hopkins University Press
All rights reserved. Published 2005
Printed in the United States of America on acid-free paper
9 8 7 6 5 4 3 2

The Johns Hopkins University Press
2715 North Charles Street
Baltimore, Maryland 21218-4363
www.press.jhu.edu

Library of Congress Cataloging-in-Publication Data

Adler, Elizabeth M.
    Living with lymphoma : a patient's guide / Elizabeth M. Adler ; introduction by Michael R. Bishop.
        p. cm.
    Includes bibliographic references and index.
    ISBN 0-8018-8179-X (hardcover : alk. paper) — ISBN 0-8018-8180-3 (pbk. : alk. paper)
    1. Lymphomas—Popular works. I. Title.
    RC280.L9A26 2005
    616.99'446—dc22
                                                                                2004028264
A catalog record for this book is available from the British Library.

Illustrations by Jacqueline Schaffer

The excerpt from the poem "Cancer Garden," on page 125, is from *Dream of Order* © 1997 by Thomas Avena. Published by Mercury House, San Francisco, California, and reprinted by permission.

For

Ruthie & Eddie

& for Paul

Midway along the journey of our life

I awoke to find myself in a dark wood.

—Dante Alighieri, opening lines of *The Divine Comedy*

Contents

🌿🌿 PART III

Understanding Lymphoma 231

Preface

Journeys in a Dark Wood

In November 1996, I was diagnosed with non-Hodgkin lymphoma, a form of cancer that affects the cells of the immune system. I had recently accepted a new position at a liberal arts college and moved from Boston to western Massachusetts. I'd been very busy settling into my new and challenging job and hadn't yet developed a strong local network of friends. As a neurobiologist, I was familiar with research suggesting that a good social support system could be invaluable to cancer survivors (see Chapter 7). But there was little available in the way of support groups in my community, and weak and vulnerable to infection, I was reluctant to venture out unnecessarily during the harsh New England winter.

My brother came to the rescue. Shortly after I was diagnosed with lymphoma, he discovered a computerized mailing list devoted to people with non-Hodgkin lymphoma (NHL; lymphoma is broadly subdivided into Hodgkin lymphoma and NHL: this book addresses both types of lymphoma). This is one of several on-line support groups available to people with lymphoma. There is also a Hodgkin lymphoma mailing list, several more specialized NHL mailing lists for people with different kinds of NHL, and a more general list for people with any of the blood-cell-derived cancers: leukemia, lymphoma, or multiple myeloma. For the next year, the NHL mailing list formed my online support group.

The NHL mailing list, which was founded and managed by Scott Pallack, a

Las Vegas cabdriver and computer expert who had been diagnosed with NHL several months before I was, put me in electronic correspondence with several hundred people who either had NHL or were taking care of someone who had lymphoma. During the year I was on the NHL mailing list, I was struck by how little most of us knew about this disease and also by how the same questions surfaced again and again as new people joined the list. The main purpose of this book is to provide answers to the questions that puzzled so many of us as we learned to cope with lymphoma.

I wanted to provide detailed information about lymphoma: its symptoms, diagnosis, and treatment. I also wanted to give readers enough background in biology, and on how biology applies to lymphoma therapy, to be able to read and evaluate articles in the medical literature by themselves. I hope that this information will help readers to understand their own situations and options for treatment better and that it will also help them formulate questions to ask their physicians about their own specific treatment plan.

A note on coping strategies

One of my major strategies in coping with the disease and its treatment was to maintain a sense of humor. I don't think that I could have remained psychologically intact during the year after my diagnosis if I hadn't tried to find a lighter side to things. The idea of laughing in the face of death is something that many people who have never faced a life-threatening diagnosis find inconceivable. Shortly after I completed therapy, my husband, Paul, and I went to an end-of-the-year party for junior faculty. This was the first social occasion I'd attended in quite a while, and seeing the "$30,000 haircut" chemotherapy had given me was the first indication many of my colleagues had that I'd been ill.

Talking with my friends at the party, I was struck by how many of them felt that they needed to assume a sober and serious attitude around me. Over and over they asked the same question: "You seem so cheerful. How can you possibly be *cheerful*—and telling *jokes* about your situation—at a time like this?"

I had no real answer to give them, except to say that it was the only way I could have survived. I've been aware that I had cancer every hour of every day of the eight years since my diagnosis. It's not something you tend to forget. But living in a constant state of anxiety and fear would be intolerable. Developing a sense of humor about the disease is one way of tolerating a potentially intolerable situation. As the great physicist Niels Bohr is reported to have said, "There are some things so serious you have to laugh at them." And I've found that, once past the initial shock of the diagnosis, a surprising number of cancer survivors I know seem to have developed the same sort of black humor as a similar sort of psychological survival strategy.

The humor that you will find here and there throughout this book is meant to reflect the philosophy that it is preferable to laugh occasionally, even when faced with an overwhelmingly frightening situation, than it is to give in to despair. It is not meant to minimize or belittle the situation of anyone who has ever faced a diagnosis of cancer.

How to use this book

I wrote this book to provide information for anyone with lymphoma as well as for those who care about someone with lymphoma and may be caring for him or her. For me, one of the most distressing aspects of being diagnosed with lymphoma was the sense that I'd lost control over my life. This book was written based on the idea that if information is knowledge and knowledge is power, then anyone who's been diagnosed with cancer deserves a little empowerment.

The book is divided into three parts: "Living with Lymphoma," "Treating Lymphoma," and "Understanding Lymphoma." At different points in your journey with lymphoma, you're likely to be interested in different sorts of information. People who have recently been diagnosed with lymphoma are likely to be most interested in the first part of the book, "Living with Lymphoma." That section is intended to help you make sense of what can be a perplexing situation by discussing and explaining many of the experiences you're likely to have. It is concerned with your experiences before and during diagnosis and treatment.

Chapter 1 is an introduction to the disease. In this chapter, I tell my personal story of developing and being diagnosed with lymphoma, explain the basics of what lymphoma is, and introduce the two main forms of the disease—Hodgkin lymphoma and non-Hodgkin lymphoma (NHL). I also talk very briefly about the prevalence of lymphoma in the United States today and how this has risen over the past thirty years.

Chapter 2 deals with the initial discovery that you have lymphoma. In it I describe the symptoms that are frequently associated with lymphoma as well as the various diagnostic procedures you may encounter during this time. This chapter will be helpful in providing a general sense of what's going on and in giving you an understanding of what all the tests are supposed to show and why you need to have them. You may be interested in reading about the various procedures you're scheduled to undergo, so you know what to expect beforehand.

In the second part of the book, "Treating Lymphoma," I discuss different forms of therapy. This section is likely to be of interest to people who are about to begin treatment and to people who are considering various treatment possibilities. This is the largest section in the book because it covers all the different forms of lymphoma therapy commonly used today. I explain how these forms of therapy work, as well as what it's like to experience them.

In Chapters 3, 4, and 5, I discuss the mainstays of conventional lymphoma therapy—chemotherapy, radiation, and monoclonal-antibody-based therapies. In Chapter 5, I also cover various promising, but still experimental, forms of treatment. These include various therapies now in clinical trials, such as angiogenesis inhibitors, lymphoma vaccines, and antisense treatment. In Chapter 6, I discuss autologous and allogeneic stem cell transplants as well as the newer, reduced-intensity (or non-myeloablative) stem cell transplant. Although stem cell transplants always involve chemotherapy, and sometimes radiation and/or monoclonal antibody therapy as well, they are rarely (if ever) the first form of treatment you are likely to encounter and differ enough from the basic procedures using chemotherapy and radiation to warrant a separate discussion. Finally, in Chapter 7, I discuss unconventional cancer therapies, including nutritional, psychological, and pharmacologically oriented approaches. While a complete discussion of unconventional cancer therapies is beyond the scope of this book, I hope the material I provide here will at least give you a reasonable introduction to this complex and controversial area.

The section on treating lymphoma should be helpful in terms of letting you know what to expect if you're scheduled to undergo a certain form of treatment—say you've been diagnosed with Hodgkin lymphoma and have been told you're about to start a form of chemotherapy called *ABVD*. I talk about the mechanisms of action and side effects of many of the commonly used antilymphoma drugs, as well as describing some of the more common regimens used against different forms of lymphoma.

If your oncologist decides that the best course of action for you at present is to defer therapy and go on "watch-and-wait," you have a breathing period. You may be interested in taking this time to learn about different therapeutic approaches to your form of lymphoma—and perhaps in thinking about the possibility of participating in a clinical trial of one of the exciting new experimental therapies. Learning about the different forms of treatment around will allow you to discuss your options more knowledgeably with your physician when the time comes for treatment. Moreover, if you do decide to opt for a clinical trial, you'll have the time to seek out the people involved in developing these new therapeutic approaches.

If you've already had lymphoma for a while and are partway through a course of treatment—or, better yet, in remission—you may find that you're interested in learning more about the biology of the disease. In this case, you're more likely to want to explore the last part of the book, "Understanding Lymphoma." You may want to learn about the different types of lymphoma and what distinguishes one type from another, or you may be interested in understanding what's gone wrong in lymphoma in the context of normal lymphocytic function. You may find yourself wondering about the causes of lymphoma or why, say, follicular lymphoma is so different from Burkitt lymphoma.

In contrast to the first two parts of the book, the third part is less concerned with the practicalities of experiencing tests and treatments and more concerned with understanding the disease. It gives you a basic understanding of the biology of lymphoma—from basic cell biology and what goes wrong in cancer, to the biology of the normal immune response, to understanding the different types of lymphoma.

Chapter 8 provides a background in modern cell biology: I explain the basics of how cells grow and divide—and what goes wrong with the rebellious cells that give rise to cancer. Chapter 9 describes the immune system—the part of our bodies that protects us from disease. Lymphoma is a disease of a type of cell called a *lymphocyte*. Lymphocytes are key players in the immune response, and understanding their normal function—and how they're supposed to grow and develop—has been critical to our understanding the twisted lymphocytes that give rise to lymphoma. Since many cancer therapies influence the immune system, and because some of the newer treatment approaches *use* it, it's helpful to have a basic understanding of immune function to understand how such therapies might affect us.

Chapter 10 gives a very detailed description of the many different types of lymphoma. It explains how they are classified and why different forms of lymphoma are treated differently. This chapter covers the specific details of how lymphoma is staged to determine how far it has spread in your body. Finally, in Chapter 11, I discuss various theories about what might cause lymphoma in the first place, considering the possible roles of viruses, diet, and substances in the environment. After reading the last section of the book, not only will you have developed a basic understanding of the disease, but you'll also be equipped to read and understand any article in the medical literature that deals with lymphoma.

A word of caution

If you have cancer, your *most* important source of specific information on your disease and treatment options is your oncologist or your hematologist. An oncologist is a doctor who has received specialized training in the treatment of cancer, and a hematologist is a doctor who has received specialized training in diseases of the blood. Both are qualified to treat lymphoma. Lymphoma, like any other form of cancer, is a very serious illness, and it's very important for those of us who've been diagnosed with it to be under the care of an appropriate physician. And your oncologist or hematologist should *always* be your primary source of medical advice and information.

If, for some reason, you feel uncomfortable with your physician's treatment plan, it might make sense to consult another physician. General information from books like this, or advice from well-intentioned friends, is *never* an adequate substitute for a good physician. This book was up to date at the time it was written; however, our current approaches to cancer therapy are advancing at an explosive rate. New therapies that are just looming on the clinical horizon as I write this may be in common use by the time you read it.

Moreover, this book can only provide general information, as I am a neurobiologist, not a physician or health care provider. Your physician will be familiar with all the specific details of your particular situation and should know which approaches promise to be most successful right now and which are most appropriate for you as an individual.

However, many physicians are extremely busy, and some of them feel unable to take the time to explain background material and general information that isn't specifically relevant to your treatment. And many patients feel shy about asking too many questions—particularly if they are uncomfortable with their understanding of the "basics." This book isn't intended to supplant the information you get from your physician in any way. It *is* intended to provide a background on lymphoma and lymphoma therapy and to familiarize you with various diagnostic tests and therapeutic treatments that you may undergo.

Introduction

By Michael R. Bishop, M.D.

There is nothing that prepares an individual for the diagnosis of lymphoma—or any cancer, for that matter. When a new diagnosis of lymphoma is shared with patient, family, or friends, the response varies with each person who is hearing it. The perspective that matters *the most*, of course, is that of the person who is diagnosed with the lymphoma. The perspective of the treating physician is generally limited to technical facts and the physician's professional experience. Usually the physician can only imagine what patients and their families are going through—although a few of my colleagues either have had someone close to them experience, or have themselves experienced, being diagnosed and treated for cancer. All of them bring those experiences into their practice, but they are only a small minority of treating physicians.

In lymphoma, the treating physicians are usually medical oncologists and hematologists. They attempt to educate the patient and recommend an individualized treatment plan in a manner that they feel most comfortable with. This manner varies from physician to physician. Some physicians are very businesslike; they present just the minimal facts with a clear, straightforward treatment plan. I know many patients who prefer not to know statistics, prognosis, or other options. They just want someone to take control. Then there are physicians who provide detailed information relative to both prognosis and all available treatment options and, after having informed the patient of the treatment options and their relative efficacy and toxicities, leave the decision to the patient. Most often the physician's approach is somewhere in the middle. He or she wants to provide enough information about the patient's diagnosis to permit the patient to make an informed decision about treatment options, but not so much information that it is overwhelming. The physician will make a treatment recommendation that he or she thinks will provide the best chance of benefiting the patient, taking into account the patient's diagnosis, prognostic features, and overall physical condition, as well as the physician's perception of how much risk the patient is willing to accept relative to each treatment available and appropriate for that individual.

No matter which approach is taken and how much time is spent at the initial visit, this experience is nearly always overwhelming. No one can take in all the information provided by the physician, despite the best attempts to explain it in the clearest, simplest, and most direct way possible. Even if the patient has the most compassionate and articulate physician in the world, it is almost impossible for the patient to come away feeling that she knows everything there is to know about her disease, that all her questions have been answered, and that she is fully confident she completely understands the risks and benefits of the treatment plan presented to her. I often start my second visit with a patient by asking him to review with me what we talked about at our first visit. It is not uncommon for a patient to say, "It was so much information and so overwhelming, I barely took in half of what you told me."

Despite the physician's best efforts, there is never enough time to discuss everything that is important to an individual. In addition, because this initial experience can often be intimidating, it is often difficult for the patient to grasp what is being said. Finally, some patients are reluctant to ask questions of their physicians, not wanting to sound unintelligent or to risk insulting the person who is about to treat them. For all these reasons, patients wanting to know what it is like to be diagnosed and go through treatment for lymphoma do the logical thing and turn to the true authorities: *other patients with lymphomas.*

There are wonderful patient-derived resources available on lymphoma, such as newsletters, support groups, chat rooms. There are even a number of books written by patients providing essential information relative to the diagnosis and treatment of cancer. However, this book by Elizabeth Adler is unique in several ways. First, it deals solely with the diagnosis of lymphoma. Second, it provides comprehensive information about biology, diagnosis, staging, and treatment.

Third, the organization is different from that of other scientific texts. Fourth, and most important, it comes from Elizabeth's perspective as a lymphoma patient and survivor.

Lymphoma is not a single disease but a heterogeneous group of disorders that are linked because they originate in lymphocytes, the major components of the immune system (see Chapter 9). The differences in prognosis and treatment among the types of lymphoma are very important for the person with lymphoma. A simple approach is first to divide lymphomas into Hodgkin lymphoma (also known as Hodgkin's disease) and non-Hodgkin lymphoma (NHL). With rare exceptions, the different types of Hodgkin lymphoma are basically treated the same. The most important aspects of prognosis and selecting a specific treatment for Hodgkin lymphomas are, first, stage and, second, presence or absence of "B" symptoms (such as significant weight loss, drenching night sweats, and fever). In marked contrast, the specific type of NHL is the most important aspect of prognosis and treatment selection, although stage and to some degree "B" symptoms are also important factors in the decision-making process. The easy way to think of the NHLs is to divide them into low-, intermediate-, and high-grade categories as described by the old National Cancer Institute (NCI) Working Formulation. This categorization is useful because it provides an easy way of thinking about the biology and relative treatment options for each category and can be applied to the majority of NHLs. However, it has severe limitations for a few specific diagnoses (such as mantle cell lymphoma), which have extremely different prognoses and treatment options than other lymphomas listed in that specific category. For this reason it is very important to understand that all lymphomas and their respective treatments are not the same, and each patient needs to focus on his own specific diagnosis and stage.

I am struck by how this text is organized. Almost all medical texts, regardless of disease, generally have a standard format. They first deal with general biology and how it relates to the disease being discussed (for example, normal lung function and asthma). Elizabeth has taken the opposite approach, which, I think, is the most appropriate for patients. It may be interesting to know the biology of your disease at some point, but if I was just finding out my diagnosis, prevalence of the disease in Antarctica would be the last thought on my mind. I would want to know my prognosis and treatment options; I can read about the rest later.

Even though the format is different, the content is as comprehensive as the majority of medical texts that you may come across. The description of mechanisms of action for individual chemotherapeutic agents and lymphoma classifications is extremely detailed yet easily readable. The information is presented in such a manner that even if you have a limited scientific background, you are provided with a sufficient understanding of your respective disease and treatment, especially in regard to potential toxicities, to have an informed conversation with your treating physician. For those who have a deeper scientific background and want greater detail, especially in regard to chemotherapeutic mechanisms and biology of lymphoma, this text provides sufficient data to meet the needs of most physicians.

Most important, the data are shared from a patient's perspective. The text is laced with humor, but this is balanced with deep self-reflection. Not all of Elizabeth's experiences were pleasant or "character building." She reflects on the experiences of her diagnosis and treatments and the effects of treatment with a tremendous amount of candor. She appropriately points out in almost every case that the side effect or situation that she either did or did not experience may or may not necessarily be experienced by others. *It cannot be overemphasized that the side effects or benefits of a specific treatment are different with every single patient.* For example, in most situations nausea can be completely avoided or significantly reduced in over 80 percent of individuals receiving chemotherapy; however, that still leaves 10 to 20 percent of patients who will experience some degree of nausea. Unfortunately, most of the time it is not possible to predict who will or will not have toxicity from a specific treatment. Be careful not to assume that the experience of others with whom you may communicate will be the same for you, positively or negatively.

AS I WAS READING THE DRAFTS OF THIS TEXT, I wondered what I could do to complement this outstanding collection of information. The idea that came to me was to describe how I would approach a physician to discuss the treatment options for a specific cancer based on my own personal experiences with patients. Here are my suggestions. First, come to your initial consultation prepared and relatively familiar with your diagnosis. I would recommend that you obtain relatively general and basic information about your diagnosis at first, as the specific details can be overwhelming and frightening. Pamphlets from the American Cancer Society and the Leukemia and Lymphoma Society of America provide adequate basic information. Most patients are already aware of their diagnosis when they are referred to a hematologist or a medical oncologist, and therefore much of this initial visit is generally spent explaining the specifics of the disease, its prognosis, and the possible treatment options.

(1)   Be prepared to take home as much information as possible from your initial visit by taking notes and using a tape recorder. A good physician will readily assent to have the conversation recorded. The amount of information that is provided in this initial consultation can be large and overwhelming. As noted above, the statement I hear most often from patients is that the information was all so much, the patient just couldn't remember everything. A tape recorder makes it possible for you to slowly go back and listen to the conversation at your own pace. It is important to bring at least one person along with you, someone who can also closely listen and preferably take notes. An additional person, be it a family member, spouse, or close friend, provides three important advantages. First, this person can take notes while you concentrate on what is being said; or, if you prefer to take notes also, he can "fill in the blanks" of your notes. Second, an additional person can help in reviewing the notes and tapes and might provide a different interpretation of the same statement. Third, this person brings a semi-objective perspective to the discussion. She obviously cares about you, but as she herself does not have the cancer, she can be relatively more objective. However, patients must be careful not to let other people project their own feelings and opinions upon them.

(2)   The next important thing to do is to ask questions. I would advise you to come prepared with a list of questions, but reserve them for the end of the initial consultation, as I think you will be surprised how many of your questions will be answered during the course of your initial consultation. Two things needed to be pointed out in regard to your questions. First, you should write down all your questions. Very often, when a patient has the opportunity to ask questions, he will say, "I had a lot of questions but now I have forgotten them." Try to avoid this situation by writing down your questions. Second, and more important, all questions are important; there are no "dumb" or "stupid" questions. I often find that the questions that begin with "I know this is a dumb question, but . . ." are the most poignant and relevant questions to a patient's particular situation. The rule of thumb is that if something is bothering you, even in the slightest, then it is important.

(3)   Finally, it is extremely important to realize that it is only in very rare situations that decisions need to be made immediately. Even though most patients want to have started treatment yesterday, the initiation of therapy can be delayed in most cases without any effect on outcome. You should take your time, review all the information, and address all your questions before making any decision in regard to treatment. I tell all my patients that they need to go home, review

everything we have discussed, discuss our consultation with their family and their primary physician, and then write down all their questions and come back to have those questions answered or to review options again before making any decision about therapy.

Sometimes this process is not sufficient, and patients need to seek a second opinion. If you are not comfortable with a physician's recommendations, do not hesitate to seek a second opinion. A good physician will not be insulted by your desire to seek a second opinion and will often help facilitate setting up the consultation. I would be wary of a physician who attempts to dissuade you from seeking another opinion. In the majority of cases, the second (or third) opinion will echo what you heard before, or you may hear of an alternative option or a different perspective on a treatment option that was presented before. It is important for you to know that different physicians will have different approaches to the same problem. This is generally a reflection of how aggressive they are relative to treatment.

My particular approach to the treatment of lymphoma is very aggressive. I view the treatment of lymphoma as a war, with the ultimate goal being cure. In that process of attempting to achieve cure, I will often recommend treatments that are potentially associated with a higher incidence and severity of toxicity that may be associated with an increased risk of death but offer a higher chance of cure. At the same time, I present treatment options that may be less toxic but that offer less of a chance of cure. As long as I am relatively assured that patients are well aware of the potential risks and benefits of a specific treatment and that all their treatment options have been presented, I am comfortable with providing the aggressive treatment option to them. Alternatively, some physicians may be less aggressive or believe that the toxicities of a specific treatment do not justify any potential benefit. When there is a difference in opinion, it is imperative to ask the physician why he or she specifically disagrees with an alternative recommendation. It may be necessary to return to the initial consulting physician or even seek a third opinion to get answers to satisfy all your questions.

The bottom line is that the choice of treatment is your decision. Probably the question I am most often asked by a patient or a family member is "Dr. Bishop, what would you do if this was your wife or mother?" My standard response is "That is not a fair question." Now, I can visualize all of you readers stopping right there and proceeding to read Elizabeth's excellent book, but, please, give me a chance to explain. My mother and my wife are two different people. My immediate response would be selfish, in that I would want both of them to have the treatment that would provide them with the best opportunity to be with me as long as possible, regardless of risk. However, is that what they want or are willing to accept? My mother, who is a cancer survivor, tends to be very aggressive, but she was unsure about accepting a particular surgical procedure because of the effect it would have on her quality of life. My wife, whom I love dearly, I am relatively sure would do anything that would provide her with the opportunity to see our daughter grow up. However, I would do the same thing that I do for all my patients, and that is present all options with their risks and benefits and let them choose based upon their own personalities and beliefs. Usually I provide my patients with an opinion as to what options I think are reasonable or unreasonable, but sometimes, especially with recurrent disease, there are no clear options, and the decision ultimately falls upon the patient, with sympathetic and compassionate guidance from the treating physician.

My mantra for all my patients is that the best patient is the educated patient. By "educated" I mean knowledgeable about your specific disease and treatment options. It has nothing to do with level of education. The more you know about your disease and your treatment options, the easier it is to make treatment decisions. The more you know about your specific treatment and its toxicities, the better overall experience you generally will have. You will be able to help identify potential problems earlier—and the earlier problems are identified, the easier they are to take care of.

The book that Elizabeth Adler has written for your use is invaluable in helping you understand the entire lymphoma experience. It is a stand-alone text for lymphoma patients. Keep it at your side along with all the questions you have (written down, of course), and come prepared to every visit, knowledgeable about your disease and your treatment.

You need to be an active participant to enhance the chances of successful treatment of your disease. Knowledge is power. Elizabeth Adler has provided you with an invaluable resource to ensure that you are knowledgeable about your disease. Congratulations, Elizabeth.

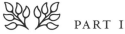 PART I

Living with Lymphoma

Learning you have cancer is never easy. Different people have different reactions: some are devastated, while others are angry; some are overwhelmed with a sense of loss, while others feel greater appreciation for what they do have; some are determined to fight to the utmost, while others resolve to accept whatever happens with grace. All of these reactions are normal and are influenced by your personal style, by where you are in your life, by the degree of support you receive from others, and by your perceptions of your chances for long-term survival. Nearly everyone, though, finds a cancer diagnosis scary and discovers that it creates significant changes in his or her life.

When I was diagnosed with lymphoma, I felt shocked and confused. The diagnosis seemed terrifying but oddly unreal. Adding to my sense of unreality was my uncertainty about exactly what lymphoma was—I didn't have the same sense of familiarity with my lymphoid tissues as with, say, my stomach or my lungs—and what was likely to happen. Like many people, I regained a sense of control over my life by learning everything I could about the disease and its treatment.

Part I of this book is intended to ease the transition as you learn to cope with the changes that take place in your life following a diagnosis of cancer. In Chapter 1, I describe my own experience with diagnosis, introduce the group of diseases known as "lymphoma," and give some general information on the prevalence of lymphoma in the United States. In Chapter 2, I discuss the events that are likely to surround the diagnosis: the symptoms that announce "something's wrong" and the various medical tests and procedures intended to give your doctor as much information as possible about the disease so it can be most effectively treated.

CHAPTER I

What Is Lymphoma?

My story

I am a neurobiologist. In 1994, I obtained an academic position at a liberal arts college in a beautiful area in the Berkshire Mountains of western Massachusetts. After many years spent working in the laboratory, I found the combination of teaching and doing research to be very challenging: both exciting and stressful. I was putting in sixteen-hour workdays and going short on sleep to get everything done. I lost weight, and I felt tired. At the end of May, after the academic year was over, I got married. In fact, the ceremony took place at the same time as the final exam for a large introductory course that Paul, my husband, and I had taught together. We spent our official honeymoon grading exam papers, but we were able to take a few weeks off later in the summer after I got my laboratory set up.

In November 1995, I had elective gynecological surgery to clean up some fibroids and endometriosis that my doctor and I thought might be interfering with my ability to become pregnant. A month later, after I passed my postsurgical checkup, Paul and I went out to dinner to celebrate. I got food poisoning. After several days of uncontrollable vomiting, I ended up in an emergency room on Christmas Eve. Unexpectedly, the blood test taken in the emergency room, to see if all that vomiting had disturbed my blood chemistry values, showed that I was marginally anemic—my blood iron levels were a little bit low. This anemia could not be attributed to vomiting.

I was very surprised: through multiple bouts of fibroids (accompanied by very heavy menstrual periods) and three gynecological surgeries, I had never shown the slightest tendency toward anemia. Indeed, my surgeon liked to say that my postsurgical blood iron levels were higher than most women's presurgery numbers. However, noting that anemia in women of childbearing age was very common, my primary care physician indicated that anemia was not a matter for great concern. Ninety-five percent of the time, he told me, it simply had to do with menstrual blood loss. This seemed unlikely to me—after all, I had been menstruating for many years without any sign of anemia—but I thought the anemia might be related to blood loss during my recent operation. My doctor started me on iron supplements and told me to come in for a repeat blood test in a month.

Over the next few months I became progressively more anemic, began to feel more and more tired, and started losing weight. I did everything I could think of to increase my iron supplies. I increased the amount of iron supplements I was taking, started taking these supplements with foods that didn't interfere with iron absorption, and incorporated more iron-rich red meat into my diet. Vaguely remembering that anemia was associated with deficiencies in folic acid, a B vitamin, I increased the level of the folic acid supplements I was already taking in anticipation of becoming pregnant. None of this seemed to affect how I felt.

By the end of the spring semester, I felt more exhausted than I could ever recall. I would arrive home from work and collapse. My typical weekend was spent lying in bed. Again, I was puzzled: the second year in my job had been far less stressful than the first. On the other hand, I had wrenched my back while lugging around equipment to set up a teaching lab, and a third-year colleague told me that she, too, had felt overwhelmingly exhausted at the end of her second year of teaching. And many women told me about their bouts with anemia and how awful it made them feel. I wondered how so many women could possibly go around feeling like this and ever manage to get anything accomplished. But I decided that what I was experiencing *must* be normal, and I became caught up in the excitement of getting back to the laboratory for the summer.

My May blood test showed the anemia was getting worse, and I was still exhausted, even after a two-week vacation. When I realized I was getting out of breath every time I climbed a flight of stairs, I decided it was time for another visit to my doctor. Sensing my concern, he reassured me that this wasn't the beginning of the long slide down. I admitted that I was beginning to feel as if I were falling apart and that it was hard to believe that this degree of exhaustion was simply due to anemia. I had never felt so weak and tired in my entire life, and the joints in my arms and legs ached all the time.

He pointed out that I had been under a great deal of stress and asked about exercise. I admitted that since I had strained my back I hadn't been getting much exercise. He suggested that I switch to a different iron preparation that might be more easily absorbed and that I start working out. He still thought my anemia was likely due to menstrual blood loss but decided to investigate a little further. He ordered a blood test to check my thyroid function and gave me materials to perform a guaiac test on my stool—to look for hidden loss of blood from the gastrointestinal tract (GI tract—the stomach, intestines, and associated structures). He told me to come back in a month to turn in the guaiac test and to get another blood test.

A combination of several factors meant that it was a couple of months before I returned to turn in the guaiac test and get the follow-up blood test. But when the test results arrived, my doctor called to tell me that the anemia was worse and the guaiac test was positive. That meant that I was probably losing blood from my gastrointestinal tract. He told me that he had decided to refer me to a gastroenterologist, a doctor who specializes in problems of the GI tract.

By this time I was convinced that the anemia was not due to menstrual blood loss. My periods were no heavier than they had ever been, and there was no reason for them to suddenly start making me anemic. However, I *had* been taking a lot of aspirin because of my constantly aching joints. I would take aspirin daily during the first half of my menstrual cycle and then quit for the last two weeks so that the aspirin wouldn't hurt any potential newly conceived babies. The disappointment that I felt each month at not becoming pregnant was slightly mitigated by the freedom to start taking aspirin again for another two weeks.

Large amounts of aspirin can lead to bleeding from the gastrointestinal tract, and I had secretly suspected for some time that this might be causing my anemia. Therefore, I was surprised and worried to learn that the guaiac test turned out positive even *after* I had stopped taking aspirin for a week. It was about this time that I began to wonder if there might be something seriously wrong. I tried to push the feelings aside as hypochondria. After all, it was clear that my doctor thought that there was nothing really seriously the matter.

The gastroenterologist's office informed me that it would be nearly a month before I could see him. Concerned that the combination of weakness, fatigue, persistent anemia, pronounced weight loss, and bleeding from the gastrointestinal tract might be symptomatic of colon cancer, I called my general practitioner

(GP) and asked whether this delay in seeing the gastroenterologist might be dangerous. He replied that it was extremely unlikely that I had colon cancer and that it was no more urgent for me to see the gastroenterologist than anyone else on his waiting list.

A month later, the gastroenterologist took a thorough medical history. He was concerned about both the anemia and the weight loss and scheduled me for a colonoscopy and a gastroendoscopy (procedures that involve a visual examination of the large intestine [colonoscopy] and the stomach [gastroendoscopy] through a long, flexible tube) the next week. After reading the usual release form explaining the possible risks of these procedures, I asked about his policy on blood transfusions, in the unlikely event that I was injured and started to bleed heavily. He said that if someone starts bleeding, the surgical staff keeps track of the hematocrit (a measure of red blood cell volume) and starts a transfusion only if it drops below 30.

After the endoscopies were completed, the gastroenterologist explained that he had found a slightly abnormal area in my large intestine where the blood vessels were very close to the surface, and he thought that this might explain the blood that showed up on the guaiac test. He did not, however, believe that this area—called angiodysplasia, which is just a fancy way of saying "abnormal growth of blood vessels"—could cause enough blood loss to account for the degree of anemia I was experiencing.

He recommended that as a next step I have an X-ray procedure called a small bowel follow-through. This involves drinking barium, which is opaque to X-rays, and then having a fluoroscopic examination of the bowel, to visualize areas of the intestinal tract that are too narrow to be easily reached with an endoscope. I scheduled the small bowel follow-through even though I wasn't happy at the idea of undergoing a diagnostic procedure that would involve X-rays.

I continued to feel weaker and more debilitated. Dutifully attempting to follow my general practitioner's advice to get more exercise, I went for a hike in the woods with my husband. As someone who had habitually walked five miles a day for years, I was alarmed to discover that I was barely able to complete a three-mile hike, collapsing in exhaustion about halfway through. I was also disturbed to have developed a vaginal yeast infection for the first time in my life. When two rounds of over-the-counter medication failed to clear it up, I consulted with my GP. He sent me to a gynecologist, who prescribed a prescription cream; two rounds of this cream also failed to have any effect on the infection.

I was getting more and more worried. I had been taking my morning temperature, to determine when I was ovulating, and had discovered that it seemed to be slightly elevated unless I had taken an aspirin the night before. This seemed peculiar, almost as though I had a chronic, low-grade fever. The weight loss was accelerating, and I got out of breath at the slightest exertion. And I was worried about the yeast infection because I knew that very stubborn yeast infections can be a sign of a weakened immune system. Embarrassed at sounding like an utter hypochondriac, I tried to bring this up to the gynecologist. He pooh-poohed the notion. "Yeast infections are *very* common in women," he said, "and the over-the-counter creams aren't always strong enough to knock out the stubborn ones."

Weight loss, fatigue, anemia, fevers, and now a stubborn yeast infection. Moreover, the information that it was standard procedure to start a blood transfusion if the hematocrit fell below 30 had scared me. My last hematocrit had registered 27. Although I knew that this was below what was considered normal, this was the first time I realized that my anemia was severe enough to be considered serious in and of itself. Although the school year had started by this time, I decided that the situation had become sufficiently serious to warrant getting another opinion. I made an appointment with my former internist, who practiced out of a major teaching hospital in Boston. Seeing him involved making a three-hour drive in each direction, but he was very smart, very experienced, and one of the best doctors I had ever known. He looked startled when he saw me and said, "You've lost a *lot* of weight." I replied that I was happy to have lost the weight but was also concerned because the weight loss was unintentional and I had *never* been able to lose weight in the past without a major effort. I then went on to explain the history of my anemia. He looked over all the blood test results and the report from the endoscopies.

He told me that everything looked as though it had been handled correctly and explained my hematocrit results to me (see Chapter 2). My hematocrit was only 27. That meant that the red cells took up only 27 percent of the total blood volume instead of the normal 35 to 45 percent. However, the *number* of red cells was normal: the decrease in total red cell volume was due to a decrease in the size of individual cells. If my iron levels were too low, my body would be unable to manufacture sufficient *hemoglobin*—the iron-bearing pigment that carries oxygen throughout the body to deliver it to every individual cell. Since red blood cells are filled with hemoglobin, a reduction in the amount of available hemoglobin will lead to smaller red blood cells. Since my hemoglobin levels and iron stores were also low, my internist interpreted this decrease in average red cell volume as due to a deficiency in iron.

My internist thought that the reduction in iron values and hemoglobin content was so pronounced that, whatever else might be going on, I had likely developed a problem with iron absorption. Since he believed that my anemia could easily drop into a critical range where I would require a blood transfusion, he recommended that I get an intravenous infusion of iron and arranged for me to see a hematologist, who would oversee the procedure. He also thought that it was important for me to undergo the small bowel follow-through, although he agreed with the gastroenterologist that it was unlikely that we'd find any small bowel abnormality. Shortly thereafter, I underwent both the iron infusion and the small bowel follow-through.

Iron infusion is a relatively rare procedure; mine was performed in a wing of the hospital set up for people who required blood transfusions—which utilize the same basic equipment. Everyone else in the room looked pale and drawn, and I felt like a fraud with my piddling problem with iron absorption. My temperature rose a little after the iron infusion. I told the nurse that I thought I'd been running a low-grade fever for several months. She brought this to the attention of one of the doctors.

"Nothing to worry about," he said; "you should be feeling *much* better soon."

I was relieved that a plausible and relatively innocuous explanation had been found for my persistent anemia and that no major problems had been uncovered, and I was looking forward to feeling stronger and more energetic as soon as the iron became incorporated into my hemoglobin and my anemia cleared up.

Several weeks after I underwent the small bowel follow-through, I received a letter from the gastroenterologist explaining that the exam had indicated that my small bowel function appeared perfectly normal. Almost as an aside, he mentioned that the radiologist reviewing my films had noticed a pleural reaction. I knew that the word *pleural* referred to the membranes around the lungs, but I had never heard of a pleural reaction. Neither had Paul. I called the gastroenterologist to ask what a pleural reaction was.

He apologized for alarming me and said that the pleural reaction was most likely meaningless. He said that if I had any symptoms of a pulmonary (lung) problem, I might want to have a chest X-ray. However, he thought that if I didn't have any pulmonary symptoms, I should just forget about it.

Did I have pulmonary symptoms? I had felt short of breath for months. But I knew that that was a classic symptom of anemia, since the oxygen-carrying capacity of the blood, which depends on the hemoglobin content of the red blood cells, is reduced. I had had a slight cough for a week or two. But it was November, and so did Paul, most of my students, and nearly everyone else I knew.

But I thought about the fatigue and the weight loss, and the possibility that I might have TB or pneumonia occurred to me. I wasn't concerned about my own ability to handle either of these diseases—I rarely got colds or the flu and had therefore always believed that I had a strong immune system. But we were planning to visit my elderly parents for Thanksgiving, and the thought of exposing them to TB or pneumonia scared me. In a fit of hypochondria-by-proxy, I called my GP to ask him to schedule a chest X-ray. Since I wanted to make sure that any possibly infectious condition was treated and cured before Thanksgiving, I asked to have the X-ray scheduled as soon as possible.

That night, I felt particularly achy and took a hot bath before I went to bed. I woke up in the middle of the night soaking wet. Bewildered, I got up to get a towel. Confused and still half asleep, I could only conclude that I had been so tired that I had forgotten to dry myself off from the bath before getting into bed. Suddenly, Paul appeared by my side.

"Are you OK?" he said. I asked him how he knew that anything was wrong. He told me that he had reached out to me, found that I was gone, and discovered that the sheets where I had been lying were so thoroughly soaked that he thought I must have vomited in my sleep. I explained my bath idea. Puzzled, we changed the sheets and went back to bed.

I went in for the chest X-ray the following afternoon, after teaching my morning class. Around seven that night, I got a phone call from my GP.

"Your chest X-ray was really strange," he said. "I wasn't sure how to interpret it, so I took it over to the radiologist." His voice was shaking, "There seems to be some kind of mass in the chest cavity. The most likely explanation is that it's lymphoma. You need to come in to the hospital for a CAT scan tomorrow."

"Lymphoma?" I said, stricken with a sudden combination of bewilderment and dread. "Isn't that a kind of cancer?"

What is lymphoma?

Lymphoma *is* a kind of cancer. Cancer means that a population of cells in your body—usually starting with a single malignant (cancerous) cell—becomes abnormal and starts to accumulate without the normal restraints that govern cell growth. These cells can start dividing too rapidly, or they can divide at the normal rate but live far beyond the normal life span for that kind of cell. This abnormal accumulation of cells leads to the development of the lumps—or tumors—that are often the first sign that something is amiss. All tumors result from an abnormal accumulation of cells, but not all tumors are malignant. In addition to their unrestrained growth, cancer cells have other peculiarities.

Cancer cells can have a bizarre appearance when you look at them under a microscope, and they behave in an abnormal manner. Malignant cells can invade and destroy normal, healthy tissue in areas adjacent to the site at which they originate and can sometimes travel through the blood and lymphatic system to colonize and attack distant sites in the body. It's this invasion and destruction of normal tissue that makes cancer so dangerous and that distinguishes it from benign (noncancerous) tumors—like fibroids or lipomas—which don't invade the surrounding tissue or travel through your body.

Different forms of cancer are distinguished from each other based on the normal populations of cells from which the malignant cells first arose. Thus breast cancer arises from the cells of the breast, and lung cancer arises from cells of the lung. Although the malignant cells are abnormal, they often retain some of the properties of the cells they came from and can still be recognized as being of a given cell type, even if they are found in distant parts of the body. Therefore, a cancer that has spread to a distant site in your body is still named for the tissue where it originated. A breast cancer cell found growing in your kidney is still considered breast cancer and not kidney cancer.

Lymphoma is a cancer of a class of cells called *lymphocytes.* Lymphocytes are key players in the normal immune response. This means that lymphoma, together with the leukemias and multiple myeloma, is unusual among cancers in that it represents a malignancy of the immune system—the very system of the body that's supposed to protect and defend our bodies from infection and, some believe, from cancer.

There are many different varieties of lymphoma. Currently there are two broad divisions of the group of diseases known as lymphoma: Hodgkin lymphoma (formerly known as and still frequently called "Hodgkin's disease") and the non-Hodgkin lymphomas (NHLs; formerly known as "non-Hodgkin's lymphomas"). This simple division into two clinical entities—two diseases that differ from each other in terms of the appearance and behavior of the malignant cells—represents a vast oversimplification of the actual situation because there are over a dozen distinct diseases that fall into the category of non-Hodgkin lymphoma and even Hodgkin lymphoma includes several specific disease entities.

All these different types of lymphoma are related to each other, since they are all cancers that arise from lymphocytes. However, they differ widely in how rapidly they progress, in who is most likely to get them, in the appearance of the malignant cells under a microscope, and in how they respond to therapy.

It's important to recognize that the term *lymphoma* actually encompasses a group of diseases. That means that the best therapy for you may be very different from the best therapy for someone else with a different form of lymphoma. In this book I am mostly concerned with the various forms of lymphoma—both Hodgkin lymphoma and the non-Hodgkin lymphomas. Multiple myeloma and the leukemias are closely related to the lymphomas and are sometimes grouped together with them; however, these related diseases are generally classified separately and are frequently treated with quite different therapies. Therefore, I do not discuss multiple myeloma in this book and discuss only those forms of leukemia that arise from lymphocytes and overlap clinically with the lymphomas.

How common is lymphoma?

I'd hardly ever heard of lymphoma when I was first diagnosed. I was surprised to learn that what I had thought was a rare and unusual disease was actually one of the ten most common forms of cancer in the United States. According to the American Cancer Society, approximately 63,740 new cases of lymphoma will be diagnosed in the United States in 2005, and about 20,600 people will die of the disease (19,200 of NHL and 1,400 of Hodgkin lymphoma).

Of the different types of lymphoma (Hodgkin lymphoma and the various forms of NHL), Hodgkin lymphoma is the most common (accounting for approximately 7,350 of those new cases); however, most cases of lymphoma involve one of the many different forms of NHL (over 56,000 new cases). NHL is now the seventh most common malignancy in the United States. Furthermore, the incidence of non-Hodgkin lymphoma increased more than 80 percent from the early 1970s through the 1990s. In other words, people are almost twice as likely to get NHL today as they were thirty years ago.

This increase in incidence was most pronounced for some of the more aggressive forms of the disease. On the good news front, the overall incidence rates for Hodgkin lymphoma declined over the same time period. At least some of this apparent decrease has to do with improved diagnostic procedures, so that more lymphomas are now correctly identified as NHL rather than misdiagnosed as Hodgkin lymphoma. However, some of it may be real. And the increase in NHL incidence finally began flattening out toward the end of the 1990s.

Among the forms of cancer tabulated by the National Cancer Institute's Surveillance, Epidemiology, and End Results (SEER) program, the rate of increase in incidence of NHL over the last half of the twentieth century was surpassed only by the rate of increase in incidence of melanoma and lung cancer in women. We have a pretty good idea why the incidence of melanoma and lung cancer in women rose. Statistics suggest that getting melanoma, which is a form of skin cancer, is associated with having gotten repeated, blistering sunburns as a child or a teenager. Therefore, the increase in incidence of melanoma is probably related both to the thinning of the ozone layer and to increases in our leisure-time sun exposure. The increase in the incidence of lung cancer in women is almost certainly related to the increase in the number of women who began smoking after World War II.

In contrast, the increased incidence of lymphoma is something of a mystery. While several factors that may increase the likelihood of developing lymphoma have now been identified (these factors are discussed in Chapter 11), the cause(s) of lymphoma remain(s) largely unknown.

SUGGESTIONS FOR FURTHER READING

Information about the incidence of the different forms of lymphoma in the United States, as well as about the incidence of other forms of cancer and trends in cancer incidence over time, is available from the National Cancer Institute's Cancer Surveillance Program. The most recent publication of these statistics is:

Ries LAG et al., eds. *SEER Cancer Statistics Review, 1975–2001.* Bethesda, Md.: National Cancer Institute. www.seer.cancer.gov/csr/1975_2001/.

Although I include them as references only for Chapter 1, these four comprehensive medical texts dealing with lymphoma, published in the late 1990s and early 2000s, contain information relevant to every aspect of lymphoma—symptoms, diagnosis, causes, and treatment. These four books are written for physicians and will be difficult reading for anyone without a background in biology or medicine. The material in Part III of this book should give you a strong enough background in lymphoma to read them:

Canellos GP, Lister TA, Sklar JL, Lampert R, eds. (1998). *The Lymphomas.* Philadelphia: W. B. Saunders.
Covers both Hodgkin lymphoma and NHL.
Magrath IT, ed. (1997). *The Non-Hodgkin's Lymphomas.* 2d ed. New York: Oxford University Press.
Mauch PM, Armitage JO, Diehl V, eds. (1999). *Hodgkin's Disease.* Philadelphia: Lippincott Williams & Wilkins.

Mauch PM, Armitage JO, Harris NL, Dalla-Favera R, Coiffier B, eds. (2003). *Non-Hodgkin's Lymphomas*. Philadelphia: Lippincott Williams & Wilkins.

This book is focused on learning about and understanding the medical and biological aspects of lymphoma. Many other issues of interest to people with lymphoma, and cancer patients in general, are not covered: finding a good oncologist (or hematologist), making informed decisions about treatment, deciding whether to enter a clinical trial, dealing with job discrimination, the emotional and psychological issues associated with being diagnosed with cancer, and so forth. Some excellent books written for cancer patients that include information on some of these topics include:

Buckman R. (1997). *What You Really Need to Know about Cancer*. Baltimore: Johns Hopkins University Press.

Coleman CN. (1998). *Understanding Cancer: A Patient's Guide to Diagnosis, Prognosis, and Treatment*. Baltimore: Johns Hopkins University Press.

Dollinger M, Rosenbaum EH, Cable G. (1997). *Everyone's Guide to Cancer Therapy*. Kansas City, Mo.: Andrews McMeel Publishing.

Harpham WS. (1995). *After Cancer: A Guide to Your New Life*. New York: HarperPerennial Library.

Harpham WS. (1997). *Diagnosis Cancer: Your Guide through the First Few Months*. New York: W. W. Norton.

Johnston L. (1999). *The Non-Hodgkin's Lymphomas: Making Sense of Diagnosis, Options and Treatment*. Sebastopol, Calif.: O'Reilly & Associates.

National Coalition for Cancer Survivorship. (1996). *A Cancer Survivor's Almanac*. Hoffman B, ed. Minneapolis: Chronimed Publishing.

Women's Cancer Group. (1997). *Songs of Strength*. Sydney: Macmillan Australia.

The Internet is a wonderful source of information. Unfortunately, it can also be a wonderful source of misinformation as well. The Internet sites I reference in this book are sites that I have found to be accurate and reliable. They are not intended to provide a comprehensive list, and my omission of any particular site is not meant as a mark of disapproval. All these sites were active as of January 2005. Since they have all been running for some time, I expect them to still be active for at least the next few years. Material posted on the Internet comes and goes, however, and it's possible that one or more of these sites may have vanished by the time you read this book.

SEER on-line: www.seer.cancer.gov/

Mike Barela, a Hodgkin lymphoma survivor, provides perhaps the most comprehensive lymphoma information site on the Net at the Lymphoma Information Network: www.lymphomainfo.net/

Lymphoma Focus also provides a highly comprehensive site, which includes Webcasts by leading lymphoma specialists: www.lymphomafocus.org/

The Lymphoma Research Foundation: www.lymphoma.org/

The Leukemia and Lymphoma Society: www.leukemia-lymphoma.org/hm_lls

Kidney cancer survivor Steve Dunn's CancerGuide provides lots of strategies for researching cancer: www.cancerguide.org/

The American Cancer Society: www.cancer.org/

Association of Cancer Online Resources (sponsors of many lymphoma-related mailing lists): www.acor.org/about/

The University of Pennsylvania's Oncolink site: www.oncolink.upenn.edu/disease/lymphoma1/

Bloodline is a tremendous (if highly technical) source of information on lymphoma and other blood-related disorders: www.bloodline.net/

Hematology, a set of reviews published annually by the American Society of Hematology (ASH), is available at www.asheducationbook.org/

CHAPTER 2

Symptoms and Diagnosis

Being diagnosed with cancer can be overwhelming. Even the word itself is ominous. And almost always, the diagnosis is followed by a plunge into an unfamiliar world of medical tests and procedures. None of these procedures is fun; some of them are frightening, bewildering, or intimidating. And always, in the background, the threatening drumbeat,

"What are they looking for? What are they going to find? Am I going to die?"

If you start treatment immediately, you may feel as if you have lost control of your entire life. That's what happened to me: I left my class one morning to have a chest X-ray, telling my students that they might have trouble reaching me that afternoon. I never returned to that class. I never saw those students again. I started a grueling round of diagnostic tests, and within a few weeks I began chemotherapy.

Or, instead of starting therapy right away, your oncologist may tell you that you're going to "watch and wait." This surrealistic scenario involves first learning that you have cancer and then learning that you aren't going to start treatment. You have cancer and you're not supposed to do anything about it? Nothing? What does *that* mean?

If you've just been diagnosed with lymphoma, you may be feeling frightened and vulnerable. You may feel as though you've lost control of your body and of your life. This chapter, on diagnosis, is intended to help you regain control and make sense of what's going on. On the other hand, if you have been living with lymphoma for a long time, this chapter may help you better understand what was going on in those early days when you first heard the word *cancer* applied to you.

Symptoms

Sometimes lymphoma is diagnosed during a routine checkup. Maybe a chest X-ray shows a mass, or maybe some abnormal results appear on a blood test. Most people, though, have some symptoms. The wide variety of lymphoma symptoms reflects the many possible manifestations of the disease. Both the specific type of lymphoma you have and the location of the growing mass of cancer cells will influence what symptoms appear, since lymphocytes—and hence lymphoma—can be found anywhere in your body and symptoms are in part determined by what normal structures are adjacent to the mass. The symptoms may seem deceptively innocuous—maybe a "swollen gland" on the side of the neck or generalized, inexplicable itching. Symptoms may be vague and nonspecific—none of the symptoms described here would, by themselves, cause a physician to announce, "Aha! Lymphoma!" Nonetheless, certain symptoms are common and fall into recognizable patterns.

Enlarged lymph nodes

The most common symptom of lymphoma is painless enlargement of one or more *lymph nodes*. In fact, in over two-thirds of persons with lymphoma, visible enlargement of lymph nodes is the symptom that sends people to the doctor. Lymph nodes are small, bean-shaped organs found at junctions in the *lymphatic system*—a series of interconnected vessels that carry a colorless fluid called *lymph* through your body (see Chapter 9). In both Hodgkin lymphoma and NHL, lymph node enlargement, or *lymphadenopathy,* is most frequently noticed in the lymph nodes of the neck. Nodes in the groin and armpit are commonly enlarged in NHL as well. Slowly growing forms of NHL—often called low-grade or *indolent* NHL—often involve widespread lymphadenopathy affecting multiple nodes.

It's important to note that lymph nodes can be enlarged for many reasons other than lymphoma and that not all strange lumps are lymph nodes. Lymph nodes can swell up, for example, as they fill with rapidly dividing lymphocytes as part of the normal immunological response to infection. They can also become enlarged due to the spread of other forms of cancer, as a result of various diseases in which there is abnormal activity of the immune system, or even in response to certain drugs (notably Dilantin and carbamazepine, two drugs used to treat epilepsy). In fact, the vast majority of people with enlarged lymph nodes—about 99 percent—have completely benign conditions.

Lymph nodes that grow in response to infectious disease tend to be tender (painful to the touch), and the skin in the vicinity of the enlarged node may appear inflamed. Lymph nodes that are enlarged because of the spread of forms of cancer other than lymphoma tend to be very hard, like little pebbles; frequently, they are fixed to underlying tissues and aren't moved easily with your finger. In lymphoma, lymph nodes are not tender, they are usually movable, and they tend to feel firm and rubbery. In several types of indolent lymphoma, the involved nodes can wax and wane in size spontaneously. They can grow larger and then shrink for no apparent reason. Thus, partial shrinkage of a suspicious node doesn't rule out the possibility of lymphoma.

In general, if you have an enlarged lymph node that is greater than 1 or 2 cm (about half an inch to a little less than an inch) in diameter and no cause can be established within a month's time, it should be biopsied. For a biopsy, a sample of tissue is cut out and examined under the microscope. Biopsy isn't necessary every time someone has a swollen lymph node (especially in the presence of a plausible cause such as mononucleosis, mumps, or flu!). On the other hand, it is not a good idea to ignore a swollen lymph node indefinitely because it is possible that a malignancy would go undetected.

In deciding whether to do a biopsy, the physician considers the physical characteristics of the enlarged node (painful vs. nonpainful; rubbery vs. soft; and so forth), how long it has persisted, and where it's located. It's common to have enlarged nodes in the groin following infections or leg and foot injuries, whereas enlarged nodes right above the collarbone are more frequently a cause for concern.

Other localized symptoms

While enlarged lymph nodes are an early symptom of the disease in many persons with lymphoma, tumors—which can be nodal, meaning they arose inside a lymph node, or extranodal, meaning they arose from lymphocytes outside the lymphatic system—may not always be visible. When I first became concerned about my anemia, fatigue, and weight loss, I wondered if I could possibly have AIDS. I decided that this was impossible because AIDS is characterized by lymphadenopathy, and no enlarged lymph nodes were apparent in my neck or armpits or groin. Meanwhile, a tumor the size of a football was quietly growing inside my chest cavity, starting from an area under the breastbone known as the mediastinum. The symptoms of such hidden masses depend on their location and what the neighboring structures are. Since extranodal lymphomas may arise virtually anywhere in the body, the possible symptoms of such masses are too varied and numerous to enumerate. In this section I describe the symptoms characteristic of some of the more commonly involved sites of disease.

Large mediastinal masses like mine are more common with Hodgkin lymphoma. They occur in about 20 percent of patients with NHL as well—most commonly with T cell lymphoblastic lymphoma and primary mediastinal large B cell lymphoma. Both of these forms of NHL tend to strike a relatively young population. Primary mediastinal large B cell lymphoma tends to affect women in their thirties, while T cell lymphoblastic lymphoma is most common in men in their late teens and early twenties.

Mediastinal masses can cause persistent cough, hoarseness, chest pain, and shortness of breath. In some cases, mediastinal masses can compress the *superior vena cava*, the large blood vessel that returns blood from the head, neck, arms, and upper chest to the heart. Since this interferes with blood returning from these regions to the rest of the circulatory system, pressure on the superior vena cava can lead to swelling of the face, neck, and arms and swollen veins in the neck and upper chest.

Large masses in the abdomen, on the other hand, can lead to chronic abdominal pain that just won't go away, a sensation of abdominal fullness, or feeling full after eating only a small amount of food. Lymphoma in the gastrointestinal tract can cause diarrhea or weight loss because of problems absorbing nutrients.

Sometimes, gastrointestinal lymphomas can lead to an abdominal emergency. Severe abdominal pain, distention, and tenderness; abdominal hardness and rigidity; severe bleeding that won't stop; and severe nausea and vomiting are all symptoms of an abdominal emergency. This means that something's wrong that needs treatment right away, and you need to get to an emergency room. Large masses in the abdomen can also cause back or leg pain, and lymphoma in the groin lymph nodes can cause your feet and legs to swell if lymph drainage from these sites is impeded.

Cutaneous T cell lymphomas show up as skin lesions, which are typically extremely itchy. At early stages of the disease the lesions tend to come and go and may be misdiagnosed as a noncancerous condition such as eczema. As the disease advances, they may appear as reddened patches, raised plaques, purplish tumors, or a generalized reddening of large areas of the skin.

Systemic symptoms

Sometimes the initial symptoms of lymphoma may be *systemic*. Rather then being localized to the specific site where the tumor is growing, systemic effects are widespread. While local symptoms depend on direct, physical effects of the tumor—I had trouble breathing because my lymphoma was crushing one of my lungs—systemic symptoms like fever depend on substances released by the tumor or from other cells responding to the tumor.

Three of these systemic manifestations of lymphoma—fever, weight loss, and night sweats—are known as the Ann Arbor "B" symptoms. The "B" symptoms are included as part of the *staging* workup, which is intended to determine how widely the lymphoma has spread throughout your body (see Chapter 10).

The "B" symptoms occur in about 30 percent of people with Hodgkin lymphoma and about 20 percent of people with NHL. With Hodgkin lymphoma, "B" symptoms are more common with widespread disease. Therefore, people who have "B" symptoms are generally treated with chemotherapy—which reaches all the cells in the body—even if other signs of the disease suggest it's relatively localized. Systemic symptoms occur more frequently with the rapidly growing forms of NHL—called intermediate or high-grade or aggressive disease—than with the low-grade, indolent forms of the disease.

The "B" symptoms are probably related to *cytokines*, the chemical messengers by which one cell type conveys information to another and signals that something needs to be done. Cytokines play an important role in coordinating the normal immune response (as well as many other aspects of bodily function). In lymphoma, the normal balance of cytokines circulating in the body can be disrupted. The malignant lymphocytes, which resemble normal lymphocytes in many ways, sometimes make the same chemical messengers that normal lymphocytes produce. And sometimes the immune system recognizes the cancer as dangerous and tries to destroy it. Both of these situations can lead to increased levels of cytokines, which in turn can cause symptoms like fever and night sweats, which resemble aspects of the normal immunological response to infection.

Fevers may be relatively low grade (less than 100°F) and persistent (lasting for days or weeks or months), or they may follow a fluctuating pattern of high fevers that last for several days or weeks alternating with several days or weeks of normal body temperature. Night sweats are drenching ("drenching" means that you have to change the sheets). When I first developed night sweats, right before my diagnosis with NHL, I woke up feeling as though someone had dumped a pail of water on me in my sleep. I began sleeping on a towel, which I needed to change several times a night, to avoid having to change sheets.

Weight loss is a common symptom of lymphoma as well as other forms of cancer. Dramatic weight loss and malnutrition occurring in cancer patients is called *cancer cachexia*. Cachexia can involve both indirect factors that depend on circulating substances and the direct effects of a growing mass. Cytokines released from both the tumor and the immune system can cause you to feel ill and lose your appetite; abnormal responses to certain hormones can influence how you metabolize your food. Tumors can also cause weight loss more directly: if there's a tumor pressing on your gut, so you feel full after you've eaten only a little food, you'll probably lose weight just because you're eating less. And the growing mass of cells in the tumor will themselves consume calories.

Perhaps because of the prevailing attitude in our society that you can't be "too thin or too rich," many people who experience unexplained weight loss feel pleased that they are getting into better shape, becoming concerned only as they slide precipitously past their "ideal weight." And it is sometimes difficult to get doctors—who, after all, are subject to the same social influences and attitudes as the rest of us—to take unexplained weight loss seriously. After I lost about a third of my initial weight, bottoming out at around 90 pounds, one of my doctors brushed off my concerns about weight loss with the airy comment "Maybe you're not eating as much."

It's important to remember that dramatic, unintentional weight loss can be a sign of many very serious illnesses and should never be taken lightly (as it were). Weight loss is counted as a "B" symptom if it is unexplained (you're not on a diet, exercising more than usual, or going short of sleep) and if you lose more than 10 percent of your initial weight over a period of six months or less. So, if you weighed 150 pounds and went down to 135 or less over six months, it would count as a "B" symptom, but if you dropped to only 140, it wouldn't. While the number is arbitrary, it distinguishes weight loss that's a signal that something's going on from the small fluctuations of weight that occur normally in all of us.

Other systemic symptoms of lymphoma include intense, unexplained itching (*pruritis*) of the legs or feet, fatigue, *malaise* (a general sense of lack of well-being), weakness, and, with Hodgkin lymphoma, pain in the affected lymph nodes after drinking alcohol.

As I learned, anemia is occasionally the first symptom of lymphoma. Indeed, children with lymphoblastic lymphoma are frequently diagnosed when their parents take them to a doctor because they are pale and easily fatigued—symptoms of anemia. About one-third of people with NHL are anemic at the time they are diagnosed; anemia is also common with advanced stages of Hodgkin lymphoma. If your bone marrow is involved, you may experience a generalized decrease in the numbers of the different types of blood cells. If platelet synthesis is affected, you may bleed and bruise easily, and tiny purple spots called *petechiae* may appear on your skin.

Both Hodgkin lymphoma and NHL can disrupt immune function, probably as a response to cytokines released by the malignant cells, which can inhibit the production and function of normal, healthy lymphocytes. In both cases, immune system dysfunction can make a person more susceptible to infections, such as colds or yeast infections. However, Hodgkin lymphoma and NHL generally affect different aspects of the normal immune response. Hodgkin lymphoma is most commonly associated with impaired T cell function, while NHL is more frequently associated with deficits in B cell function (see Chapter 9).

Diagnosis

Lymphocytes are found throughout the body, so lymphoma can arise virtually anywhere and can have many different effects. And as the discussion of symptoms indicates, lymphoma can "announce itself" in many different ways. The specific diagnostic procedures used for any individual will depend, to some extent, on the specific details of his or her disease. A discussion of every diagnostic procedure that might be useful for every manifestation of lymphoma is beyond the scope of this book. In this section, however, I describe those procedures that are most commonly used in diagnosing lymphoma, including some that are usually performed only under specific conditions.

What are they looking for?

There are three main goals of diagnosis. The first is determining what's wrong: in this case determining whether you have lymphoma and, if so, what kind of lymphoma you have. This is critically important because different types of lymphoma typically follow very different courses (some progressing extremely slowly and others progressing very rapidly) and respond to different therapeutic treatments. While a history, physical, and various diagnostic tests (see following sections) may *suggest* that you have lymphoma, lymphoma can be definitively diagnosed only by taking a biopsy.

The severity of your illness depends not only on what kind of lymphoma you have but also on how far it has spread throughout your body. Thus, the second goal of diagnosis is staging the disease. Staging (discussed in more detail in Chapter 10) defines how far the disease has spread. Staging the disease, like classifying it, is critical to determining the optimal treatment plan.

Stage I disease is the most localized. With Stage I disease, the lymphoma is restricted to a specific lymphatic region of your body—for instance, the lymph nodes of your left armpit. Stage II disease involves two or more lymph node regions on the same side of your diaphragm (midriff section). The involved nodes can be all above the diaphragm (head, neck, arms, chest) or all below (belly, pelvis, legs). Stage II disease can be *contiguous* (the involved regions are touching each other) or *noncontiguous*—the involved regions are separate. Stage I and contiguous Stage II are sometimes called *localized disease.*

In Stage III and Stage IV, sometimes called *advanced disease,* the lymphoma has spread more widely than in Stage I and Stage II. In Stage III, the disease has spread to lymph node regions on both sides of the diaphragm. In Stage IV disease, lymphoma has spread throughout one or more organs—the liver or bone marrow, for example—that aren't part of the lymphatic system. (A *small* area of extranodal disease outside the lymphatic system is not necessarily considered Stage IV.)

Staging is achieved through techniques that allow the physician to "see" inside the body, such as X-rays, CT scans, PET scans, and MRIs, as well as through techniques that involve examining small samples of different tissues, such as bone marrow biopsies and lumbar punctures. The presence or absence of the Ann Arbor "B" symptoms (see above) is considered during staging as well.

The third goal of diagnosis is concerned with assessing your overall condition. Diagnostic tests are performed to determine how the disease has affected normal bodily functions (for example, are you anemic?) and whether these effects of the disease require treatment (do you need a blood transfusion?). Evaluating the general condition is important for the overall treatment plan. For instance, people with heart conditions may not be able to take certain drugs; people with poor lung and kidney function may not be able to undergo a bone marrow transplant.

Biopsying the node

I learned that I had cancer when a chest X-ray disclosed a large, abnormal mass inside my rib cage. A computerized axial tomography (CAT or CT) scan confirmed the results of the chest X-ray, showing that an enormous tumor filled the right half of my chest, crushing the right lung completely flat and reaching malignant tendrils into the supraclavicular nodes above my left collarbone. While it was clear from the outset that the mass was malignant—no benign process would have produced anything so big in that location—and probably lymphoma, the specific classification was uncertain.

A local oncologist kindly fit me into his schedule the very evening that first CT scan was performed. He was certain that I had Hodgkin lymphoma. He thought that the enormous mediastinal mass, the apparent lack of involvement elsewhere, my youth, and the presence of "B" symptoms were all consistent with Hodgkin lymphoma rather than NHL. And he had just seen another young woman with Hodgkin's who had also gone undiagnosed for a year. The oncologist spent a long time reassuring me about how treatable Hodgkin lymphoma was. "Cure rates approaching 90 percent for all but the most advanced cases! If you have to have cancer, it's a good kind to have!" As for NHL . . . well . . . he didn't think I had NHL.

I felt reassured by this meeting, but, after thinking things over, I decided that I wanted to be treated in a major medical center, where the doctors had extensive experience with lymphoma. I asked my internist to refer me to an oncologist in Boston. The second oncologist also told me that Hodgkin lymphoma was highly treatable. But while she was unwilling to commit herself one way or another as to what *I* had, she was inclined to think it was NHL. In that case, things were a bit less rosy.

The only way to distinguish between the two possibilities was with a biopsy. Lymphoma is diagnosed by biopsying an enlarged lymph node (or other suspicious tissue, if a suspect mass is located outside the lymphatic system). The biopsy allows the pathologist to determine whether lymphoma is present and, if so, to identify the specific type. Usually a lymph node biopsy can be performed under a local anesthetic. An intravenous sedative may be injected into a vein in your arm, and the area around the enlarged node will be sterilized and numbed. The surgeon will make an incision and try to remove the entire affected lymph node.

For the initial diagnosis, this sort of biopsy, called an *excisional biopsy,* is generally preferable to a *fine needle biopsy,* in which a needle is inserted into the suspicious mass and a small sample of tissue is withdrawn. With a fine needle biopsy, a small area of cancer surrounded by normal lymphocytes reacting to it could be missed (in Hodgkin lymphoma, for instance, malignant cells constitute only a small fraction of the total tumor mass). Moreover, an excisional biopsy allows the physician to determine the pattern of cell growth. Fine needle biopsies can sometimes be useful later on to evaluate a mass remaining after therapy or to investigate a possible relapse.

Samples of the biopsied tissue are cut into very thin sections, stained with special dyes, and examined under a microscope. In order to cut the very thin slices of tissue necessary to visualize the cells under the microscope, the sample must first be treated so that it is hard. (If you've ever tried to cut very thin slices of something that's soft and mushy, you'll understand why.)

There are several ways to go about this. In one method, small blocks of tissue are rapidly frozen, and *frozen sections* are prepared. This has the advantage of being extremely rapid, so that tissue samples can be examined while the patient is still on the operating table. However, frozen sections aren't permanent, and it's more difficult to visualize the cells than in permanent sections, which have undergone extensive processing to make all the tiny structures in the cells as distinct as possible.

Preparing *permanent sections* entails a more involved procedure: the tissue is *fixed* with formaldehyde, so that all the small structures that make up the cells remain in place during treatment, and it is then soaked in liquid paraffin wax to harden it. After the sections of paraffin-infiltrated tissue are cut and placed on a microscope slide, they are treated with special dyes, which stain the different structures inside the cells. A *pathologist*, a doctor who specializes in interpreting and diagnosing abnormalities in the appearance of tissue, examines the slides.

The disease is classified on the basis of the microscopic appearance—or *histology*—of the cells in the biopsy. This classification depends both on the pattern of cell growth and on the appearance of individual cells (size, appearance of the cell's nucleus, and so forth; see Chapter 10). It is common to make both frozen and permanent sections of different pieces of the same biopsy. This allows for both an immediate impression (do the cells look cancerous?) and a more leisurely detailed analysis (is it Hodgkin lymphoma or NHL? what subtype?) as well as providing a permanent record of the appearance of the malignant cells.

Because the mass in my chest extended into my supraclavicular lymph nodes, I was able to have a lymph node biopsy rather than undergoing a more complex procedure to biopsy the main tumor mass inside my chest. The report of the frozen section came back while I was still lying on the surgical table. Having been given intravenous Versed—a sedative similar to Valium—I was in a daze, and most of the conversation between the surgeon and his assistants flew right over me. However, suddenly, clearly, cutting cleanly through the haze like the iceberg that sinks your ship looming ominously through the fog, I heard a voice saying: "No Reed-Sternberg cells."

I had already done some reading, and I knew what that meant. Reed-Sternberg cells were pathognomonic for Hodgkin lymphoma. So, if you have Reed-Sternberg cells, it means that you have Hodgkin lymphoma. The good kind of lymphoma. The curable kind. No Reed-Sternberg cells meant I had the awful, the dreaded, the not-very-rosy NHL. The bad kind of lymphoma. Lying there on the table, I began to cry. A kindhearted resident tried to reassure me, "It's only the frozen section," he said. "You only need one Reed-Sternberg cell. They can be very infrequent. They're easy to miss on a frozen section. They may very well find some in the paraffin section."

But lying there, like the evening spread out against the sky, I knew it was NHL.

Immunophenotyping

While an experienced pathologist can obtain a good deal of information simply by examining the biopsied tissue under a microscope, it is often desirable to supplement this visual examination with specialized tests to determine the *immunophenotype* of the malignant cells. The immunophenotype is the specific repertoire of proteins displayed on the cell surface. The methods used to determine the tumor's immunophenotype are immunofluorescence, flow cytometry, and immunohistochemistry.

All these techniques utilize *antibodies,* which are proteins made by cells in the immune system that recognize and bind to specific substances. We make antibodies to substances that the immune system recognizes as foreign. This helps the immune system defend us against disease-causing organisms. For instance, we have antibodies that recognize the poliovirus, antibodies that recognize the smallpox virus, and antibodies that recognize the measles virus. Different antibodies recognize and bind to different substances. They are amazingly selective; an antibody that recognizes poliovirus would waltz right past a smallpox virus.

The techniques of immunofluorescence, flow cytometry, and immunohistochemistry rely on the ability of antibodies to recognize and bind to specific proteins. The specimen of biopsied tissue is exposed to a solution of antibodies that bind to a protein found only on a specific class of cells. Such proteins are called *markers* or *marker proteins* because they can be used to mark whether a cell is a member of a specific class.

For example, the pathologist might expose a specimen on a slide to antibodies that recognize CD20, a protein found on certain normal lymphocytes as well as in some forms of lymphoma. The antibodies can be visualized by attaching a label to the antibody—for example, *immunofluorescence* uses a label that will glow (fluoresce) when exposed to light.

If the malignant cells do carry CD20, the antibodies will bind to the CD20 molecules, and the cells light up with fluorescent antibodies like Times Square after dark. If the cells don't have CD20, however, the antibodies will simply wash away. If the cells carry many CD20 molecules, they will appear bright, while if they only carry a few, they will fluoresce only dimly.

Flow cytometry also uses fluorescently labeled antibodies to look for the presence of specific marker proteins. It differs from immunofluorescence in that individual cells from the specimen float in fluid, rather than sitting in a section of tissue on a microscope slide. A thin stream of the fluid containing the cells is forced through a hole, so that individual cells pass through a laser beam one at a time. If the cell bears labeled antibodies, they will fluoresce, and a light-sensitive counter called a *cytometer* will detect this fluorescence. By labeling antibodies to different proteins with different molecules that fluoresce when they are exposed to different wavelengths of light (different colors of light), the presence (or absence) of several proteins can be evaluated simultaneously.

Immunohistochemistry is similar to immunofluorescence, except that instead of using a fluorescent label, the antibodies are attached to an enzyme that causes a colorless substance to become colored so that it can be readily visualized under a microscope.

Bone marrow biopsy

In addition to getting a lymph node biopsy, most people also have a bone marrow biopsy to determine whether there's any lymphoma in the bone marrow. Bone marrow involvement is very common in indolent NHL (the slowly growing, "low-grade" form) but less common in Hodgkin lymphoma and aggressive NHL. If there are lymphoma cells in the bone marrow, one is automatically considered to be at Stage IV, regardless of how little disease is present elsewhere in the body.

Bone marrow biopsies are one of those procedures that have a bad reputation. During the time I was presumed to have a simple iron deficiency anemia, I knew that a bone marrow biopsy was supposed to be the "gold standard" for evaluating that type of anemia (small, pale red blood cells). I refrained from pointing this out to my doctor because I was afraid of having a bone marrow biopsy. I had

E.

heard that bone marrow biopsies were horribly painful, and if he didn't think one was warranted, *I* certainly wasn't going to bring it up.

If I'd known then what I know now, I'd have asked for a bone marrow biopsy, and we'd have discovered that I didn't have a simple iron deficiency anemia. The truth of the matter is that I needn't have been afraid. A badly done bone marrow biopsy can be excruciatingly painful, but, properly handled, bone marrow biopsies are uncomfortable but don't need to be painful at all.

During the procedure, patients may lie on their stomach or curled up on their side. The doctor will insert an instrument that's a cross between a very small apple corer and a largish needle into the center of the hipbone and use it to remove a small plug of bone. (Occasionally, bone marrow may be removed from the breastbone.) A sample of liquid marrow is withdrawn through a needle as well. Sometimes people need to undergo bilateral bone marrow biopsies—one on either side—since the cancer isn't necessarily evenly distributed throughout the entire bone marrow and it's possible that a single biopsy could miss hitting any cancerous regions.

It is important to be adequately medicated beforehand (as long as there is no medical reason to avoid such premedication), particularly if you are young and athletic and have strong bones. Premedication can sometimes include an antianxiety drug—such as Versed—and/or a painkiller like morphine. My doctor scheduled my bone marrow biopsy for a few hours after the lymph node biopsy so that I'd still be a little groggy. She cleaned the area well with antiseptics. Before inserting the apple corer and aspiration needles, she injected local anesthetics all around the area to numb the entire region (just like getting Novocain during dental work). My husband, Paul, stood nearby to hand her things.

"I once knew someone who used to do bone marrow biopsies without enough anesthetics, and his patients would lie there screaming," she remarked. "After seeing that, I've always made sure to inject a lot of local anesthetic and to give proper medication beforehand."

I felt a twinge of pain during the marrow aspiration, but only at about the level of a two or three on a one-to-ten scale, where one is the mildest sensation you would consider painful and ten is the most excruciating pain you can possibly imagine. The dreaded bone marrow biopsy was over.

Lumbar puncture

It's very uncommon for low-grade lymphoma to affect the *central nervous system* (abbreviated CNS and consisting of the brain and spinal cord), but this can happen with the more aggressive forms of the disease. It's not uncommon with AIDS-related lymphomas. If there's any reason to believe that someone diagnosed with aggressive lymphoma may have lymphoma in the CNS, such as neurological symptoms that cannot be otherwise explained, the physician may perform a *lumbar puncture*, also known as a spinal tap. This procedure involves withdrawing a small sample of fluid from around the spinal cord in the lumbar region of the lower back. People with lymphoblastic lymphoma and Burkitt lymphoma (formerly known as "Burkitt's lymphoma") may undergo lumbar punctures even if they do not have any neurological symptoms because if these aggressive forms of the disease have invaded the CNS, it is critical to bring them under control as rapidly as possible.

The doctor may want to perform a lumbar puncture in the absence of any obvious signs of CNS involvement with other forms of aggressive lymphoma as well, particularly if the bone marrow, the sinuses, or the testes are involved, since the presence of lymphoma in these sites increases the likelihood that the disease will spread to the CNS. Lumbar punctures are also frequently performed in preparation for bone marrow transplants.

During the lumbar puncture, the patient lies on his or her side rolled up into a ball, with the neck bent and the knees drawn up to the body. The lower back will be carefully cleaned with antiseptic solutions, and, as in the bone marrow biopsy, local anesthetics will be injected into the area. A needle will be inserted into the spinal canal so that a sample of *cerebrospinal fluid*, the clear liquid that bathes the brain and spinal cord, can be withdrawn and examined. If lymphoma has invaded the CNS, malignant cells will show up in the sample of cerebrospinal fluid. It's very important to remain lying down for about an hour after the procedure to avoid getting a severe headache.

History

The microscopic appearance and immunophenotype of the cells in the biopsy will identify the specific type of lymphoma. Is it Hodgkin lymphoma or NHL? If it's NHL, is it a B cell lymphoma or a T cell lymphoma or one of the rare NK cell lymphomas? Is it a slowly growing, indolent form or a rapidly progressing aggressive form? What's the specific version of the disease? This information is critical to developing an optimal treatment plan. However, it is also important to determine the extent of the disease and its impact on your overall well-being. This requires evaluating very different information than the sort you can obtain by examining a specimen of tissue under a microscope.

The first step is to obtain a *history*—indeed, your doctor almost certainly took a history, as well as performing a complete physical exam, when you first came in with the symptoms that suggested that you might have lymphoma. When you are first referred to an oncologist or hematologist, he or she will want to go carefully over all this background information again. The physician will want to hear all about your experience with the disease. If you have visibly enlarged lymph nodes, he or she will want to know how long you have been aware of them, how rapidly they've enlarged, and whether they've ever gotten smaller. The physician will ask whether you've experienced the Ann Arbor "B" symptoms of unexplained weight loss, unexplained fevers, and night sweats. He or she will want to know if you've experienced other lymphoma symptoms like intense, unexplained itching and pain in the affected nodes after drinking alcohol. Strange flu-like aches and pains? The physician will also ask about symptoms that might suggest localized involvement of certain specific sites outside the lymphatic system, such as the skin or the gastrointestinal tract.

The physician will also inquire about your family. Has anyone in your immediate family (parents, brothers, sisters, or children) ever had cancer? If so, what kind? He or she may also try to determine what may have increased the likelihood you would develop this disease. Knowing that I was a biologist, the first oncologist I saw asked what chemicals I had worked with, while the second asked if I had worked with any viruses.

When my dog developed lymphoma as well (several years after I was diagnosed), my oncologist asked if the two of us had been exposed to high levels of pesticides or herbicides. As far as I know we hadn't; indeed, when I was growing up, my parents were resented by their neighbors for letting their lawn run to weeds and wildflowers. I've sometimes thought that I was exposed to fewer herbicides or pesticides than 99 percent of people who grew up in suburbia.

Physical

In addition to taking a history, the physician will perform a *physical examination.* The physical will include a careful examination of all lymph node regions for signs of lymphadenopathy (fig. 2.1). Referred to by longtime lymphoma patients as "the grope," this part of the exam involves feeling for enlarged nodes in the neck, armpits, and groin. The physician will look for involvement of your tonsils and adenoids (which are lymphatic structures), any sign of liver and spleen enlargement, any extralymphatic lumps and bumps, suspicious-looking areas of skin, and swelling of the ankles (which could reflect dysfunction of the lymph nodes in the groin). He or she will listen to your heart and lungs with a stethoscope and measure your temperature, blood pressure, and weight.

These seemingly mundane "doctor rituals" can be surprisingly informative. As someone whose work involved doing biomedical research, I have a number of personal friends who are physicians. Upon hearing the story of my diagnosis, they universally responded by gasping: "You had shortness of breath and nobody listened to your chest with a stethoscope?"

All I could say was that everyone assumed that my shortness of breath re-

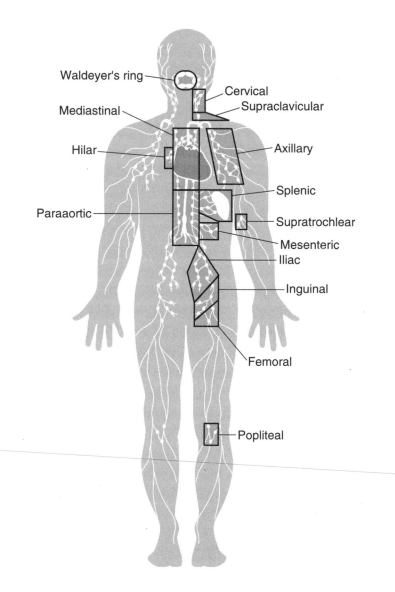

sulted from my anemia—moreover, my internist and all the specialists assumed that my GP had done this during the initial workup. Once it had been *determined* that I had a mass in my chest, it seemed as though every doctor in Boston came rushing up to put a stethoscope to my chest. A complete physical performed during the months before my diagnosis would likely have uncovered the lymphoma significantly earlier.

Blood work

In addition to the history and the physical examination, the doctor will order various blood tests. The most common blood studies are described below.

Complete blood count

Blood consists of white cells (*leukocytes*), red cells (*erythrocytes*), and platelets (*thrombocytes*) floating in a fluid called *plasma*. Plasma contains salts (like sodium, potassium, and chloride, which constitute the blood *electrolytes*), proteins, and various other physiologically useful substances such as vitamins and hormones. The complete blood count (CBC) determines the total numbers of white cells, red cells, and platelets found in a microliter (μl, a fraction of a typical drop) of blood.

The CBC is usually determined automatically; a known volume of blood is diluted and placed in an automated cell-counting machine. The cells pass through a small hole and, depending on the type of counter, either interrupt an electrical current running from one side of the hole to the other or deflect a beam of light. This provides an "event" that the counter can record. The counter keeps

---

Figure 2.1. *Lymph node regions.* The different lymph node regions define areas in the body in which lymph nodes cluster. The number of lymph node regions affected by lymphoma—and whether they are on the same side or different sides of the diaphragm—help define the stage of the disease. Waldeyer's ring consists of a ring of lymphoid tissue (the tonsils and adenoids) that circles the back of the throat. Other lymph node regions above the diaphragm include the cervical lymph nodes in the neck, the supraclavicular lymph nodes above the collarbones, the axillary lymph nodes in the armpits, and the mediastinal and hilar lymph nodes in the chest. Lymph node regions below the diaphragm include the paraaortic and mesenteric lymph nodes and the spleen, which are found in the abdomen; the iliac lymph nodes in the pelvis; and the inguinal lymph nodes of the groin. Femoral lymph nodes are found in the upper leg, popliteal lymph nodes are found behind the knee, and supratrochlear lymph nodes are in the crook of the elbow.

track electronically of the number and size of the cells in the blood sample. It records the total number of white cells, red cells, and platelets in the sample and the range of sizes of the red cells. Some counters can also distinguish one type of white cell from another.

Standard values for the CBC are:

Red cells (erythrocytes): 4.1–4.9 million cells/μl blood
White cells (leukocytes): 4,300–10,800 cells/μl blood
Platelets (thrombocytes): 130,000–400,000/μl blood

White cell differential count

In addition to the basic information on total cell number, it's useful to have a breakdown of the percentages of the different *types* of white cells present in the sample. This is called a white cell *differential.* (Chapter 10 describes what the different types of white cells do.) Large laboratories have automated cell counters that can discriminate between the different types of white cells. Alternatively, a drop of blood can be smeared across a microscope slide so that it forms a layer that is only one cell thick. The smear is then stained, and the white cell differential is determined manually by examining the slide under a microscope, counting one hundred cells and noting the numbers of each type.

In addition to providing the differential count of normal leukocytes, the smear is also useful for detecting abnormal cells. Chronic lymphocytic leukemia (and those cases of small lymphocytic lymphoma in which there are some malignant cells circulating in the blood) is characterized by fragile cells that break down during preparation of the smear into what is called a "*smudge cell*"; abnormal immature lymphocytes, called *lymphoblasts,* characteristic of the acute leukemias, may be seen in smears from people with acute lymphoblastic lymphoma.

Standard values for the white cell differential are:

Neutrophils: 45 to 74 percent (up to 4 percent may be neutrophils in the next-to-last stage of maturation, called *band cells* because of the shape of the cell nucleus)
Eosinophils: 0 to 7 percent
Basophils: 0 to 2 percent
Lymphocytes: 16 to 45 percent (about 80 percent of the circulating lymphocytes are T cells)
Monocytes: 4 to 10 percent

The absolute numbers (and therefore the relative percentages) of the different types of white cells may vary under certain conditions. Some of these conditions are pertinent to lymphoma; both the disease and its treatment can affect your white cell counts. The differential provides information on the underlying disease and also gives critical feedback on the effects of the treatment. Conditions affecting your white cell differential that are directly related to lymphoma or its treatment are described below. Other conditions that might affect your white cell counts are included in table 2.1.

An increase in the production and numbers of circulating neutrophils is called *neutrophilia*. Neutrophils play an important role in the response to bacterial infection (see Chapter 9), and neutrophilia is most commonly seen in infections. It also occurs in some malignancies; a mild to moderate neutrophilia is sometimes present in Hodgkin lymphoma. Certain drugs, such as the glucocorticoids, a class of steroid hormones used in some antilymphoma chemotherapy regimens, also cause neutrophilia: this will show up if someone takes prednisone or dexamethasone before undergoing a blood test.

Neutropenia is a reduction in the number of circulating neutrophils; it may result either from decreased production of cells or from increased destruction of circulating leukocytes. Since neutrophils, like all blood cells, are produced in the bone marrow, neutropenia can result when malignant cells, which can crowd out the precursor cells necessary for replenishing the supply of healthy white cells, invade the bone marrow. Neutropenia can also result when malignant cells release inhibitory cytokines inappropriately, telling the bone marrow to slow down neutrophil production.

The rapidly dividing cells in the bone marrow, which give rise to all the different blood cells, are very sensitive to many drugs used to treat cancer. Therefore, most drugs used in chemotherapy suppress blood cell production. Since neutrophils have a very brief lifetime, their levels can drop quickly in response to bone marrow suppression—which inhibits the production of new cells to replace those that have died. Susceptibility to bacterial infection increases dramatically when the levels of circulating neutrophils drop below 500 cells/μl of blood; therefore the neutrophil count needs to be monitored carefully when a person is undergoing chemotherapy. Sometimes drugs that stimulate blood cell production are given to combat severe chemotherapy-induced neutropenia (see Chapter 3).

Eosinophilia, an increase in the levels of circulating eosinophils, is found in a number of conditions, including Hodgkin lymphoma and some forms of NHL,

Table 2.1. Factors That Can Affect White Cell Counts

Cell Type and Abnormality	Some Possible Causes
Neutrophil:	
increased levels (neutrophilia) more than 10,000/µl of blood	infection (particularly bacterial infection) malignancies: leukemia (and some others), mild to moderate neutrophilia is sometimes present with Hodgkin lymphoma drugs: *glucocorticoid hormones (may be given as part of some chemo regimens)*, lithium (used to treat certain psychiatric conditions) colony-stimulating factors (see Chap. 3) given to treat chemotherapy-induced neutropenia may cause a neutrophilic "rebound" vigorous exercise and stress may mobilize neutrophils ordinarily found along the walls of small blood vessels in the lungs and spleen, so that there is a temporary increase in those circulating in the blood
decreased levels (neutropenia) less than 1,500 cells/µl of blood	drugs: *many chemotherapy drugs* disease: *some autoimmune diseases (lupus, rheumatoid arthritis) that may predispose to lymphoma*, following some infections vitamin deficiency: folic acid, B_{12} *lymphoma: direct effect (bone marrow invasion), indirect effect (inhibitory cytokines)*
Eosinophil:	
increased levels (eosinophilia) more than 500 cells/µl of blood	allergic responses parasitic infections disease: *some autoimmune diseases (lupus, rheumatoid arthritis) that may predispose to lymphoma* malignancies: *including Hodgkin lymphoma and some forms of NHL*
decreased levels (eosinopenia) less than 50 cells/µl blood	drugs: *glucocorticoid hormones (may be given as part of some chemotherapy regimens)* acute stress: including severe bacterial infection Cushing syndrome (an endocrine disorder that affects glucocorticoid levels)
Monocyte:	
increased levels (monocytosis) more than 800 cells/µl of blood	infections: tuberculosis, malaria malignancies: leukemia, preleukemic conditions, *sometimes lymphoma*
decreased levels (monocytopenia) less than 100 cells/µl of blood	drugs: *many chemotherapy drugs, glucocorticoid hormones (may be given as part of some chemotherapy regimens)*

Table 2.1 (continued)

Cell Type and Abnormality	Some Possible Causes
	acute stress: including severe bacterial infection
	Cushing syndrome (an endocrine disorder that affects glucocorticoid levels)
	malignancy: some forms of leukemia
Lymphocyte:	
increased levels (lymphocytosis) more than 5000 cells/μl of blood	malignancies: *chronic lymphocytic leukemia lymphoplasmacytoid lymphoma, splenic lymphoma with villous lymphocytes (splenic marginal zone lymphoma), mild lymphocytosis with other indolent lymphomas and leukemias*
	infection: typhoid, tuberculosis, mononucleosis, *early stages of HIV*
	drugs: Dilantin, carbamazepine
decreased levels (lymphocytopenia) less than 1000 cells/μl of blood	malignancies: *lymphoma (mostly Hodgkin lymphoma)*
	radiation therapy: may be very prolonged
	drugs: certain chemotherapy drugs (fludarabine and cladribine), glucocorticoid hormones (may be given as part of some chemotherapy regimens)
	biological therapies
	AIDS and certain other infections
	severe malnutrition
	hereditary

Note: This table includes common causes of abnormalities in white cell levels; it is not exhaustive. Causes that are most relevant to people with lymphoma are *italicized*.

and may be associated with severe itching. *Eosinopenia,* or lowered levels of eosinophils, occurs in response to treatment with glucocorticoids (opposite to the effect on neutrophils).

An increase in the number of monocytes, termed *monocytosis,* sometimes appears in conjunction with malignancies, including lymphoma. But don't worry if you have a slightly elevated monocyte count while you're undergoing chemotherapy. Drugs that cause neutropenia by suppressing bone marrow function tend to cause monocytopenia as well. Monocytes tend to recover from this suppression a little faster than the other cell types, and this may show up as a slight monocytosis during the time your marrow is recovering. Like eosinopenia, monocytopenia occurs in response to elevated levels of glucocorticoids.

The white cell of most interest to those of us with lymphoma is, of course, the lymphocyte. In most forms of lymphoma, the malignant lymphocytes tend to congregate in the lymph nodes and other lymphoid tissues or simply in various solid tissues of the body. However, in chronic lymphocytic leukemia, as well as in other, less common, indolent leukemias, such as hairy cell leukemia and splenic lymphoma with villous lymphocytes, people develop *lymphocytosis*, an increase in the number of circulating lymphocytes. Lymphocytosis is frequently seen in lymphoplasmacytoid lymphoma.

While it is not uncommon to find a few malignant lymphocytes circulating in the blood in other forms of lymphoma—particularly the other indolent lymphomas—these are rarely associated with a pronounced lymphocytosis at the time of diagnosis (counts may go up later in the course of the disease). Malignant lymphocytes that are clearly abnormal can be found circulating in acute lymphoblastic lymphoma, adult T cell leukemia/lymphoma, and some cases of mycosis fungoides.

Lymphocytopenia (reduced levels of circulating lymphocytes), like monocytopenia and eosinopenia, can be caused by high levels of glucocorticoids. It may also occur in Hodgkin lymphoma. Radiation therapy and some forms of chemotherapy (fludarabine and cladribine) can cause a profound and long-lasting lymphocytopenia (predominantly of T cells), and some of the antibody therapies affect levels of normal circulating lymphocytes as well as the malignant cells they target. People who experience sustained lymphocytopenia may need to take antibiotics to avoid the risk of certain infections.

Red cell values
Hematocrit

Unlike white cells, there's only one kind of mature red cell, the erythrocyte. The function of the erythrocyte is to bring oxygen to all the different cells in the body. The oxygen is carried by *hemoglobin*, an iron-containing protein that is synthesized by the red cells and gives them their red color.

The *hematocrit* is a test that measures the fraction of blood that is composed of red cells. It can be determined by placing a known volume of blood in a small graduated tube and spinning the tube in a centrifuge. Since blood cells are heavier than plasma, they will settle to the bottom of the tube, leaving the cell-free plasma on top, and the percentage of the total volume that is taken up by the red cells can be measured. The normal hematocrit in adult men lies between 42 and 52, which means that red blood cells make up 42 to 52 percent of the total volume of blood in the sample; in women, the hematocrit lies between 36 and 46. If the hematocrit lies below this normal range, the person is said to be *anemic*.

Either excessive loss or diminished production of red cells can result in anemia. You lose red cells when you lose a lot of blood or when there's abnormal destruction of red cells (*hemolytic anemia*). Red cell production can decrease for a number of reasons. These include suppression of the bone marrow by certain drugs, insufficient iron, kidney disease (the kidneys produce *erythropoietin*, a chemical growth factor that stimulates the production of red cells), and infiltration of the bone marrow by malignant cells. Since the total red cell volume determines the hematocrit, either a reduction in the size of individual cells or a decrease in the total number of red cells can cause anemia.

Iron deficiency anemia occurs when the amount of dietary iron absorbed isn't sufficient to replace iron lost from the body in blood. Since the erythrocytes will contain only a portion of their normal hemoglobin content, this leads to production of small, pale red blood cells (*microcytic, hypochromic* anemia). Iron deficiency anemia is fairly common in otherwise healthy menstruating women; however, iron deficiency anemia in *men* should prompt a search for an ongoing source of blood loss.

The anemia of chronic disease, which can result from malignancies (including lymphoma), as well as some chronic infections, involves cytokines that create abnormalities in iron handling; this kind of anemia can sometimes mimic iron deficiency anemia (as in my case). It can usually be distinguished from a true iron deficiency anemia by measuring iron stores in the blood and bone marrow. These stores will be low in iron deficiency anemia but not in the anemia of chronic disease.

In people with lymphoma, anemia most frequently occurs in response to suppression of red cell production by certain forms of chemotherapy—especially the high-dose therapies given in preparation for a bone marrow transplant. The resulting anemia can be exacerbated by excessive blood loss if the platelet production is suppressed as well, in which case the blood doesn't clot properly.

However, anemia can result from the disease as well as its treatment. Some forms of lymphoma can lead to hemolytic anemias, caused by excessive red cell destruction, if the immune system misidentifies the red cells as foreign and starts attacking them. The anemia of chronic disease can occur with both Hodgkin lymphoma and NHL. If someone's bone marrow is heavily infiltrated by cancerous cells that crowd out the normal cells destined to become erythrocytes, he or she is likely to become anemic.

Whatever the cause, reduced hemoglobin content and total red cell volume lead to a condition of oxygen deficiency. The person is breathing in enough oxygen, but not enough is being delivered to his or her cells. This will cause short-ness of breath because the brain interprets the lack of oxygen as an inadequate supply and signals that the person needs to breathe in more air. This will be par-ticularly apparent after any physical exertion, since the more a person exercises, the more oxygen the body needs.

Other symptoms of anemia include fatigue, loss of stamina, and an increase in heart rate as the heart tries to circulate more blood to oxygen-starved tissues. People who are anemic are typically pale because it's the iron in the hemoglobin that gives blood its red color. The ancient Greeks knew enough to treat anemia with solutions prepared from iron swords left to rust in water. They believed that iron, which was symbolic of Ares, the powerful red god of war, would counter-act the typical anemic symptoms of pallor and fatigue. They were right, even if we no longer agree with their reasons.

A blood test may also provide values for MCV, MCH, and MCHC. These somewhat obscure letters stand for *mean corpuscular volume, mean corpuscular hemo-globin,* and *mean corpuscular hemoglobin content.* The MCV refers to the average size of a red cell (also known as a corpuscle). It's a useful measure in evaluating the anemias, since it can be used to distinguish between the microcytic anemias, associated with diminished red cell size; the normocytic anemias, associated with normal cell size; and the macrocytic anemias, associated with enlarged red cells.

Mean corpuscular hemoglobin, which is calculated from the total hemoglo-bin in a sample divided by the number of red cells, shows whether individual cells contain sufficient hemoglobin, as does mean cell hemoglobin concentra-tion, which is calculated from the total hemoglobin divided by the hematocrit and thus takes cell size into account as well as cell number. Normal red cell val-ues are:

Hemoglobin:	130–180 grams/liter (adult men)
	120–160 grams/liter (adult women; this may be higher after menopause and is usually somewhat lower during the third trimester of pregnancy)
Hematocrit	42–52 (adult men)
	36–46 (adult women)
MCV	86–98 femtoliters
MCH	28–34 picograms/cell
MCHC	32–36 grams/liter

Erythrocyte sedimentation rate

While the hematocrit measures the volume of blood taken up by the red cells, the *erythrocyte sedimentation rate* (ESR) measures the speed with which red cells, which are the heaviest component of blood, settle out of a sample of blood in a tube. This has to do with the presence of excess blood proteins, which cause the red cells to clump up and fall out of suspension more rapidly. The ESR is a relatively nonspecific test, as the rate of sedimentation can be elevated in a variety of inflammatory conditions. It's sometimes elevated in lymphoma and may provide a convenient measure by which to monitor responses to treatment. It is more frequently used to monitor Hodgkin lymphoma than NHL.

Serum protein electrophoresis

Moving out of the cells and into the plasma, the fluid cell-free portion of the blood, we come to the serum protein electrophoresis (SPEP) test. This test detects the presence of high levels of abnormal immunoglobulins. Since lymphocytes produce immunoglobulins (see Chapter 9), certain forms of lymphoma in which the malignant cells continue to manufacture and secrete immunoglobulins are characterized by abnormalities in the SPEP.

Here's how the test works. As mentioned earlier, the blood contains extracellular proteins. The most abundant of these proteins are albumin, fibrinogen, and a group of proteins called the globulins. Serum, which is the fluid portion that is left after the blood clots, is similar to plasma except that fibrinogen (which is involved in clotting) and several related proteins have been removed. However, serum still contains albumin and the globulins.

If an electrical current is run through a sample of serum placed on a solid support, the different proteins present in the serum will migrate at different rates, depending on their size and electrical charge. Those with the greatest positive charge will migrate most rapidly in one direction; those with the greatest negative charge will migrate most rapidly in the other. The proteins in serum separate into characteristic bands, which can be classified as albumin, and the α_1, α_2, β_1, β_2, and γ globulins. The more abundant a particular protein species, the more dense its associated band. If the density of each of the different protein bands is graphed, peaks appear that indicate how much of each specific kind of protein is present (fig. 2.2). The antibodies (or immunoglobulins) are found in the γ globulin fraction. The γ globulin peak is typically rather broad and shallow as all the different forms of immunoglobulin spread out. In those types of lymphoma where the

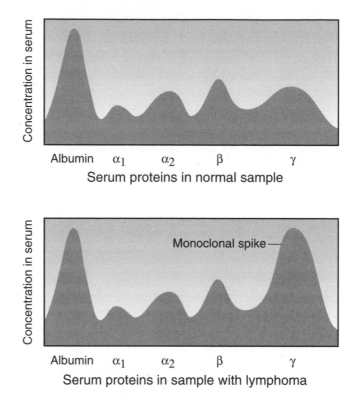

Figure 2.2. *Serum protein electrophoresis.* This blood test can reveal the presence of forms of lymphoma in which the malignant cells secrete antibodies. The results of a normal serum protein electrophoresis test can be graphed as peaks that correspond to the serum concentration of albumin and to the α, β, and γ globulins (after the first three letters of the Greek alphabet). The γ globulin peak contains all the antibodies (immunoglobulins) found circulating in the blood. Because different antibodies will migrate at slightly different rates in response to an electric current, the normal γ globulin peak tends to be broad and low. In someone who has multiple myeloma or a form of lymphoma in which the malignant cells secrete antibody, the malignant cells are clonal: they are all descended from a single parent cell, and they secrete identical antibodies. All these monoclonal antibodies will migrate at the same rate, and this will show up as a monoclonal spike in the γ globulin fraction.

malignant cells synthesize and secrete immunoglobulin, the molecules of immunoglobulin made by the cancer cells will all migrate together, since all the malignant cells are descended from a single malignant clone and make an identical form of immunoglobulin. Therefore, that immunoglobulin will show up as a single sharp peak on the SPEP. This peak is referred to as a *monoclonal spike.*

The SPEP will also show if there is a reduction in the level of other immunoglobulins (*hypogammaglobulinemia*), which can lead to enhanced susceptibility to infection. Hypogammaglobulinemia can occur if the malignant cells send out cytokine signals that inhibit the production of normal lymphocytes. Sometimes in lymphoma the albumin peak is suppressed as well.

LDH and β_2 microglobulin

Lactate dehydrogenase (or lactic dehydrogenase, LDH) and β_2 microglobulin are two proteins found in serum that are frequently measured in patients with lymphoma. LDH is an enzyme (actually a group of enzymes) that plays a role in metabolizing carbohydrates (sugars and starches) to extract energy. This process takes place inside the cytoplasm of cells. When a cell is damaged or destroyed, its LDH leaks out and shows up in the serum.

Therefore, serum LDH rises under conditions involving massive cell damage and death (like a heart attack). Growing tumors frequently display a rapid rate of cell turnover and cell death. Since large tumors contain more cells than small tumors, the LDH released by dying cells is an indirect measure of total tumor size. Higher LDH levels correlate with more extensive disease, and lower LDH levels correlate with less extensive disease. A tumor mass's response to chemotherapy can be monitored by measuring the serum LDH levels: a drop means a decrease in tumor size.

As you might expect from the name, free β_2 microglobulin is one of the serum proteins that migrates in the β globulin band during serum protein electrophoresis. It is a protein that is associated with the MHC protein molecules and helps stabilize their structure (see Chapter 9). Serum β_2 microglobulin is elevated in most forms of lymphoma (except primary mediastinal large cell lymphoma) and, like LDH, is often used as a marker for tumor mass.

Other blood tests

Calcium

Lymphoma, like several other forms of cancer, can lead to an increase in levels of serum calcium. This condition, called *hypercalcemia*, is caused by *resorption* of calcium from the bones: the calcium is reclaimed from bone and dissolved back into the blood. While we ordinarily think of our bones as eternal and unchanging, they are actually constantly undergoing a process of formation and resorption. In adults, about 20 percent of the calcium in bone turns over each year. That means we essentially rebuild our entire skeleton about every five years! This process of calcium turnover depends on the activity of two kinds of cells: the osteoblasts and the osteoclasts ("osteo" refers to bone).

Osteoblasts build bone, while *osteoclasts* resorb calcium and erode bone. Both of them labor continuously at their jobs. Sometimes people with lymphoma develop a relative increase in activity on the part of the osteoclasts, either because of local invasion of the bone marrow by lymphoma cells or in response to circulating cytokines released from the malignant cells. In either case, there's net loss of calcium from the bone and a rise in serum calcium. Since hypercalcemia can be dangerous if left uncontrolled, it's common to test serum calcium levels in people with lymphoma.

Liver and kidney function

People with lymphoma generally have blood tests to evaluate kidney function (creatinine, uric acid, the electrolytes sodium, potassium, and chloride) and liver function (various liver enzymes as well as bilirubin). These tests help determine whether lymphoma has invaded (or impinged on) the liver or the kidneys, and they may also influence therapeutic decisions.

Both the liver and the kidney play important roles in clearing toxic substances from the body. The liver is involved in excretion of various substances (drugs, hormones, metabolic end products) and also converts some substances into different forms. This enzymatic conversion is important as a mechanism for inactivating some poisons, and, conversely, can turn some inert drugs (including some used in chemotherapy) into a therapeutically useful form.

Before a patient starts chemotherapy, it's important to determine whether the liver is functioning normally. This is to make sure that drug levels in the body will be therapeutically appropriate. The doctor will want to be certain that drugs that are normally cleared out of your body by the liver won't build up to potentially toxic levels and that drugs that need to be turned on by liver enzymes will, in fact, be converted to the active form.

The kidneys clear various substances out of blood so they can be excreted in the urine. One such substance is uric acid, which is released into the blood whenever cells are destroyed. Occasionally, when you have a large tumor mass, therapy can lead to the synchronized death of numerous tumor cells, so that large quantities of uric acid flow into the blood. If the levels of uric acid get too high, it can crystallize out of the blood in the joints and kidneys, causing a condition called gout. The sharp little crystals of uric acid can be extremely painful and can be damaging.

In persons with normal kidney function, this condition, called *tumor lysis syndrome*, can be controlled with *allopurinol*, a drug that reduces the formation of uric acid, or with *rasburicase*, a drug that accelerates uric acid breakdown. In people with impaired kidney function, it may be necessary to set up for dialysis before starting chemotherapy. Then, if blood uric acid levels start to rise, the excess uric acid can be removed with a dialysis machine before concentrations get high enough to create a problem. The kidneys also clear certain dyes out of the body that are commonly used in CT scans (see below); consequently it is desirable to determine renal function before a person undergoes a CT scan.

Imaging techniques

If our skin and muscles were transparent, it would be easy to visualize lymphoma tumors. We could see how big they were, where they were located, and how well they responded to therapy. That isn't possible, of course, so people have had to devise alternative ways to view the inside of the body. Various techniques are used to obtain images of internal structures. The most common of these techniques involve X-rays.

Procedures involving X-rays

In November 1895, almost exactly 101 years before I had my first CT scan, the German physicist Wilhelm Roentgen was experimenting with a cathode-ray tube in an opaque container and was astonished to notice some glowing fluorescent material nearby. (A cathode-ray tube is a vacuum tube through which a high-voltage electric current is passed.) Fluorescent materials glow when they are stimulated with external radiation (including visible radiation—or light), but Roentgen couldn't see any light rays that could excite the glowing material. He discovered that invisible radiation generated in the tube passed through opaque materials and that these rays could expose film or make a fluorescent screen glow. He named these mysterious rays X-rays.

He found that X-rays passed more readily through less dense material and discovered that he could use them to take a picture of the bones of his hand. X-rays were used for medical diagnostic purposes within months of their discovery and for therapeutic purposes shortly thereafter. (As a modern biomedical researcher, I found the speed with which X-rays were adopted into common use the most unfamiliar part of this story.) For discovering X-rays, Roentgen received the first Nobel Prize in Physics, in 1901.

The techniques involved in passing X-rays through the human body and capturing the resulting shadows on film have been refined a bit since Roentgen's time. For instance, we now filter out low-energy X-rays (which are readily absorbed by the body) and use a fluorescent screen to magnify the signal that reaches the film to limit our X-ray exposure. (One of the earliest radiographs, a picture Roentgen took of his wife's hand, required an exposure time of about thirty minutes. Such long exposures would now be considered unacceptable.) However, the basic idea remains unchanged and provides a useful means of obtaining pictures of what's going on inside our bodies.

Most people with lymphoma get chest X-rays as part of the diagnostic procedure. Views are taken through your chest from back to front, as well as from the side. Chest X-rays show intrathoracic disease, such as mediastinal tumors and involvement of the lungs. If you look at one of your chest X-rays, the dark areas, where many X-rays made it through your body to expose the film, represent low-density regions like your lungs; high-density regions, like your ribs, will look white. Your heart, which is pretty dense, shows up light as well.

Like me, many people discover that they have a thoracic tumor following a chest X-ray. In my case, the lack of any dark film along one side of the chest was the tip-off that something was amiss. However, plain X-rays give less information about what's going on in the abdomen, which is filled with different structures of similar density.

In order to evaluate abdominal disease, a CT (pronounced "see-tea") scan of the abdomen and pelvis (abdominopelvic CT scan) is generally performed. The CT scan (or CAT scan, for *computerized axial tomography*) is a refined version of the

Figure 2.3. *Computerized axial tomography (CT).* As you pass through the CT scan machine, a very narrow X-ray beam produced by an emitter ("E") rotates around your body, passing through a thin cross-sectional "slice." Detectors ("D") on the other side pick up whatever radiation passes all the way through your body. In this way, the tissue density at all the possible different angles through the slice can be measured and recorded. Once a particular slice has been completed, such as the shoulder-level slice shown in the top part of the figure, you advance through the scanner so that tissue density of the next slice can be computed. Slice by slice, a three-dimensional picture of the entire region of the body being scanned can be built up. The top part of this figure gives a view looking down on someone who is passing through the CT scan machine, who is now having a shoulder-level slice scanned. The bottom shows the CT scan machine. The person undergoing the scan lies down on the platform, which carries the person along as it advances through the scanner.

LIVING WITH LYMPHOMA

X-ray that can give more detailed information about internal structures. In a CT scan, a very narrow X-ray beam rotates around your body, passing through a thin cross-sectional "slice." Detectors on the other side of your body pick up whatever passes through. In this way, the tissue density at all the possible different angles through the slice can be measured and recorded (fig. 2.3).

The information from the scan is fed into a computer. Then, you move a little farther through the CT machine (see below) so that a new "slice" of your body is exposed to the beam. All the images of sequential "slices" are fed into a computer to build an amazingly detailed three-dimensional picture of your internal structures, based on the exact map of differences in tissue density. Most people

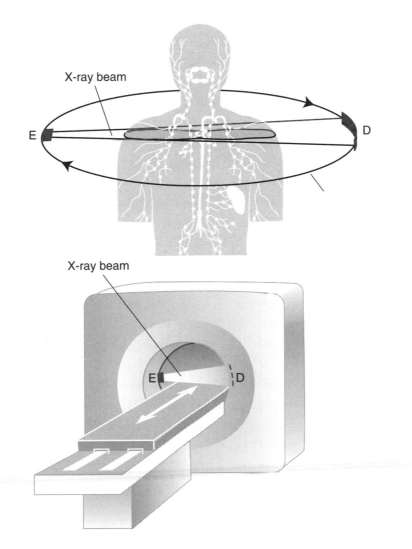

with lymphoma get an abdominopelvic CT scan as part of the diagnostic workup; many people need CT scans of the chest or head as well, depending on where the lymphoma is located.

As far as you're concerned, the process is very simple. The CT scanner is shaped something like a giant plastic doughnut. You lie quite still on a movable slab that goes through the center of the doughnut. Periodically, the technician running the machine (or a disembodied machine voice, in a fancy facility) instructs you to breathe in and then hold your breath as the rotating beam scans your body.

This is important: movement of the chest and abdomen during normal breathing would blur the images in the CT scan. As you're being scanned, you can see the X-ray equipment whirling around in a thin transparent band on the inside of the doughnut ring. Then it stops whirling and you're allowed to breathe as the machine moves you into position for the next set of scans.

If, like me, you have a large mass in your chest, you may find it difficult to hold your breath. In this case, do the best you can, and when you *absolutely can't* hold your breath anymore, let it out slowly and then slowly draw in a new breath. When I had my first scan, I told the technician that I couldn't hold my breath very well. I explained that I had shortness of breath because I was anemic and said I hoped this hadn't interfered with the scan. At the time, I had no idea I had a tumor so large that I could only use one lung, and it was only after I saw the scan that I understood why she patted my arm and looked so sad.

Generally, patients drink a chalky solution before undergoing an abdominal CT scan; this fills the inside of the gastrointestinal tract with a dense material (barium) that is opaque to X-rays. This makes the intestines clearly distinguishable from the rest of the abdominal *viscera* (organs) and improves visualization of abdominal structures. Patients are generally asked to avoid eating for at least several hours before the procedure so that the stomach and intestines are empty of food and can fill up with the barium contrast solution.

A high-contrast solution containing iodine is sometimes injected into a vein as well. Again, this is to improve visualization. The iodine contrast solution can cause a brief unpleasant sensation of heat, an increase in heart rate, and a strange taste; occasionally it can cause nausea or pain. In addition to a pounding heart, I generally experience such an intense flash of heat in my groin as to be mildly painful. Fortunately, it doesn't last very long.

It's important to start the scan right after injecting the contrast, before the kidneys start clearing it out of the body. The first time I had a CT scan, the technician had me lie down, gave me the injection, and then raced out of the room as fast as she could to start the apparatus that would load me into the scanner. Another time, a resident had me lie in the scanner with my arm sticking out awk- wardly so he could inject the contrast at the last possible minute. More recently, I have gotten an IV line inserted in my arm beforehand. That way, the techni- cians can inject the dye into the IV right before they're ready to start the scan. This procedure seems to work the best.

While you're not supposed to eat before an abdominal scan, it's a good idea to drink enough fluids to avoid becoming dehydrated. Otherwise your veins can flatten out, making it harder to inject the dye. This is particularly important if you get your scans at a facility that tends to get backed up so that you need to wait a long time before getting your scan. After you've been given an intravenous contrast medium, it's also important to drink lots of water for the rest of the day to flush it out of your system.

People who are allergic to shellfish or iodine, or who have severe allergies in general, should inform the CT personnel before undergoing the CT scan. They will likely decide to use a different kind of contrast medium to avoid the possi- bility of an allergic reaction. This form of contrast, called nonionic contrast, is also preferable for people with diabetes and for people with impaired kidney function.

While chest X-rays and abdominopelvic CT scans are standard procedure for virtually everyone with lymphoma, other imaging procedures are sometimes used as well. The *lymphangiogram* is another procedure in the basic family of radi- ology (the branch of medicine concerned with the use of X-rays for diagnostic or therapeutic procedures). In a lymphangiogram, contrast medium is injected into the big toe. This radio-opaque dye spreads through the lymphatic vessels in the lower portion of the body over a period of several hours, and the lower lym- phatic system can then be visualized by means of X-rays.

Lymphangiograms can occasionally pick up early involvement of abdominal lymph nodes that aren't yet enlarged and could therefore be missed by a CT scan. Therefore, while lymphangiograms are much less common now than formerly, they are sometimes performed when the doctor suspects that there is unidenti- fied abdominal disease and such abdominal disease would change the treatment plan. For instance, someone who appeared to have localized Hodgkin lymphoma in his or her chest might get a lymphangiogram if the presence of abdominal dis- ease would change the proposed course of therapy from radiation alone to chemotherapy *and* radiation.

Lymphangiograms can also be useful in identifying involvement of the lymphatic system of the legs.

Radioisotopic scans

Shortly after Roentgen discovered X-rays, the French physicist A. Henri Becquerel, intrigued by Roentgen's results, began investigating the properties of fluorescent compounds. He began working with an ore of uranium to see if sunlight could excite the uranium into giving off X-rays. One cloudy day, when he couldn't perform any experiments, he left some uranium in a drawer with some film. He was amazed to discover that he got a picture of his uranium crystals in the absence of any sunlight (and hence any fluorescence). That meant that the uranium was *spontaneously* emitting some sort of radiation that exposed film. He had discovered radioactivity, for which he shared a Nobel Prize with Marie and Pierre Curie in 1903.

Many elements exist in several forms in which the atoms differ slightly in weight from one another because their nuclei contain more or fewer neutrons. These different forms are referred to as *isotopes*. *Radioisotopes* are unstable isotopes: they undergo what is called *radioactive decay* into another substance by giving off radiation. Radiation can consist of small particles as well as the "rays" we typically associate with the term. The emission of radiation by a radioisotope is called a *radioactive disintegration*.

Because radioisotopes are constantly undergoing radioactive decay, they don't last forever but eventually break down into the second substance. Different radioisotopes characteristically decay at different rates. The rate at which a given radioisotope breaks down defines its *half-life*, which is the amount of time required for a given amount of isotope to decay by half. So, if you had a radioisotope with a half-life of two days, half of it would be gone in two days. Half of what remained would be gone in another two days, leaving you with a quarter of the initial amount after four days, and half of *that* would be gone in another two days, leaving you with an eighth of the initial amount, and so forth. Typically, the radioisotopes used in radioisotopic imaging have short half-lives, so patients don't carry around radioactive substances for very long.

Nuclear medicine is the branch of medicine that uses radioisotopes to obtain images of internal structures and to treat certain conditions. Many different radioisotopes are used in nuclear medicine. In some cases, a given substance has an affinity for a particular tissue. For example, the thyroid accumulates iodine, which is a component of thyroid hormone. Since the thyroid cannot distinguish between radioactive and nonradioactive iodine, any free radioiodine a person ingests ends up in his or her thyroid. A scan of someone who had eaten radioiodine would show radiation emanating from the thyroid.

In other cases, nonradioactive compounds that are used by a specific tissue are "tagged" with a radioisotope. When the tissue of interest takes up the tagged compound, the radioisotope goes along for the ride. This allows that tissue to be visualized. It's a procedure that's essentially analogous to James Bond attaching a tiny radio transmitter to the diamond bracelet he gives to the beautiful enemy agent whose movements he wants to track.

Although both radiology and nuclear medicine use invisible forms of radiation to obtain images of structures that we wouldn't be able to see otherwise, the two fields are different in that one involves passing radiation through the body from an external source, while the other involves taking a small amount of some radioactive substance into the body.

Many people are concerned about taking radioisotopes. This is natural: we've all learned to be cautious about radioactivity. The very word conjures up visions of atom bombs and fallout. It's important to remember that, in these diagnostic tests, only tiny doses of radiation are used. While they're certainly nothing you'd want to do just for fun and repeating the tests over and over and over could lead to a certain amount of cumulative damage, nuclear medicine imaging tests are an instance of a procedure in which the benefits clearly outweigh the risks.

When I needed to undergo radioisotopic scans, though, I wondered whether I could pose a danger to other people—for whom there were no benefits. Since radiation, like chemotherapy, does more damage to dividing cells, I was particularly concerned about being around children, whose cells divide more frequently than those of adults. Shortly after being injected with radioactive gallium, I started to get into a crowded hospital elevator. A mother with a small child got on after me. Looking down at the little child standing innocently next to me, oblivious to the deadly rays I pictured pouring from my body, I was overcome with fear. I imagined him getting leukemia in a few years and never knowing why. I got off the elevator and walked downstairs.

As it turns out, I might as well have stayed on that elevator. In all the tests discussed in this chapter, this is *not* a matter for concern. Any radiation that other people around you might encounter is negligible. When I asked a radiologist whether someone waiting for a gallium scan might pose a danger to other people he replied, "I'd feel perfectly comfortable sleeping next to my pregnant wife after being injected with radioisotope for a diagnostic text." (Procedures that use radioisotopes as therapy to destroy the malignant tissue, rather than in diagnosis, are a different story.)

Some substances used in radioisotopic imaging, like gallium, are secreted in milk; ask your doctor about this if you are breastfeeding at the time you need to undergo a nuclear medicine scan.

Several diagnostic tests involving radioisotopic imaging are commonly used in people with lymphoma. Some of these tests use substances that are accumulated by the malignant tissue and are useful in determining the extent of the disease and the response to therapy. Other tests use substances that are selectively accumulated by specific organs. These tests are used to determine whether that organ is functioning normally. An abnormal result on one of these tests may indicate involvement of that organ by the disease or may rule out certain therapeutic regimens.

Gallium and thallium scans

Gallium and thallium scans fall into the category of tests used to determine the extent of disease and the response to therapy. *Gallium* is a metal that's picked up by the tumors of Hodgkin lymphoma and most aggressive (intermediate and high-grade) non-Hodgkin lymphomas. Gallium is also accumulated by inflammatory tissue—when there's some sort of major immunological response going on—and bone.

It is not clear why lymphoma cells should want to sop up gallium, although it's possible that they mistake the gallium for iron. (If that's the case, then red cells and the hematopoietic cells in the bone marrow are perceptive enough to avoid this mistake.) Whatever the reason, gallium accumulation by malignant lymphocytes provides a useful tool for determining the response to therapy. Since gallium accumulation is much less consistent in low-grade NHL, it's not as useful in evaluating indolent disease.

Gallium scans are sometimes used to evaluate abnormal tissue that may remain following a standard treatment regimen. These "residual masses" can be detected by CT scan and are frequently found in people who had large tumors at the time of diagnosis (referred to as "bulky disease"). However, a CT scan alone, which simply measures the density of the tissue the X-rays passed through on their way to the detector, can't discriminate between active disease and scar tissue left behind by the dying tumor.

It's critically important to make this distinction: with Hodgkin lymphoma and aggressive NHL, the best hope for a cure lies in knocking the disease out completely in the first round of treatment. People with relapsed disease *have* gone on to attain cures, but it's a longer, tougher road. If active disease is present at the end of the initial therapeutic regimen, the oncologist will likely switch to a more aggressive treatment plan. On the other hand, it would be undesirable (to say the least) to continue hammering an innocuous mass of scar tissue with ever more aggressive regimens of chemotherapy, none of which will ever make it go away completely. A gallium scan can frequently distinguish between residual disease and plain old scar tissue; areas of active disease should take up gallium, while scar tissue should not.

Since gallium is absorbed poorly from the gastrointestinal tract, the radioactive isotope ^{67}gallium is given intravenously. Typically the scan is performed two days after the patient receives the gallium injection. (Gallium has a half-life of a little over three days and is eliminated from the body rather slowly, so there's still enough radioactivity left at this time to perform the scan.) This timing provides the optimal "signal" (gallium in the tumor) to "noise" (gallium in normal tissue) ratio, although, if necessary, the scan can be performed successfully between six hours and five days after injection.

Gallium is excreted both in the urine and in the stool. Therefore, the patient usually takes a laxative the night before the scan in order to eliminate radioactive gallium waste from the intestines. The results of the laxative are the most unpleasant part of the whole procedure. However, it's important to go through with it, since a gallium signal inside the gut could confound the interpretation of abdominal results.

The gallium scan utilizes computerized tomography to measure the frequency of radioactive disintegrations (proportional to the amount of radioactivity) in vertical "slices" of the body. Only a small dose of radioactive gallium is administered to begin with, so these radioactive emanations are infrequent even in areas of the body that have accumulated gallium. Since it's necessary to measure enough radioactive disintegrations to obtain an accurate picture of where the gallium is localized, gallium scans can take a long time. The patient needs to lie still during the scan (often with hands over head), and it can sometimes get uncomfortable. The good news is that people don't usually need to get gallium scans very often.

People with bulky disease, who are likely to have a residual mass after completing therapy (whether or not their disease has been cured), may undergo a gallium scan before starting treatment. This is to make sure that the tumor is, in fact, one of the majority (in aggressive NHL and Hodgkin lymphoma) that do accumulate gallium. Without a pretreatment scan verifying that the tumor took up gallium prior to therapy, it's impossible to interpret a negative scan after therapy with complete certainty. It's always possible that this represents a false negative—a rare tumor that couldn't accumulate gallium in the first place.

Because I had a large tumor, it was likely that I would be left with some residual abnormality. Since I was having other diagnostic radioisotopic procedures performed that couldn't be run along with a gallium scan, and because my oncologist thought that it was critical to start treatment as soon as possible, she decided to skip the pretreatment scan. Later on, I found myself haunted by her decision when I couldn't take the reassurance from the gallium-negative postchemo scan of a residual mass that a positive pretreatment scan would have provided.

Sometimes people undergo gallium scans midway through therapy, since a negative scan at this time (assuming it was positive in the first place) is a very good sign. While a negative gallium scan at the end of the initial chemotherapy regimen is a good thing, a positive scan isn't always bad news. Occasionally, people show false positives; likely this is due to healthy lymphocytes and macrophages attacking the last of the dying cancer cells. In this case, a repeat scan, performed after the inflammatory response has subsided, should convert to negative.

Although the names are similar, and *thallium*, like gallium, is a metal, the two substances are quite different. Thallium is used to image indolent lymphoma, since, unlike gallium, it is accumulated by low-grade malignancies (as well as certain other forms of cancer). People started using thallium in tumor imaging after physicians using thallium in a cardiac function test (similar to the MUGA test described below) realized that it was being taken up by tissue that turned out to be undiagnosed lung cancer!

Although thallium scans are relatively uncommon, they are sometimes used to evaluate the extent of low-grade disease and the response to chemotherapy. They are also used to evaluate a benign condition called *thymic rebound*, which can sometimes resemble active disease in the mediastinal region. Thallium scans aren't usually used to evaluate abdominal disease because normal cells in the gut secrete thallium.

PET scans

PET (*positron emission tomography*) scanning has had a tremendous impact on various aspects of medicine. That's because it measures metabolic activity and can therefore detect *functional* abnormalities even in the absence of any gross anatomical changes. Even small regions of cancerous cells that wouldn't show up on a CT scan could light up with a PET scan.

In most PET scans, a positron-emitting isotope is attached to a substance that resembles sugar. (A positron is a positively charged electron; when it encounters an electron in the neighboring tissue, the two become annihilated in the matter/antimatter burst beloved of science fiction writers. This burst can then be detected.) The tagged sugar is similar enough to real sugar that cells are fooled into taking it up, but different enough that it cannot be used.

Since cancer cells are typically more metabolically active than other cells, they accumulate more of the tagged sugar substitute in an attempt to get more fuel. Therefore, it's possible to detect even a very small region of malignant tissue by "bursts" resulting from the high levels of radioactive sugar substitute. PET scans, like gallium scans, can help distinguish scar tissue from malignant cells remaining after treatment, and recent studies have indicated that negative PET scans midway through chemotherapy are an encouraging sign. In fact, PET scans may be even more sensitive than gallium scans in detecting residual disease. Additionally, PET scans may be useful in staging some kinds of indolent lymphoma, as well as in evaluating aggressive NHL and Hodgkin lymphoma. As PET scans are becoming more widely available, they are gradually replacing gallium scans in lymphoma diagnosis and in evaluating the response to therapy.

Bone scans

If the physician suspects that the bone may be involved—either because the patient is experiencing bone pain or because blood levels of a certain enzyme (alkaline phosphatase) are elevated—he or she may order a bone scan. Bone scans utilize a very short lived isotope of technetium (half-life of six hours) coupled to a substance called methylene diphosphonate. Methylene diphosphonate binds tightly to bone and becomes concentrated in regions where bone is rapidly turning over. The radioactive technetium acts as a marker, so that an image of the skeleton—showing any areas of abnormal bone activity—can be visualized.

A blood test showed that I had elevated levels of alkaline phosphatase. Alkaline phosphatase levels go up if the liver is malfunctioning and can also indicate abnormal bone activity. Since my liver seemed to be OK otherwise, my oncologist went ahead and ordered a bone scan.

Since technetium has such a short half-life, the bone scan is performed three or four hours after administration of the radioactive technetium–methylene diphosphonate. The scan itself takes about twenty minutes. The radioactive technetium is eliminated through the kidneys, so the scan looks like a perfect little Halloween decoration of an orange skeleton with kidneys. (Don't be surprised if one of your kidneys is higher than the other; mine was, and the technician assured me that this was perfectly normal.) About 70 percent of the technetium is eliminated from the body within six hours. In someone with normal kidney function, only about 3 percent of the radioactivity will remain in the body twenty-four hours after the scan.

Oh yes, my alkaline phosphatase. As with many people who have elevated alkaline phosphatase, both my liver function and my bones turned out to be fine. We chalked it up to "unknown reasons."

MUGA scans (heart scan)

Radioactive technetium is also used in the MUGA—for *multiple-gated cardiac blood pool*—scan. In a MUGA scan, technetium is used to label the patient's own red blood cells! A sample of blood is removed from an arm, mixed with radioactive technetium, and injected back into a vein. Then an electrocardiogram—an electrical measure of heart activity—is performed while the radiation emitted by the technetium is recorded. Using the electrocardiogram as a signal (this is the "gate" in MUGA), the MUGA scan shows how much of the blood in the heart is ejected with each beat. This provides a measure of the strength of the heart and of how well it is functioning. The whole procedure—from removing the sample of blood to completing the scan—should take only a couple of hours.

People frequently undergo MUGA scans before starting chemotherapy with the drug Adriamycin (also called doxorubicin or hydroxydaunomycin). Adriamycin is a very effective drug that is often used in chemotherapy regimens for aggressive NHL and Hodgkin lymphoma (see Chapter 3). But at high doses, Adriamycin can cause heart damage. Although heart damage is very rare at the doses used in first-line chemotherapy regimens, it could become a problem if someone needs to undergo further chemotherapy utilizing Adriamycin after completing the initial treatment. Since radiation can *also* cause cardiac damage, people with widespread thoracic disease who undergo radiation therapy to the chest as well as a chemotherapy regimen utilizing Adriamycin should be particularly aware of this potential complication.

It's a good idea to evaluate cardiac function before starting therapy to determine if the heart is weak to begin with. If that's the case, the oncologist may recommend a regimen featuring a different drug. If someone has a weak heart and *needs* to take Adriamycin, or needs dosages beyond those usually considered safe (in a second round of treatment), he or she can take a cardioprotective drug called Zinecard (dexrazoxane). Since it's possible—but not known at present—that Zinecard could partially protect the *cancer* cells from Adriamycin, Zinecard isn't used routinely but only when there's particular reason to be concerned about cardiac damage.

MRI

Nonradioactive diagnostic imaging procedures may be performed as well. The most common of these is magnetic resonance imaging (MRI), also known as nuclear magnetic resonance (NMR). When certain atoms are exposed to a strong magnetic field, their nuclei become aligned with the field like so many tiny compasses all pointing to the North Pole. Among the atoms that behave this way are hydrogen atoms, which, together with oxygen, make up water—which is the chief constituent of living tissue. If these lined-up hydrogen nuclei are subjected to a brief pulse of energy in the form of radio waves, some of them will be knocked out of alignment. After the radio waves are turned off, the nuclei will gradually return to their aligned positions, giving off little bursts of energy as they do so. This energy can be detected and used to create an image of internal structures.

The information obtained from an MRI is complementary to that obtained by a CT scan. While MRIs are rarely used on a routine basis (they are far more expensive than CT scans), they may be desirable in certain situations. MRI appears to be particularly helpful in assessing hidden involvement of the bone marrow (other than in the sample biopsied) and in evaluating disease in the brain and spinal cord. It can also be useful when it's necessary to take a "closer look" at a particular region that appears ambiguous on a CT scan. For example, it was unclear from my CT scan whether my tumor was simply pressed up against my chest wall or had actually invaded it, and I had an MRI scan of the chest to try to clarify this. Some studies suggest that MRI may also be useful in evaluating residual masses remaining after therapy.

An MRI takes longer than an equivalent CT scan and usually requires that the patient be enclosed in the magnetic chamber. Periodically during the scan the patient hears hammering sounds: it's a bit like being inside a mineshaft, listening to people trying to break through to rescue you. Other times it sounds like the loudest and most obnoxious of busy signals. Sometimes, there is a slight sensation of warmth in the area being imaged. Since an MRI involves being enclosed in a tube, people with claustrophobia can have a tough time. Wearing a sleep mask to avoid seeing the machine can help. (There are newer "open" MRI machines that eliminate this problem, but these are less sensitive and still relatively uncommon.)

Unlike CT scans, MRI doesn't involve any form of radiation and uses a different kind of contrast. MRI is considered an extremely safe procedure. However, you cannot carry credit cards or ATM cards with magnetic strips into the chamber because of the strong magnetic field. Similarly, MRIs can be hazardous for people with cardiac pacemakers, metal aneurysm clips, metal heart valves, post-cataract-surgery metal lens clips, or permanently tattooed eyeliner. Be sure to tell the technician if any of these situations apply to you or if you have *any* other metal implants in your body. Implants that contain iron can move when they're subjected to a magnetic field, and even nonmagnetic metals can heat up during MRI and damage delicate tissues.

Laparoscopy and laparotomy

Occasionally, it may be necessary to perform a surgical procedure such as a *laparoscopy* or a *laparotomy* so the surgeon can directly evaluate disease in the abdomen. A laparoscopy is a minimally invasive procedure that involves making a small incision in the navel so that a lighted viewing instrument called a *laparascope* can be inserted into the abdomen. One or two additional small incisions may be made in the abdomen if it is necessary to insert surgical instruments to take a biopsy. The laparoscopy may be performed either under general anesthesia or with local anesthetic, and the patient can usually go home the same day.

A staging laparotomy is somewhat more involved. A larger incision is needed so the viscera can be examined and biopsies can be taken of the liver and of lymph nodes. Sometimes the spleen is removed during a staging laparotomy as well (*splenectomy*). Since losing the spleen makes a person more susceptible to certain infections, however, doctors try to avoid removing it, unless this is necessary for therapeutic reasons or discovering that there was lymphoma in the spleen would change the therapeutic plan.

The size and location of the laparotomy incision will depend on the specific areas to be biopsied. Laparotomies are performed under general anesthesia and generally require several nights' stay in the hospital. Usually, the patient is catheterized (a tube is inserted into the bladder to drain the urine). The patient generally feels tired and weak after the procedure and finds it painful to cough for a few days. As with any other abdominal surgery, it's important to avoid lifting heavy objects.

Although staging laparotomies used to be performed as part of the routine staging of most people with Hodgkin lymphoma (except those with obvious Stage IV disease), they're much less common today and are only very rarely performed on people with NHL. One exception occurs when NHL involves the stomach and intestines, where laparoscopies and laparotomies are frequently performed for both diagnostic and therapeutic reasons. In general, laparoscopies and laparotomies are performed in cases of apparently localized disease if radiation therapy alone is an option, and the presence of more widespread disease would significantly alter the treatment plan.

Conclusion

After completing this exhaustive (and possibly exhausting) battery of diagnostic tests, you and your physician will have learned a lot about your lymphoma. You will have identified your specific type of lymphoma, you will have determined how far it has spread through your body, and you will have uncovered any other medical conditions that could influence your treatment. You will have obtained all the information necessary for the next step in your lymphoma journey—undergoing treatment.

SUGGESTIONS FOR FURTHER READING

An excellent review article covering lymphoma symptoms and diagnosis:

Labson LI I, Armitage JO. (1999). "Current approaches to the lymphomas (Hodgkin's disease and non-Hodgkin's lymphomas)." *Patient Care* 33:65–82.

This broad review has a section on the use of PET scans in Hodgkin lymphoma:

Meyer RM, Ambinder RF, Stroobants S. (2004). "Hodgkin's lymphoma: Evolving concepts with implications for practice." *Hematology* 2004:184–202.

Helpful online resources include:

Dr. Ed Uthman's sites on blood cells and disease: web2.iadfw.net/uthman/blood
_cells.html and on pathology reports: web2.iadfw.net/uthman/biopsy.html
Dr. David Weissmann's page on immunophenotyping lymphomas: pleiad.umdnj
.edu/~dweiss/immuno/immuno.html

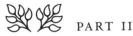 PART II

Treating Lymphoma

While chemotherapy and radiation therapy continue to be mainstays of lymphoma treatment, more selective "magic bullet" approaches—particularly those involving antibodies directed against proteins found on lymphoma cells—have become frequent components of lymphoma therapy as well. Surgery is a rare option in some forms of lymphoma, and stem cell transplants are becoming more common. The choice of treatment depends on such factors as the type of lymphoma you have, the extent of disease, the presence or absence of painful or dangerous symptoms, and your overall condition. In Chapters 3, 4, 5, and 6, I describe the different conventional approaches to lymphoma therapy in turn, both treatments in common use and experimental treatments.

Chapter 3 describes how chemotherapy works, some of the regimens used in treating the different kinds of lymphoma, and specific drugs. Chapter 4 addresses radiation therapy and surgery, Chapter 5 covers the newer, more selective therapies such as monoclonal antibodies, and Chapter 6 describes the procedures involved in undergoing a stem cell transplant. Since many people are interested in nontraditional therapies, I discuss these approaches as well, in Chapter 7. These chapters will give you an idea of what to expect from treatment and of how to cope with some of the side effects. These chapters will *not* tell you which therapy is right for you. Every person with lymphoma is unique, and only an oncologist or hematologist who is familiar with that person's case can determine the optimal treatment for any given individual. Only a physician on the scene can establish what's best for you. However, the information in these five chapters *will* help you speak knowledgeably with your physician about your choices.

General approaches

Localized Hodgkin lymphoma without "B" symptoms (Stage I and contiguous Stage II—which means that the affected lymph nodes are in contact with each other) and localized indolent NHL are sometimes treated with radiation alone. Before chemotherapy, radiation was used to treat most lymphoma. Radiation can be delivered precisely to a defined location, like the chest, while chemotherapy is systemic—it goes everywhere and can affect every tissue in the body. Because of this, radiation was initially viewed as "milder" than chemotherapy in terms of overall effects on health.

When it first became apparent that both localized Hodgkin lymphoma and localized indolent lymphoma were sometimes curable with radiation alone and that chemotherapy could be administered later in the event of a relapse, treating localized disease with radiation had more appeal than using chemotherapy, since doctors and, especially, patients are concerned with minimizing the chances of dangerous or unpleasant complications of treatment. Recent research, however, suggests that chemotherapy can be as successful in controlling early-stage Hodgkin lymphoma as radiation. And concerns have started to surface about the long-term effects of radiation on Hodgkin's survivors. Thus, the initial approach to treating localized Hodgkin lymphoma may well shift toward chemotherapy, particularly as less toxic chemotherapy regimens are developed.

Most aggressive non-Hodgkin lymphomas are treated with chemotherapy from the start. Chemotherapy and radiation may be used together; in this case radiation is given to affected areas (if you have localized disease) or to areas of bulky disease (if you have generalized disease with a specific cancer "hot spot" that involves a large tumor). Chemotherapy may also be given in combination with antibodies. The combination of different forms of treatment—such as chemotherapy and radiation or chemotherapy and antibodies—is frequently called "combined modality therapy."

Advanced Hodgkin lymphoma (some Stage II, most Stage III, all Stage IV, and "B" symptoms at any stage) is generally treated with chemotherapy as well, sometimes supplemented with radiation.

With the possible exception of aggressive therapies involving bone marrow transplants or peripheral stem cell transplants, no therapy currently available has been demonstrated to cure advanced stages of indolent NHL. Since different chemotherapy regimens may be preferable for different individuals and none are clearly curative, people diagnosed with advanced stage indolent NHL may be offered one of several initial treatment options.

Because no current cancer therapy is completely without unpleasant side effects or risk of complications, it makes sense to hold off delivering such treatments to people who are likely to survive for a long time even without therapy if they remain asymptomatic and are enjoying a decent quality of life. This is consistent with the "first do no harm" principle embodied in the Hippocratic oath that doctors take upon graduating from medical school. Therefore, people with advanced-stage indolent NHL who are asymptomatic and in a disease "holding pattern" frequently go on "watch-and-wait." Treatment is deferred until it becomes necessary.

Deferring treatment doesn't make sense, however, if your condition is getting worse. You will start some sort of therapy if you have advanced-stage indolent NHL and are experiencing dangerous or distressing symptoms, if your disease is progressing rapidly, or if you simply can't bear the idea of sitting back and doing nothing. Generally, you will start with relatively mild regimens that may include treatment with monoclonal antibodies, some form of chemotherapy, or both and move on to more aggressive regimens if you have a relapse or if your disease becomes unresponsive to treatment. If long-term studies prove that stem cell transplants do, in fact, cure or prolong life in a substantial number of people with advanced-stage, indolent NHL, this strategy may change, and stem cell transplants may become more common as a *front-line treatment* (the first approach used to treat a disease) rather than as *second-line treatment*, to be used in case of a relapse.

The goals of treatment: cures and remissions

Ideally, the result of all cancer treatment would be cure. You'd take some medicine and the lymphoma would vanish forever. You'd forget you ever had lymphoma and get on with your life. Unfortunately, we haven't reached that point yet. Some forms of lymphoma appear to be incurable with our current approaches to therapy. And even with forms that are considered curable, some physicians are uncomfortable using the word *cure* to imply a permanent eradication of lymphoma. Cancer can lie low only to reappear after many years (generally considered a *relapse*). Some oncologists prefer terms like *long-term progression-free survival* or *durable remission* rather than *cure*.

Cancer can reappear even after years have passed, *and it's important for every cancer survivor to get follow-up care for the rest of his or her life.* With curable forms of lymphoma, though, these late recurrences are uncommon. Moreover, it's hard to be sure that cancer showing up after such a long time represents a recurrence of the same disease; it may be a new disease. Lightning *can* sometimes strike twice.

My own feeling as far as the *good* "C word" is concerned is that, if I live out the rest of my life without a recurrence, I'll consider myself to have been cured. Indeed, it's now been long enough since my treatment that I hope and believe that this is the case. Somehow, I'd rather think about a "cure" than a "long-term event-free survival" or a "durable remission." And with Hodgkin lymphoma, aggressive NHL, and localized indolent NHL, once you make it past a certain time, chances are that the lymphoma will never come back. In this book, I use a definition of *cure* that I've seen several times: the chance that someone who is considered cured will get lymphoma again is equal to that of someone who never had lymphoma developing it. How much time must go by before you are considered unlikely to have a recurrence varies with the specific type of lymphoma, but it is generally a matter of years. As a rule, the more aggressive your disease, the shorter the interval before you are considered to have made it home free.

The first goal in lymphoma treatment is known as a *remission*. In a remission, your body returns toward its normal, healthy condition. There are different kinds of remission, which are described by different terms. You can have either a *partial remission* or a *complete remission.* In a partial remission, your lymphoma responds to treatment but doesn't disappear completely. A tumor that started out the size of a grapefruit might shrink to the size of a lemon. Or if your bone marrow biopsy showed 50 percent normal cells and 50 percent cancerous cells before you started treatment, the percentage of cancerous cells might drop to 5 or 10 percent after therapy. You're better off than you were, but there are still signs of disease. Or you can have a complete remission, in which all signs of the disease disappear. A complete remission means that evidence of lymphoma can no longer be detected in your body. No signs of a tumor. Your CT scans are normal, your lumps and bumps go away, and your bone marrow is free of abnormal cells.

Oddly enough, obtaining a complete remission doesn't necessarily mean that you have been cured of the disease, while obtaining a partial remission doesn't necessarily mean that you *haven't*. With a complete remission, all *visible* signs of the disease vanish. However, cells are microscopic. A small number of malignant cells may not be detected by physical exam or even the most sensitive imaging techniques, but they can multiply in your body and cause a relapse.

Relapses are very common in people diagnosed with widespread indolent disease—even those who have attained a complete remission. This is one of the puzzling things about low-grade lymphoma. As my oncologist put it:

"Everybody loves patients with lymphoma. They respond so beautifully to therapy. But, then, the disease so frequently recurs." (I used the first sentence as my personal mantra, whenever I felt depressed, for about a year.)

This pattern of recurrence is probably related to the slow progression of these forms of lymphoma. If there's a population of malignant cells or abnormal premalignant cells that reproduces very slowly, they may never be hit at just the right moment by chemotherapy drugs, which are typically most active against rapidly dividing cells. Or a few malignant cells may remain in "privileged regions" of the body, where drugs can't penetrate.

Even with the aggressive forms of lymphoma, in which the cancer cells divide rapidly, so that it's more likely that the chemotherapy will hit when they're vulnerable, a few stray malignant cells may remain, even without signs of disease. Therefore, treatment is generally continued even after a complete remission has been obtained, since it's necessary to eliminate *all* the malignant cells in order to cure the disease.

Recently, researchers have used very sensitive tests to look for individual diseased cells. A technique called the *polymerase chain reaction,* or PCR, can be used to detect the abnormal DNA characteristic of certain types of lymphoma in blood or bone marrow samples that contain only a single malignant cell among a million normal cells. The presence of such abnormal DNA in someone in an apparent complete remission is called *minimal residual disease.* The absence of any detectable abnormal DNA is called a *complete molecular remission.*

The significance of minimal residual disease *versus* a complete molecular remission to an individual person's health isn't completely clear. Sometimes even people who have obtained a complete molecular remission will relapse. And sometimes perfectly healthy people have the DNA abnormalities associated with minimal residual disease. However, people who receive their own bone marrow in a transplant are less likely to relapse if the marrow they receive shows no signs of disease at the molecular level. And following a bone marrow transplant, the absence of detectable DNA abnormalities is strongly associated with freedom from relapse.

Just as a complete remission doesn't necessarily imply a cure, a partial remission, determined by a chest X-ray or CT scan, doesn't necessarily signify active disease. While I was undergoing chemotherapy, my tumor shrank dramatically. Football! Deflated football! Softball! Fist! Fist. Fist. At the end of my scheduled chemo treatments, chest X-rays and CT scans showed a residual mass the size of my fist.

Since my chest X-rays and CT scans were still abnormal, I hadn't attained a complete remission. However, there was no way to tell by an X-ray or CT scan or physical examination whether this mass represented active tumor—in which case I would have needed more chemotherapy—or simply scar tissue. Even a biopsy would have been inconclusive, since parts of the mass might have consisted of scar tissue with active tumor cells present elsewhere.

This presented a dilemma. If I had active tumor, I would have required more chemotherapy: probably, a high-dose regimen followed by a stem cell transplant. However, it would be undesirable (to say the least!) to subject me to a stem cell transplant if the disease was gone.

Since my gallium scan was negative, I was categorized as having obtained a *gallium complete remission* (see the section of Chapter 2 on imaging techniques, and note that PET scans are gradually replacing gallium scans for this purpose), and we took a middle course. We stopped chemotherapy and moved on to radiation to kill any lurking malignant cells.

In a general sense, lymphoma therapy is designed to help as many people as possible. However, "help" can mean different things to different people. Many people with localized indolent NHL, as well as many people with localized or widespread Hodgkin lymphoma and localized or widespread aggressive NHL, can now be cured. The goal of treatment for someone with potentially curable disease is to cure that person while minimizing the risk of any dangerous side effects of therapy. For the group of people with potentially curable disease, the treatment attempts to eradicate all malignant cells. Cancer starts with a single malignant cell, and it is only after all malignant cells have been routed from your body that you can be considered cured.

The majority of people with widespread indolent NHL cannot be cured with currently available therapies. Therefore, with this group of people, a good partial remission, in which a particular lymph node that is causing trouble is significantly reduced in size and halted in its progression, may be considered a satisfactory response to treatment. The goals of treatment for people whose disease is not yet curable are to keep them alive as long as possible and to maintain as good a quality of life as possible during this time. We can continue to hope that most people who now have widespread indolent disease will survive long enough for a real cure to come along.

CHAPTER 3

Chemotherapy

How chemotherapy works

Chemotherapy is the use of drugs—chemicals—that are toxic to malignant cells to treat disease. In some cases, chemotherapy is used with the intention of trying to cure cancer. When a cure is not considered possible, chemotherapy may be used to alleviate symptoms of disease and prolong life. Chemotherapy that is used simply to relieve symptoms and improve quality of life is sometimes referred to as *palliative*. The drugs used to treat cancer, known as *antineoplastic agents*, are usually taken by mouth or injected into a vein. Since this means that your whole body will be exposed to these drugs, not just the regions that contain cancer cells, chemotherapy is considered a *systemic treatment*. Monoclonal antibodies, another form of systemic therapy used to treat lymphoma, are discussed in Chapter 5.

In the never ending battle against disease, one general principle in selecting therapeutic drugs is to exploit differences between the harmful cells, which you are trying to eliminate, and the innocent cells, which you want to protect. It's like using an herbicide on a beautiful garden that has been invaded by weeds that are rapidly taking over and choking out all the flowers. You need to find a weed killer that is strong enough to kill (or at least control) all the poison ivy but selective enough to leave the roses and the peonies alone. The tricky part is figuring out what differences between cancer cells (the weeds in the cancer garden) and healthy cells (the flowers) might make the cancer cells susceptible to treatment.

Perhaps the most striking difference between most cancer cells and most healthy cells is unrestrained growth. Therefore, many antineoplastic drugs are designed to target rapidly dividing cells. Actively growing and dividing cells pass through several distinct stages in what is known as the *cell cycle* (see Chapter 8). Some antineoplastic drugs not only act preferentially against actively dividing cells but also act at specific steps in the cell cycle. Another feature that characterizes cancer cells is their failure to undergo *apoptosis*—a form of programmed cell death used to eliminate cells that are no longer useful—under the appropriate circumstances. This failure to undergo apoptosis allows populations of malignant cells to accumulate. Although different antineoplastic drugs work in different ways, many of them ultimately work by triggering apoptosis, so that the damaged cells commit suicide.

In the following discussion, I've classified drugs used to treat lymphoma into five basic groups: four As and a C. The five groups are the *antimetabolites*, the *alkylating agents*, the *anthracyclines*, the *antimitotics*, and the *corticosteroids*. These categories are used to distinguish different types of drugs by how they work—in other words, by their mechanisms of action. Most of the drugs used to treat lymphoma fall into one of these five categories. If you're not interested in learning how the drugs work right now, which requires reviewing some basic cell biology, feel free to skip ahead to the section on side effects. You can always come back to the section on drug mechanisms.

Antimetabolites

With very few exceptions, all of our cells contain DNA, a large molecule that comprises the genetic material that acts as blueprint to specify how to construct and maintain a living being. Actively dividing cells need to duplicate their DNA, so that each of the daughter cells will have a copy of the DNA. As discussed in more detail in Chapter 8, this process of DNA duplication takes place during the S, or *synthesis*, phase of the cell cycle and uses various DNA components that the cell has amassed previously.

The class of antineoplastic drugs known as antimetabolites interferes with DNA synthesis. Some of these drugs inhibit the production of the compounds that make up DNA. Others mimic such compounds well enough to be mistakenly incorporated into DNA. Both of these actions inhibit DNA synthesis. Antimetabolites used in treating lymphoma include methotrexate, fludarabine, cytarabine (cytosine arabinoside), pentostatin (2'-deoxycoformycin), and cladribine (2-chlorodeoxyadenosine).

Alkylating agents

Another class of antineoplastic drugs, the alkylating agents, adds a specific type of chemical group called an *alkyl group* to inappropriate sites on other molecules. The alkylating agents, which include mechlorethamine, cyclophosphamide, ifosfamide, chlorambucil, carmustine, lomustine, procarbazine, and dacarbazine, bind avidly to DNA and damage it. In some cases, they bind to two separate sites and form a bridge, inappropriately linking strands of DNA together. This is called *crosslinking* and interferes with the normal function of DNA molecules.

Alkylation can take place at any phase of the cell cycle; however, DNA strands that are undergoing replication are more susceptible to attack. This means that alkylating agents are more likely to act against dividing cells. Moreover, the DNA damage induced by alkylation triggers intracellular pathways (series of linked chemical reactions that take place inside cells) that lead to cell death when the damaged cell enters S phase. Resting cells have more time to repair their DNA before they get to S phase than cells that are rapidly cycling and are therefore more likely to survive such damage.

Although it is not an alkylating agent, cisplatin, a platinum-containing complex that is often used to treat relapsed lymphoma, binds to DNA and crosslinks strands of DNA in a similar manner. This inhibits DNA replication, inhibits the synthesis of RNA, and promotes breakage of the DNA strands.

Mechlorethamine, cyclophosphamide, ifosfamide, and chlorambucil are members of a group of alkylating agents known as the *nitrogen mustards.* They are related chemically to the mustard gas (sulfur mustard) used in chemical warfare during the First World War. Doctors discovered that soldiers who had been exposed to mustard gas had decreased levels of circulating white cells and badly damaged bone marrow and lymphoid tissue. These observations led them to try testing similar chemicals against leukemia and lymphoma.

Amazingly, people treated with these chemical warfare–like drugs went into remissions! Chemicals developed for use in war against humans were diverted to the war against cancerous cells. The nitrogen mustards are still used in front-line therapies against lymphoma. Mechlorethamine is a component of one of the regimens used to treat Hodgkin lymphoma, while cyclophosphamide and chlorambucil are frequently used to treat NHL.

Anthracyclines and other drugs utilizing similar mechanisms

The group of antineoplastic agents known as the anthracyclines damages DNA. These drugs, which are derived from a fungus, *Streptomyces peucetius*, include doxorubicin, daunorubicin, idarubicin, and mitoxantrone. They bind to DNA, becoming incorporated into its structure, and interfere with an enzyme, *topoisomerase II*, that breaks and then repairs strands of DNA during the processes of DNA replication and RNA synthesis. When topoisomerase II is inhibited by the anthracycline compounds, it can no longer repair breaks in the DNA strands, and, as a result, the long DNA strands become chopped up into pieces and fragmented, leading to cell death.

The anthracyclines also promote the generation of *free radicals*, highly reactive and destructive compounds that can damage DNA and other components of the cell. The production of free radicals is stimulated by iron. Anthracyclines are most effective during the S phase of the cell cycle.

Etoposide, a drug derived from the mayapple, which was used in folk medicine to promote purging and vomiting, also binds to DNA and inhibits topoisomerase II. Bleomycin, derived from the fungus *Streptomyces verticillus*, interacts with iron and oxygen to cause fragmentation of DNA.

Antimitotic drugs

This class of antineoplastic agents is unlike the others discussed so far in that these drugs don't act against nucleic acids like DNA and RNA. Instead, they interfere with the function of structures called *mitotic spindles* that are found inside dividing cells and pull apart the chromosomes during *mitosis* (cell division; see Chapter 8). The mitotic spindles are mostly made up of microtubules, which contain a protein called *tubulin*. Tubulin can exist either as individual molecules floating free in the cell's cytoplasm or joined together to create a microtubule, similar to pop beads forming a necklace. The linked tubulin beads in the assembled microtubule "necklace" are in a state of equilibrium with the individual tubulin beads in the cytoplasm so that beads of tubulin are constantly popping off the microtubule and then joining back up.

The vinca alkaloids, vincristine and vinblastine, which are derived from the Madagascar periwinkle, bind to the individual free-floating beads of tubulin and prevent them from assembling into microtubules. This interferes with the formation of the mitotic spindle and prevents the cell from dividing, leading the blocked cell into apoptosis. Paclitaxel and docetaxel, which are derived from the bark and needles of the Pacific yew, have the opposite effect on microtubules. They promote tubulin polymerization and block microtubule disassembly into individual tubulin monomers. This, too, disrupts the function of the mitotic spindles, blocks cell division, and eventually leads to death of the cell.

Corticosteroid hormones

Another group of chemotherapeutic agents commonly used to treat lymphoma is the corticosteroid hormones. Corticosteroid hormones are produced naturally by the outer portions of our adrenal glands (the adrenal cortex); they play a critical role in our response to stress, and they influence nearly every system in the body. The corticosteroids are divided into two classes. *Glucocorticoids* influence carbohydrate, protein, and fat metabolism, while *mineralocorticoids* regulate the handling of substances like sodium and potassium and water. The three synthetic corticosteroids used in treating lymphoma are prednisone, methylprednisolone, and dexamethasone. All three act as glucocorticoids.

Like other glucocorticoids, prednisone, methylprednisolone, and dexamethasone reduce inflammation and suppress the immune response. This is part of their role in protecting the body during conditions of stress, since, left unchecked, high levels of the powerful cytokines released during a major inflammatory response could lead to collapse of the circulatory system, massive clotting, and death.

The glucocorticoids inhibit these potentially hazardous immune responses. They bind to specialized sites inside their target cells, called intracellular receptors, and regulate the production of various intracellular proteins. As part of their immunosuppressive activities, they inhibit the production and release of various cytokines. High levels of glucocorticoids reduce the numbers of circulating lymphocytes and the total mass of lymphatic tissue in the body. This anti-lymphocytic activity appears to be even more pronounced against the malignant lymphoid cells found in lymphoma than it is against normal lymphocytes.

Side effects

The idea of exploiting differences between harmful cells and normal cells going peacefully about their business works beautifully in theory; in practice, however, most drugs aren't absolutely selective. Rather then acting only against the targeted population of bad cells, they damage some normal, healthy cells as well. This lack of selectivity leads to unwanted drug side effects.

The more similar the cells you are trying to destroy and the cells you are trying to protect, the more difficult it will be to find a drug that can differentiate between them. Antibiotics that are active against fungal infections, for instance, tend to be more toxic to people than those that are active against bacterial infections because (unwelcome as this thought might be) we are more similar to fungi than we are to bacteria.

This difficulty in distinguishing between good cells and bad cells reaches its ultimate expression in cancer. A cancer cell is much more like the rest of the cells in your body than is a bacterium or a fungus. This makes it very difficult to design effective antineoplastic agents that don't cause undesirable side effects.

Many drug side effects are unpleasant. At high doses, some can become dangerous. The sort of side effect that is so dangerous that it puts a cap on the amount of drug that can be safely administered is called the *dose-limiting toxicity* of a drug. Dose-limiting toxicity can be acute, limiting the amount of drug that you can safely take at any one time, or it can be chronic, limiting the cumulative dose that you can take over your whole lifetime. For many antineoplastic drugs, the acute dose-limiting toxicity is bone marrow suppression.

Since many antineoplastic drugs specifically target rapidly dividing cells, it isn't surprising that rapidly proliferating populations of healthy cells can be affected. The stem cells in your bone marrow, the epithelial cells that line your mouth and gastrointestinal tract, and the cells in your hair follicles all divide rapidly, and all of these cell types are frequently affected by chemotherapy. Therefore, such side effects as hair loss, bone marrow suppression, and mouth sores can occur with many different antineoplastic agents. To a certain extent, these side effects are unavoidable.

Additionally, certain drugs have side effects that depend on their specific mechanism of action; for example, microtubules not only form mitotic spindles but also transport substances down the length of nerve cells. Therefore, drugs like vincristine that interfere with microtubule function have side effects related to the disruption in the transport of substances in nerve cells.

If you expect to undergo chemotherapy, please don't feel intimidated by the list of potential side effects. Keep in mind that the following discussion concerns things that *may* happen, not things that *will* happen, and that few people experience *all* the side effects described. Moreover, even in the group of people who experience a certain side effect, the degree to which different individuals are affected varies tremendously. If you have a difficult time with chemotherapy, you may be reassured to know that what you are experiencing is normal. However, you may find, as I did, that you experience only a few side effects while you are undergoing chemotherapy. Indeed, most of the time I was on chemo I felt far better than I had for the year preceding my diagnosis.

If you should experience any painful or alarming side effects while undergoing chemotherapy, don't hesitate to call your oncologist, hematologist, or treatment nurse. This is one time where it's truly better to be safe than sorry. Even if it turns out to be nothing serious, it's part of your physician's and nurse's job to reassure you.

Hair loss, nail ridges, and dry or discolored skin

Everybody knows that chemotherapy can cause hair loss, more formally known as *alopecia*. Not only the hair on your head but hair anywhere on your body may fall out (yes, pubic hair, too). I ended up losing all my hair except for some of my eyebrows and eyelashes. Many people find the loss of their hair to be profoundly disturbing. Indeed, some people consider hair loss the most traumatic side effect of chemotherapy. If you plan on getting a wig (your insurance may cover this if your doctor writes a prescription for a "scalp prosthesis"), it makes sense to choose one early on so you can match it to your own hair. While alopecia is one of the most common side effects of chemotherapy, it doesn't occur with all the drugs used in treating lymphoma, and some people keep their hair even while taking drugs that generally cause hair loss.

Hair generally grows back, often while you are still undergoing chemotherapy. Two years postchemo, my hair reached down below my shoulders. It was thicker and seemed to grow faster than it ever had before! Frequently, the new hair has a different texture than before (usually curlier); sometimes it is a different color as well.

It usually takes a few weeks before your hair starts to fall out; I didn't lose mine until after my second treatment, when I had started to think that I might escape with my hair intact. Your hair may fall out gradually, or it may come out in clumps. It's easier to cope with falling hair if you cut it short as soon as it starts coming out. It's not as messy, and you don't have to deal with waking up to find huge clumps of hair on your pillow. If you lose your hair during the winter, you'll find that you need to cover your head when it's cold out. On the other hand, if you lose your eyebrows during the summer, you may find it difficult to keep sweat out of your eyes. This can be a problem while driving! And eyelashes tumbling into your eyes are a real nuisance at any time of year.

Although I'd had long hair all my life and had dreaded losing it, when it actually happened, I found losing my hair to be profoundly unimportant. In the context of fighting for my life, losing my hair seemed trivial. While I generally covered my head when I went out in public and wore a wig when I wanted to look dressy, I discovered that I liked the hairless look: I felt like an exotic Star Trek character. Three months after I completed chemotherapy, Paul and I took a vacation on the West Coast, and I actually received many compliments from strangers on my avant-garde, crewcut "do." (Well, a $30,000 haircut really *ought* to generate a few compliments.)

There's some evidence that wearing a shower cap filled with ice while you're receiving chemotherapy, which decreases blood flow to the cells in your hair follicles and minimizes their exposure to the chemo drugs, reduces hair loss. Unfortunately, there's a small chance that a malignant cell lurking near the hair follicles could also be saved from destruction. As a guaranteed safe alternative, you may find that interesting scarves, caps, hats, turbans, earrings, or paste-on tattoos can compensate for the lost hair. Remember, it *will* come back.

Chemotherapy also interferes with the growth of your nails, a less widely recognized (and usually less upsetting) side effect. I developed six horizontal bands on my nails—like tiny little tree rings—corresponding to my six rounds of chemo. Your nails may become very brittle and break; it helps to trim them quite short and to wear gloves when you are doing anything that might cause nail trauma.

Chemotherapy can also cause dry, itchy, or reddened skin. Taking short, warm baths and showers rather than long, hot ones and using nonperfumed creams and lotions can help alleviate this. Dry skin should not be confused with sudden, severe itching or hives, which could indicate an allergic reaction and should be reported to your doctor at once.

Occasionally, chemotherapy can cause darkening of your skin, called *hyperpigmentation.* This can appear all over, like a chemical-induced tan (somehow, I don't think this form of artificial tanning will ever catch on), or as localized spots. I developed "age spots," large, pale freckles on my face, neck, and forearms. My oncologist thought they would fade away, but, eight years later, they are still there.

Mouth sores and diarrhea

Because the cells lining your mouth, throat, and gastrointestinal tract are constantly renewing themselves and proliferating, they are quite susceptible to chemotherapy-induced damage, which can lead to mouth sores and diarrhea. Because your ability to fight infection may also be reduced during chemotherapy (see the section "Bone marrow suppression," below), and because your mouth is normally a hotbed of germs, mouth sores can become infected with bacteria or fungi. This can be quite painful.

There are precautions you can take to avoid mouth sores and things you can do to help deal with any that do develop. If you have time, it's a good idea to see a dentist before starting chemotherapy. The dentist can clean your teeth and identify and treat any hidden infections.

It's preferable to take care of this before beginning chemotherapy so that any minor injuries heal before you start any regimens that could enhance the likelihood of infection. If necessary, though, you can see a dentist while chemotherapy is ongoing. I developed a slight gum infection during the second or third cycle of chemo and saw a dentist prior to my fourth cycle. We timed the visit so that my white cell counts had mostly recovered from the previous round of chemo and would remain high for a few days.

It's important to keep your mouth clean and avoid any trauma to your mouth and gums. You should avoid eating sharp or crispy foods that could inflict little cuts. With a stressed population of cells and an increased susceptibility to infection, such tiny injuries can develop into painful mouth sores. Most oncologists recommend using a soft toothbrush after every meal but avoiding floss while your immune defenses are weak, since flossing can introduce bacteria from your mouth into your bloodstream. My dentist was horrified:

"Your gums look awful! You're starting to get periodontal disease!" she said, "You need to keep up your flossing!"

"Hmmm," I thought, "I'd rather get periodontal disease than a blood infection. Who knows if I'll live long enough for my teeth to fall out?"

But I was careful to start flossing again once chemo was over.

Rinsing your mouth with saline, baking soda, or special antiseptics, such as chlorhexidine, may be helpful. Rinsing your mouth with diluted hydrogen peroxide can help prevent mouth sores but will irritate any that have already surfaced. If, like me, you have grayish teeth, you'll find that rinsing with hydrogen peroxide brightens your smile. Chlorhexidine, on the other hand, darkens your teeth a little.

If you develop mouth sores in spite of your precautions, most doctors will prescribe a swish-and-swallow preparation that contains something viscous to coat the surface of your mouth, combined with a local anesthetic, an anti-inflammatory agent, and an antibiotic or antifungal drug. Sucking on chips of ice may also help to numb the pain.

Carafate, a locally acting compound that speeds healing of ulcers in the small intestine, works pretty well against mouth sores too. And a "hot" tip says that candy made with capsaicin, found in chili peppers, helps alleviate pain from mouth sores.

Damage to the epithelial cells lining your throat can cause a mild sore throat: this can be treated with the swish-and-swallow preparations described above or with antiulcerative medications like Carafate. A severe sore throat, however, may be a sign of a serious infection and should be reported to your physician immediately.

Damage to the epithelial cells lining your intestines can cause diarrhea. Avoiding foods that contain a lot of roughage, eating small, frequent meals rather than large, infrequent ones, and drinking a lot of fluids to replace those that are lost may help. If diarrhea is accompanied by painful cramps or is very severe or prolonged, call your doctor.

Bone marrow suppression

All your blood cells—the red blood cells, the white blood cells, and the platelets—are descended from precursor cells that live in the bone marrow. The blood cell precursors (the cells in your bone marrow that give rise to your blood cells) are among the most rapidly dividing populations of cells in your body. Therefore, it isn't surprising that bone marrow suppression is a consequence of many (although not all) of the chemotherapy regimens used to treat lymphoma. Indeed, the anticancer potential of several classes of antineoplastic drugs was first recognized when people noticed that these drugs caused bone marrow suppression. Levels of white cells (neutrophils, lymphocytes, and monocytes), red cells (erythrocytes), and platelets may all be affected by antineoplastic drugs.

For some people, chemotherapy-induced bone marrow suppression is relatively innocuous: the worst consequences I experienced were recurrence of my yeast infection and fatigue. For others, bone marrow suppression can be more serious. This invisible side effect of chemotherapy can increase your susceptibility to severe infections or to blood problems like anemia or difficulty with clotting. It's therefore necessary to have your blood counts monitored while you are undergoing certain forms of chemotherapy.

Bone marrow suppression isn't instantaneous. Nor are all populations of blood cells affected equally; this depends on the rate of precursor cell proliferation and the life span of mature (nondividing) cells as well as the specific antineoplastic agent(s) used.

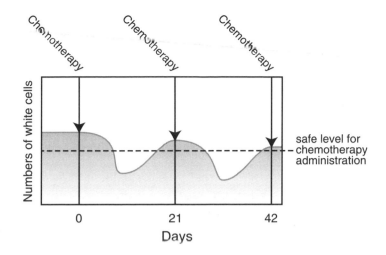

Figure 3.1. *White cell counts during chemotherapy.* Chemotherapy suppresses the rapidly proliferating cells in your bone marrow, particularly those that give rise to the neutrophils. With many chemotherapy regimens, the lowest white cell count, called nadir, occurs ten to fourteen days after chemotherapy. During nadir, you are most susceptible to infection. Once the suppressive effects of the chemotherapy drugs are gone from your system, your white cell count starts rising back toward normal levels. If the white count hasn't yet recovered to a high enough level by the time you are due for your next treatment, that cycle of chemotherapy may be delayed.

Since neutrophils are the most rapidly dividing population of white cells and have a mature life span of only a few hours, they're usually the population most severely affected by chemotherapy. Platelets are generally affected less than neutrophils, and red cells (which have a long life span) are affected the least. Lymphocyte levels are more sensitive to the corticosteroids, and the drugs fludarabine and cladribine, than they are to other agents commonly used to treat lymphoma.

With many chemotherapy regimens, the lowest white cell count occurs ten to fourteen days after chemotherapy. This lowest count is called the *nadir*. With certain chemotherapy drugs, the reduction in white cell levels is more delayed and protracted (see section on specific drugs, below). During nadir, you are most susceptible to infections. Once the chemotherapy drugs are gone from your system, your white cell count starts rising back toward normal levels (fig. 3.1). Your physician may take several samples of blood during the first cycle to monitor the pattern of your white cell response and determine exactly when your personal nadir occurs.

In any event, he or she will obtain a complete blood count before administering the next round of chemo. If your neutrophil levels are still very low, your physician may delay treatment until your cell count has returned to levels where it's safe to administer the next dose of drugs. Don't be upset if this happens: modifications in schedule are not uncommon.

Keeping track of blood cell levels matters. As discussed in Chapter 9, neutrophils play a critical role in the defense against pathogens, particularly bacteria. Therefore, neutropenia, a reduction in the levels of circulating neutrophils, increases susceptibility to infection and decreases ability to fight off bacterial invaders. The more severe the neutropenia and the longer it lasts, the greater the chance of contracting an infection. Neutropenic infections are probably the most dangerous of the common short-term side effects of chemotherapy; you need to take precautions against infection and to get in touch with your oncologist at once if you think that you may have developed one.

Your nurse or physician will give you a list of precautions to follow. These can sound overwhelming, but most are common sense, and it isn't quite as much like living in a suit of armor as it sounds. These precautions may include the following:

Avoid flossing your teeth and use only a soft toothbrush to avoid introducing bacteria from your mouth into your bloodstream.

Wash your hands frequently, but not so frequently that they get chapped.

Avoid eating uncooked "food grown in the earth" (such as raw carrots, lettuce, or celery) and raw eggs, fish, and shellfish.

Eat meat (especially hamburger) only after it has been cooked "well done."

Be gentle when wiping yourself, particularly if you have hemorrhoids, to avoid small injuries that may cause bleeding.

Avoid handling animals (or wear gloves).

Avoid getting nicks and cuts when you're shaving (not an issue if you've lost all your hair!), cutting your nails, or generally doing anything likely to lead to cuts or scrapes.

If, in spite of your efforts, you do injure yourself, clean the wound thoroughly with an antiseptic.

Don't pick your nose or stick unwashed fingers in your eyes (not that you would, anyway).

Avoid doing anything like gardening that could kick up a lot of dirt.

Wear gloves when doing housework. (I stopped doing housework altogether while on chemotherapy. I figured it was a great excuse.)

You will also want to avoid crowds, stay away from people with highly contagious diseases like chickenpox or the flu (or wear gloves and a mask), and put off getting any immunizations that utilize weakened viruses, such as polio and chickenpox vaccines, rather than dead ones. (Most immunizations given at this time wouldn't work very well, anyway.)

While it's important to take due care, and a neutropenic infection is no laughing matter, it's also possible to fall overboard into the Sea of Hypochondria (after all, you have *cancer*). Just after I had completed chemotherapy, while I was still undergoing radiation, I visited friends and learned that their baby, whom I'd been cuddling in my lap, had just received an oral polio vaccine made from a live, attenuated virus, which was shed in bodily waste. I restrained myself from hurling the baby to the floor in a mad dash to the sink, spent the rest of the evening in a state of silent horror brooding about iron lungs, and called my internist as soon as I got home. He replied, rather dryly, that he wouldn't worry about it, unless I'd eaten dinner off the baby's diaper.

If, in spite of all of your precautions, you develop signs of an infection, call your physician right away. (This is important, and not hypochondria.) Such signs may include one or more of the following:

Fever of over 100°F
Severe sore throat
Shaking chills
Redness, swelling, or tenderness, particularly near a wound or an indwelling catheter
Blood in your urine or a burning sensation when you urinate
Unusual vaginal discharge or itching

If you do have an infection, your physician will want to see you right away to put you on antibiotics and bring the infection under control as rapidly as possible.

Colony-Stimulating Factors

If the cells in your bone marrow are particularly sensitive to chemotherapy and you develop severe neutropenia, your physician may treat you with colony-stimulating factors (CSFs, also known as growth factors) during future chemotherapy cycles. CSFs are cytokines: chemical messengers that influence the survival, proliferation, and/or differentiation of specific cell types. They are called "colony-stimulating factors" because when these cells are grown in vitro (outside the body, literally "in glass"), they form little clusters called colonies. In vitro, CSFs increase the size of the cell colonies. More important, in your body CSFs increase the number of the appropriate types of cells.

In any given cycle, the CSF is started shortly after chemotherapy is administered (well before white cell nadir) and is continued until an appropriate white count has been achieved. CSFs reduce the magnitude and duration of chemotherapy-induced neutropenia, the frequency of infections, and the number of days someone on a given regimen spends recovering from neutropenic fevers. They frequently cause bone pain—probably from the effects of stimulating the marrow.

Several different CSFs are now available. *Granulocyte colony-stimulating factor* (abbreviated G-CSF; also known as filgrastim [brand name: Neupogen] and pegfilgrastim [brand name: Neulasta], which is a long-acting form) enhances the production of granulocytes (neutrophils, eosinophils, and basophils; see Chapter 9 for description of the different types of blood cells), increases mobilization of mature granulocytes and their precursors from the bone marrow into the blood, and enhances granulocyte function. *Granulocyte/macrophage colony-stimulating factor* (abbreviated GM-CSF; also known as sargramostrim [brand name: Leukine]) acts at an earlier stage in precursor cell development and promotes the production of macrophages (another cell type) as well as granulocytes.

Chemotherapy can also cause anemia, leading to fatigue, weakness, and shortness of breath (severe anemia, which can put a strain on your heart, will not suddenly appear as a side effect of chemo). Anemia can be treated with a blood transfusion or with erythropoietin (brand names: Epogen or Procrit) or the closely related darbepoetin (brand name: Aranesp), another naturally occurring substance that is produced by your kidneys and stimulates the production of red blood cells.

In some cases, chemotherapy can cause *thrombocytopenia,* a reduction in the platelet levels. Since platelets are important in blood clotting, thrombocytopenia can manifest as *petechiae*—small red spots on the skin—easy bruising, bleeding gums, or unexplained nosebleeds. Severe thrombocytopenia is treated with infusion of donor platelets or with a recently developed cytokine for *megakaryocytes* (the platelet precursor cell), interleukin-11 (abbreviated rhIL-11; also known as oprelvekin [brand name: Neumega]).

Reproduction and infertility

At the time I was diagnosed with lymphoma, Paul and I had been trying to conceive a child for over a year. We knew that the infertility had to do with me, but no one could figure out what was wrong. My oncologist figured it out. The good news was that my infertility was due to a curable malignancy. The bad news (aside from the minor point that I had a *malignancy*) was that chemotherapy would probably leave me sterile. A real Rumpelstiltskin bargain, that. The drugs required to save my life would demand, as payment, not only my firstborn but all my other children as well. Like the miller's daughter in the fairy tale, I had no real choice. If I didn't undergo chemotherapy, I wouldn't have any children, anyway. I'd be dead.

Sterility is a side effect of many antineoplastic drugs; whether it is temporary or permanent depends on the specific drug regimen, the dose you receive, the duration of treatment, your age, and your gender. Since some forms of lymphoma also cause infertility, it can be difficult to know whether post-therapy sterility was caused by the treatment or by the lymphoma. However, the alkylating agents are most clearly associated with subsequent sterility, and combinations of drugs—particularly the high-dose regimens used in conjunction with stem cell transplants—seem to have more long-lasting effects on fertility than treatment with single agents.

If you need to undergo a form of chemotherapy that will likely lead to sterility and you are interested in having children in the future, you may want to investigate the possibility of banking frozen sperm (for men) or harvesting eggs, which are fertilized with your partner's sperm in vitro and then frozen (for women).

While none of the "assisted reproduction" procedures are guaranteed, they provide a greater chance of success than simply hoping that your fertility will be spared. Women who do not have a male partner may wish to investigate having their unfertilized oocytes (eggs) frozen, although freezing embryos appears to work better than freezing unfertilized eggs. Another option would be to have your oocytes fertilized with sperm from a sperm bank prior to putting them in cold storage. Recently, researchers have investigated freezing portions of ovarian tissue, to be reimplanted and take up their job again after treatment is over. Women who are unable to preserve embryos or oocytes prior to therapy and who develop ovarian failure as a result of chemotherapy can still undergo a pregnancy using eggs donated by another woman. And, of course, adoption is an option as well.

Since most antineoplastic agents target rapidly dividing cells, researchers have investigated the possibility that hormones that suppress ovulation could protect women from incurring permanent ovarian damage during chemotherapy. The results of some studies appear promising, but others have failed to find any benefit of suppressing ovulation. Therefore, this approach has not been proved to be beneficial. Nonetheless, if you're a young woman who'd like to have children someday, it's worth asking your doctor about the current status of this line of research.

It's a good idea to use effective birth control while you are undergoing chemotherapy, even if you are receiving a form of treatment that leads to infertility or sterility. This applies to both men and women. Sperm arise from a rapidly dividing population of cells; if the antineoplastic drugs don't destroy them outright, they may sustain damage that could lead to a birth defect in any baby conceived at this time.

While pregnant women have been diagnosed with lymphoma and successfully treated (with both the mother and the developing baby coming through fine), it's not a good idea to *become* pregnant while you are undergoing chemotherapy. The rapidly dividing cells of an embryo early in development represent an easy target for many antineoplastic drugs. Chemotherapy is most toxic to the developing fetus early in pregnancy; children born to women who were exposed to chemotherapy only during the third trimester of pregnancy experienced few problems other than low birth weight and slowed growth.

Children born to parents who have cancer—or who have had cancer in the past—but who are not undergoing treatment at the time of conception (or pregnancy in the case of the mother) are no more likely to have developmental problems than children born to parents who never had cancer.

Nausea and vomiting

Nausea and vomiting, like hair loss, are side effects of chemotherapy that everyone knows about. Unlike most of the side effects we've discussed so far, nausea and vomiting are primarily caused by chemical stimulation of the vomiting center of the brain (yes, that's really what it's called) rather than by toxicity to rapidly dividing cells. This is one of the most dreaded of chemotherapy's side effects—who can sustain any sort of quality of life while throwing up? Fortunately, there are now very effective drugs available to combat nausea and vomiting. These drugs can *completely* suppress nausea for many people undergoing front-line therapy for lymphoma: the absolute *worst* I experienced in this regard was a mild queasiness for several hours after chemotherapy was administered.

Vomiting evolved as a protective mechanism: when you eat a noxious substance, it's a good idea to have some means of getting rid of it as quickly as possible, before too much is absorbed. When you eat something that irritates your stomach, esophagus, or small intestine, these organs send signals to the vomiting center—an area in the lower brain. The vomiting center then initiates vomiting.

An area of the brain called the chemoreceptor trigger zone detects noxious substances circulating in the bloodstream. Unlike most of the brain, which is kept isolated from substances in the blood by the blood-brain barrier (formed by the cells in the small blood vessels that supply blood to the brain), the chemoreceptor trigger zone is supplied by leaky capillaries. These leaky capillaries allow the chemoreceptor trigger zone to detect any potentially toxic substances in your blood. The chemoreceptor trigger zone then passes the word along to the vomiting center that it's time to go into action.

The nerve cells in the brain, like other cells in the body, communicate by means of chemical messengers that bind to specialized regions on the cell surface called receptors. When a chemical messenger from one cell binds to its receptor on a second cell, it sets off a signal in the recipient cell. In the brain, these messenger molecules are known as *neurotransmitters*, and the brain has a host of different neurotransmitters available to convey messages.

Two neurotransmitters, *serotonin* and *dopamine*, are particularly important in carrying signals to the vomiting center (dopamine also carries signals *from* the vomiting center to the gastrointestinal tract). Some of the most effective *antiemetic* agents used to combat nausea and vomiting act as serotonin or dopamine *antagonists*. (An *emetic* is something that makes you feel like vomiting; an antiemetic suppresses this sensation. An antagonist is a drug that binds to a specific cell surface receptor and prevents the neurotransmitter from binding and passing along its message.) Serotonin and dopamine antagonists act as antiemetics by preventing serotonin and dopamine from binding to their receptors, thereby keeping the "nausea" message from getting through to the vomiting center (fig. 3.2).

Different chemotherapy agents are more or less likely to cause nausea and vomiting. For example, most people who take cisplatin become nauseated, but very few people find vincristine nauseating. This probably depends on how well different antineoplastic drugs stimulate the chemoreceptor trigger zone.

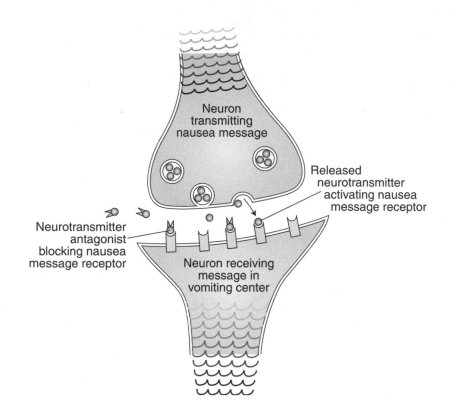

Figure 3.2. *Antiemetics act as neurotransmitter antagonists.* Neurotransmitters, such as serotonin and dopamine, carry a "nausea" message from one nerve cell (the presynaptic cell) to another (the postsynaptic cell) by binding to receptors on the postsynaptic cell. The receptors stimulate the postsynaptic cell to convey the message to the next neuron down the line. Antiemetics that bind to the receptor without stimulating it will prevent the neurotransmitter from binding and stop the nausea message from getting through.

Different antiemetic drugs are used with different chemo drugs. Dopamine antagonists, such as chlorpromazine, prochlorperazine, and perphenazine, are frequently used to combat mild to moderate nausea, as are sedatives such as Ativan, corticosteroids (such as dexamethasone), and Marinol, which is derived from the active ingredient in marijuana. The more powerful serotonin antagonists, such as ondansetron and granisetron, are used with chemo drugs that are likely to cause severe nausea and vomiting. Antiemetic drugs are frequently used in combination with one another.

Like any other drugs, the antiemetics can have side effects, and it may take a little experimentation to hit on the best combination. Some of these drugs can cause side effects like drowsiness, dry mouth, or a mild headache. The one and only time I took prochlorperazine (during the episode of food poisoning that led to the discovery of my anemia), I experienced a terrible restlessness that was almost as disturbing as the nausea and vomiting. Late at night, I was unable to sleep or even keep still. I roamed ceaselessly through the apartment from my bed, to the couch, to the bathtub, weakly retching every now and then. Finally, I collapsed in exhaustion and fell asleep.

For me, prochlorperazine wasn't a very effective antiemetic, either. It made it impossible to actually vomit but didn't affect the nausea at all. It was a horrible feeling, and I've never gone near prochlorperazine again. For many people, though, it's an extremely effective antiemetic. This underlines the fact that we're all a little different and can respond differently to any given treatment. If you experience nausea during chemotherapy and the first antiemetics you try don't work, ask for different combinations of antiemetic drugs.

You need to take antiemetics a little *before* you receive the chemotherapy. Antiemetic drugs are most effective when used preemptively, before nausea and vomiting strike. Once you're already feeling ill, they don't work nearly as well. It's also important to try to avoid these side effects in the first place. Aside from the immediate unpleasantness, nausea and vomiting can lead to a learned response.

Just as Pavlov's dog learned to salivate at the sound of the bell that rang when he was presented with food, your body can learn to associate the very *idea* of chemotherapy, or the sights and smells of the hospital ward, with the experience of nausea and vomiting. Then, next time you go to the hospital, you can start feeling nauseated even *before* you receive any drugs. You've learned to associate going to the hospital with feeling sick.

Eating small meals may help you avoid postchemo nausea, as well as eating foods that are cool or room temperature rather than hot (to avoid strong odors) or sucking on ice cubes or candy (it's probably not a good idea to suck on candy if you have mouth sores). You may also find it helps to adjust your diet, as chemotherapy can affect the way things taste. If eating makes you nauseated, you may wish to try taking an antiemetic such as metoclopramide (brand name: Reglan) thirty minutes before each meal.

It also makes sense to avoid eating your favorite foods right before the first few times you receive chemotherapy. That way, if you *do* experience nausea and vomiting, you won't develop a learned aversion to those foods (which would be a shame). People who are interested in alternative therapies may wish to consider acupuncture or acupressure. Several research studies have suggested that stimulating "P6," an acupuncture point just above the wrist, can help control the nausea associated with chemotherapy.

Habitually heavy drinkers generally have the fewest problems with nausea during chemotherapy. It isn't clear why—perhaps their vomiting centers have lost sensitivity following years of exposure to a potentially noxious stimulus, or perhaps their liver is more practiced at detoxifying things. Regardless of the reason, this is one of the few health benefits of being a heavy drinker, so, if it applies to you, you might as well enjoy it. This *isn't* an excuse to start drinking while you're undergoing chemotherapy. Alcohol, which puts stress on your liver, doesn't mix well with ongoing chemotherapy: it can affect how your body handles the chemo drugs and thereby influence their effectiveness and potential toxicity (in any event, it takes a long time to build up the tolerance to nausea).

Fatigue

Although it isn't as dramatic as nausea and vomiting, isn't as obvious as hair loss, and isn't as dangerous as bone marrow suppression, fatigue is one of the most pervasive and disruptive side effects of chemotherapy—as well as of radiation therapy and of lymphoma itself. By fatigue, I mean more than simple tiredness: fatigue refers to a state of exhaustion in which your ability to function normally is impaired by your lack of energy. More than three-quarters of people diagnosed with cancer experience major fatigue before, during, or after treatment. This is fatigue worse than any fatigue you've ever encountered before. Cancer fatigue has received very little attention until recently. After all, it isn't life threatening. But it can interfere tremendously with your quality of life.

By the time I was diagnosed with lymphoma, I needed to lie down for a moment after so much as tying my shoes. Shortly after starting therapy, things got even worse. During the first few cycles of chemotherapy, simply sitting up to eat a meal in a restaurant was so exhausting that I had to lie down for several hours afterward to recover. The word *tiredness* simply can't express this sort of exhaustion. Just as the Eskimos are said to have hundreds of different words for snow, it seems as though lymphoma survivors—particularly those who have undergone chemotherapy or radiation—should have a hundred different terms to describe fatigue.

Cancer fatigue can be acute: you'll be in the middle of doing something and will suddenly be hit with an overwhelming need to lie down and rest *at once.* I called this "aggressive fatigue" because there was no way around it: the only thing I could do was lie down. Simply lying down and taking it easy for a while can often relieve this sort of fatigue.

Or fatigue can be chronic and cumulative, creeping up on you and slowly pervading every aspect of your being until you *cannot* keep up with even the simplest routines of daily life. Your limbs may feel heavy or weak or disconnected. You may find it difficult to concentrate or to remember things. This sort of chronic fatigue can be more difficult to address than the acute kind.

Before I was diagnosed, I'd get tired from exertion. Going up a flight of stairs was exhausting. I couldn't remain standing for an entire seventy-five-minute lecture period. But this fatigue was acute—once I had a chance to lie down and rest, I could go on again. And after a weekend spent resting, I recovered enough energy to start out the new week.

When I first returned to teaching after cancer therapy and had to start keeping a normal schedule—instead of lying down whenever I got tired—I found myself in a state of chronic fatigue. Simply sitting down to catch my breath didn't help much. I was so exhausted that I couldn't concentrate or think straight. This fatigue was cumulative. It had built up over the years of illness and months of treatment, and nothing—short of sleeping for several days straight—seemed to help at all.

Chemotherapy-induced fatigue has many causes; some are well understood and can be treated, others not. If your chemotherapy involves drugs that suppress your production of red blood cells, the ensuing anemia can lead to fatigue. With anemia, you may experience decreased endurance and shortness of breath. Fortunately, anemia is treatable: you can take erythropoietin, a naturally occurring substance that stimulates red cell production, or (for a quick fix) get a blood transfusion to provide you with ready-made red blood cells.

Although anemia is often a major player in cancer fatigue, and while treating it may help you feel very much better, its importance in the overall fatigue experience can vary with the individual. I experienced massive blood loss (unrelated to my cancer) shortly after completing cancer therapy. It was only after recovering from the ensuing anemia that I could evaluate what part it played in my fatigue. I found that anemia limited my endurance during physical exertion. It left me breathless going up stairs and unable to walk for more than a few blocks at a time. But curing the anemia had little impact on my general perception of fatigue. I still needed to sleep all the time, was hit with the "aggressive tiredness" if I tried to do too much, and felt debilitated. I finally understood the mystery of how tired women with iron deficiency anemia (but not cancer) ever get anything accomplished. It has to do with different meanings of the word *tired*.

Substances liberated by the dying cancer cells, together with the increased metabolic demand imposed on your body by the need to repair or replace healthy tissue (like white cells or the cells that line the inside of your intestines) that has been damaged or destroyed by the therapy, may contribute to fatigue during chemotherapy. If you lost a lot of muscle mass before starting therapy, your muscles may not be functioning as efficiently as usual. You may need to work harder to accomplish any given physical task. This can lead to an increase in energy expenditure and consequent tiredness.

If you experience nausea, mouth sores, or alterations in how things taste as a side effect of chemotherapy, you may not be eating properly. Being diagnosed with cancer and undergoing chemotherapy can be emotionally draining, and psychological factors—such as stress and depression—may also lead to fatigue. If you are in pain or experiencing night sweats, you may not be sleeping well. All these factors can combine to make you tired.

Taking good care of yourself during this stressful time can help. Get enough sleep, limit unnecessary daily activities, try to eat a well-balanced diet with enough protein, and try to get regular exercise. Take naps if you need to. All these mundane things can really make a difference in how you feel. Meditating or practicing imagery (see Chapter 7) may help you cope with stress and feel stronger.

You may also need to set aside certain expectations of how things should be. While I was undergoing chemotherapy, there were times when my formerly beautiful apartment resembled the aftermath of a wild party. Paul tried his best to keep up with the housework, but his idea of tidiness seemed to fall short of mine. Were clean dishes, counters, and floors worth jeopardizing my physical well-being over? Clearly they weren't, and I had to give up expectations rather than exhaust myself to maintain a Martha Stewart home.

Medication is sometimes useful in combating fatigue. Stimulants such as Dexedrine may give you needed energy, and certain types of antidepressants may help alleviate chronic fatigue (the older class of tricyclic antidepressants seems to be more useful in combating chronic fatigue than the newer serotonin-uptake inhibitor Prozac-type drugs). If you've had radiation to your neck, your thyroid may become underactive (a blood test will let you know). In this case, taking synthetic thyroid hormone may help. Under the appropriate circumstances, painkillers and sleeping pills can give you a better night's sleep and alleviate some of the problems that lead to fatigue as well.

Chemo brain

Many people undergoing chemotherapy experience difficulty thinking clearly. This generally takes the form of memory loss, inability to concentrate, difficulty in solving math problems in your head, and a general sense of "cloudy thinking." Like cancer fatigue, this perception, sometimes called *chemo brain*, is something that cancer survivors talk about but physicians, until recently, have tended to minimize. That's probably because, like fatigue, such cognitive problems aren't life-threatening and are highly subjective—they're part of your perception of things and difficult for your doctor to measure.

Additionally, stress, fatigue, and depression—all of which are likely to exist while you're undergoing chemotherapy—can cause very similar cognitive disturbances. That makes it difficult to conclude that it's the chemotherapy per se that's causing any cognitive symptoms you might experience.

I certainly experienced difficulty concentrating while I was undergoing chemotherapy. And my memory of many events that occurred during that time is hazy. However, in my case, at least some of this had to do with the shock of the diagnosis; Paul later told me about several significant events that took place during the first weeks after my diagnosis that I didn't remember, and this was before I started chemotherapy at all.

However, research suggests that lymphoma survivors who have undergone chemotherapy are more likely to experience cognitive deficits than those who have undergone only radiation therapy or surgery. In a minority of cases, these problems persist after therapy is completed. While far from definitive, this research implies that there may indeed be a physiological basis for chemo brain.

Long-term effects

While all the side effects described above can be unpleasant and distressing, most of them (except for bone marrow suppression, with the consequent risk of infection) aren't really dangerous. Nobody wants to lose his or her hair or feel exhausted or nauseated or have mouth sores, but I think that most people would willingly put up with such temporary side effects for the chance of being cured of their cancer—or even the chance of a long-term remission.

However, the drugs used in chemotherapy are very powerful. Although they are far more active against cancer than against healthy tissue, they can sometimes cause long-lasting damage to normal tissue. Several of the side effects described above—notably fatigue and infertility—are potentially long-term effects of chemotherapy. Even after several years in remission I carefully hoarded my limited supplies of energy. It felt as though a miser had dealt me a daily allowance of "energy tokens." I went to bed absurdly early every night and still needed to take naps. I gave up on the idea of having children who were genetically related to me. But these are things one can adjust to. Other long-term effects of treatment are downright scary: high doses of Adriamycin can damage your heart; bleomycin can damage your lungs; cisplatin can damage your kidneys.

The most frightening potential long-term effect of chemotherapy is a secondary malignancy. This isn't surprising—many antineoplastic drugs damage DNA, and DNA disruption is what ultimately leads to cancer (see Chapter 8). Nonlymphocytic leukemia is the most common secondary malignancy following the chemotherapy regimens used to treat lymphoma. It is most frequently associated with some of the alkylating drugs. Solid tumors are less common and are more frequently associated with radiation than with chemotherapy.

While the *great majority* of lymphoma survivors—particularly those cured with a single six- or eight-cycle round of chemotherapy—do *not* go on to develop leukemia or any other treatment-related secondary malignancy, some do. Therefore, it's very important to be vigilant about your health and to keep in close touch with your doctor, even if you are pronounced cured of your lymphoma, so that, if a secondary malignancy should occur, you can catch it right away.

It's upsetting to think about battling your way through a bout with cancer only to face the possibility that the very treatments that saved your life could cause a secondary cancer somewhere down the line. It somehow doesn't seem fair. I coped with this knowledge through two psychological strategies (neither entirely satisfactory): first, the realization that, if I was alive to deal with a second cancer at some future date, I'd be better off than I would have been had my lymphoma simply run its course; second, the belief that, if and when a secondary malignancy occurred, our ability to treat cancer would have advanced to the point where it would be readily curable. As it happened, I was diagnosed with breast cancer four years after my diagnosis with lymphoma. It was detected early, in a postlymphoma CT scan, and my current prognosis is considered favorable.

Combination chemotherapy versus single-agent approaches

As noted earlier, small populations of chemotherapy-resistant cells can cause relapses and recurrences of cancer. These populations of resistant cells arise from mutations. They develop some mechanism that allows them to survive a drug that would normally be lethal. Cancer cells tend to be genetically unstable: they mutate to new forms more frequently than healthy cells do. A drug-resistant population of cells will arise when a mutation takes place that allows a cancer cell to evade the action of some antineoplastic drug.

Recognition that this sort of mutation could lead to emergence of chemo-resistant disease led oncologists to try using antineoplastic drugs in combination with each other. This approach is called *combination chemotherapy*. Since different classes of antineoplastic drugs can act through different mechanisms, cancer cells are less likely to figure out a way to resist a combination of drugs than to develop a resistance to any given drug alone. Therefore, combination chemotherapy is frequently used instead of single-drug chemotherapy, particularly when you have a curable form of lymphoma.

Unfortunately, even though combination chemotherapy has a much higher cure rate than single-agent treatment, even combination chemotherapy isn't always successful. Some mutations can simultaneously confer resistance to multiple drugs. For example, some cancer cells become adept at transporting any unwanted substances out of the cell. These cells then become *multidrug resistant*.

How chemo is administered

Some of the drugs used in chemotherapy can be taken as pills. Most antineo-plastic drugs, however, are delivered *intravenously*—by injection into a vein. Brief intravenous injections can be given through a needle attached to a syringe. This is similar to having blood taken for a blood test. Longer injections are delivered through a flexible plastic tube called an intravenous catheter line (IV line). IV lines are used when a large volume of some drug needs to be delivered or when the drug must be diluted before it reaches your veins.

With an IV catheter, a needle is inserted into a large vein (generally in your forearm or the back of your hand), and the catheter is threaded into your vein through the needle, which is then withdrawn. Since the tip of the catheter is soft, you can move your arm around without the tip piercing your vein. The other end of the catheter is attached to a bag filled with saline solution (salt water) or sugar water. These solutions help flush your kidneys and bladder (an important consideration with some chemo drugs) and also dilute irritating antineoplastic drugs before they hit your veins. Both antineoplastic drugs and supplemental medications (such as antiemetics or diuretics) can easily be injected into the catheter.

It's a good idea to drink some fluids before getting an IV line inserted. If you're very dehydrated, your veins can flatten out and be difficult to locate with the needle (ouch). The nurse will put a tourniquet on your arm to make your veins stand out and ask you to pump your fist. If your veins remain shy, the nurse may slap your arm (lightly) to irritate your veins or apply a heating pad. As a longer-term measure, exercise, if you feel up to it, tends to make your veins easier to find.

Sadly, we live in an imperfect world, in which mistakes sometimes get made. Getting the wrong chemo drug can be a fatal mistake; it's a good idea to take a look and make sure that you're getting all the correct medications (and *only* the correct medications). If you know the dose you're supposed to get, check that too. Although such mistakes are very rare—and there are safeguards in place to prevent them—there have been tragic cases where people have died from overdoses of chemo medication. Your doctors and nurses will be very sorry if this happens to you, but that won't do you much good. If you feel up to it, it's worth being proactive to make sure this doesn't happen. Or you may have a friend or relative come along to act as your advocate.

Sometimes fluid simply drips into your arm, at a rate that is determined by a clamp placed on the soft plastic portion of the catheter. When it's important to control the rate of drug delivery precisely, an infusion pump may be used: the plastic catheter line is threaded through the infusion pump, which controls the drip rate. If the bag of fluid is emptied, or if flow is blocked for some reason, the pump will send out an alert. The pumps used in my chemo unit played a cheerful three-note tune whenever the flow of solution stopped. More than anything else, hearing the characteristic "la-la-la" of blocked infusion pumps as I walk past the chemo wing of the hospital evokes that time for me.

If you experience any pain, swelling, redness, or tenderness around the site of your IV line, it's important to let the oncology nurse know right away. It could be a sign that the medication is leaking out of your vein into the surrounding tissue (if, for instance, the IV line was placed immediately upstream of the site of a very recent blood draw). Such a leak, called an *infiltration*, is not uncommon. Some antineoplastic drugs can damage tissue if they leak out of your veins; also, local leaks affect the total concentration of drug that most of your body receives. Therefore, it's important to speak up if you think that there may be a problem.

I've always hated needles. Believing this feeling was universal, I almost didn't bother to write this sentence, but Paul tells me he never minded needles. I did. When I was younger and had low blood pressure, I sometimes fainted after having blood drawn. The first time I had surgery, the prospect of getting an IV line was one of the scariest parts. Therefore, I wasn't looking forward to this aspect of chemotherapy *at all.* Moreover, the vampire (uh, phlebotomist) who took the gallons of blood required for the prediagnostic blood tests was full of dire stories about chemotherapy patients whose veins, scarred by repeated infusions of antineoplastic drugs, disappeared, making it impossible to find them. This was one of the points where anticipation was far worse than the reality. I was fortunate enough to have large, easily accessible veins that held up beautifully to chemotherapy, as well as oncology nurses and phlebotomists who specialized in painless needles (thank you, Ieva, Linda, Connie, and Gloria).

If you aren't that lucky, or if you expect to undergo a very prolonged chemotherapy regimen, you may want to investigate getting a central line, or permanent venous access device (nearly everyone undergoing a bone marrow transplant gets one of these). These devices are catheters that are inserted semipermanently (for months or even years) and feed into the large veins near your heart. Aside from avoiding repeated sticks into scarred and shrinking veins, they allow drugs to be delivered into the largest veins of your body—which are the least likely to be damaged by any caustic drugs. Central lines come in two basic flavors: external tunneled catheters and implanted ports. Placing a central line is considered a surgical procedure, but it is a relatively routine one and is done on an outpatient basis.

The external tunneled catheters include Broviac, Hickman, and Groshong catheters. These catheters are placed into a central vein and tunnel a short distance under your skin before emerging from your body. Some central catheters emerge on your chest, close to the veins into which they are inserted. A newer innovation, called a peripherally inserted central catheter, involves inserting the catheter into a vein in your arm and threading it all the way to your central veins. Either way, central catheters frequently contain several tubes running alongside each other so that several substances can be injected into different tubes simultaneously. This type of catheter can be used to withdraw blood, as well as to administer chemotherapeutic drugs, nutrient solutions, blood transfusions, or even bone marrow.

Once an external catheter has been placed, that's it as far as needle sticks. You do need to be careful not to tug on it or do anything that could displace it (for this reason, external catheters may not be a good choice for people with very small children). You will be shown how to flush it out, change the bandages that cover it, and keep it clean. It's important to be conscientious about this to avoid getting blood clots or infections.

Implanted ports, such as the Port-a-Cath or Infusa-Port, follow the same basic idea as the external tunneled catheters, except that the ends of the catheter stay inside your body: they connect to a drum-shaped port with a thick rubber membrane covering it. Injections are made into the rubber membrane covering the port. Ports, like external catheters, can be implanted either centrally or peripherally. Ports are somewhat easier to deal with than catheters: there's nothing protruding from your body, so they're more difficult to dislodge and you don't need a bandage. Moreover, they're easier to care for: you don't need to dress them, and they need to be flushed only about every six weeks and filled with a solution called heparin that keeps clots from forming in the port. On the other hand, you still need to be stuck with needles to access the drum of the port, and, once removed, they leave a larger scar.

If you're on a regimen where you need to maintain high levels of antineoplastic drugs over an extended period of time, you may get an infusion pump. These pumps allow you to receive prolonged infusions at home rather than in a hospital. They may be small portable pumps that can be carried in a pouch or in a holster attached to your belt, or you can get them implanted (usually in the abdomen). The implanted pumps, which are about the size of a hockey puck, can be refilled by an injection through the overlying tissue. These pumps are used to deliver pain medication like morphine, as well as chemotherapy drugs.

People who have central nervous system (CNS) lymphoma or are considered at risk of this may get *intrathecal* chemotherapy. With intrathecal delivery, drugs are delivered directly into the cerebrospinal fluid bathing the brain and spinal cord. A catheter may be inserted into the spinal canal, or an *Ommaya reservoir* may be placed under the skin of the scalp. This reservoir attaches to a catheter that leads to one of the large, fluid-filled ventricles inside your brain and can be filled through a needle, like an implanted port or implanted infusion pump.

Because of its action on neuronal microtubules, the drug vincristine should *never* be administered intrathecally. If you are on a regimen that involves intrathecal medication and you also take vincristine, check to make sure that no one tries to administer the vincristine intrathecally. This error has been made more than once, with tragic results.

Regimens used in treating Hodgkin lymphoma

The development of high-intensity radiation therapy and combination chemotherapy to treat Hodgkin lymphoma has been one of the great success stories of modern oncology. The majority of persons with Hodgkin lymphoma—even those diagnosed with advanced disease—can be cured. While radiation therapy alone is sometimes used to treat localized disease (Stage I, II, and rarely Stage III), combination chemotherapy is usually used for people with generalized disease and for those with localized disease that is "bulky" and/or accompanied by the Ann Arbor "B" symptoms (see Chapter 10).

Front-line combination chemotherapy for Hodgkin lymphoma revolves around two different regimens: ABVD and MOPP. These two regimens appear to be useful for all the different types of the disease. Treatment may also involve alternating the two regimens or administering hybrid regimens containing drugs from both MOPP and ABVD. MOPP, ABVD, and the hybrid therapies are all highly effective in treating the disease; the choice of which one to use to treat a given individual is often made on the basis of potential side effects.

For example, MOPP is much more commonly associated with sterility than ABVD. Over 90 percent of men and a majority of women who receive MOPP become irreversibly sterile as a result of the treatment. Permanent sterility is much less common with ABVD. MOPP has also been associated with a small risk of developing leukemia; this risk may be increased when MOPP is given in association with radiation therapy. Because MOPP treatment is associated with sterility and a risk of leukemia (even if it's a small risk) and ABVD is at least as effective in curing Hodgkin lymphoma, ABVD and related therapies are much more commonly used as front-line treatment.

On the other hand, ABVD, when used in combination with radiation to the chest, may increase the risk of radiation damage to the heart and lungs. Someone with massive mediastinal disease who already has children, who has some preexisting heart or lung condition, and who will likely need combined modality treatment involving radiation to the chest might be a candidate for MOPP.

ABVD consists of four drugs: Adriamycin (doxorubicin), bleomycin, vinblastine, and dacarbazine. As with most combination chemotherapy regimens, ABVD utilizes antineoplastic drugs from several different classes. Adriamycin and bleomycin damage DNA, vinblastine is an antimitotic drug, and dacarbazine is an alkylating agent. (See descriptions of individual drugs under "Specific Drugs," below.) In the classic ABVD regimen, all four drugs are given by intravenous injection on days 1 and 15 of a 28-day cycle.

MOPP also consists of four drugs: mechlorethamine, vincristine (also known as Oncovin), procarbazine, and prednisone. Of these drugs, mechlorethamine and procarbazine are alkylating agents, vincristine is an antimitotic drug, and prednisone is a corticosteroid. In the classic MOPP regimen, mechlorethamine and vincristine are given as intravenous injections on days 1 and 8 of a 28-day cycle, and procarbazine and prednisone are taken as pills on days 1–14. You get days 15 through 28 off from treatment and then start all over again.

In the MOPP-ABV hybrid regimen, mechlorethamine and vincristine are given intravenously on day 1; Adriamycin, bleomycin, and vinblastine are given intravenously on day 8; and procarbazine (days 1–7) and prednisone (days 1–14) are taken as pills.

Several newer regimens for treating Hodgkin lymphoma have been developed. Stanford V incorporates many of the drugs used in MOPP and ABVD and adds some new ones (Adriamycin, vinblastine, mechlorethamine, etoposide, vincristine, bleomycin, and prednisone) but uses a distinct dosing schedule and a briefer course of chemotherapy. Stanford V appears to have an effectiveness similar to that of MOPP and ABVD and may have fewer long-term side effects. Recent research suggests that BEACOPP (bleomycin, etoposide, Adriamycin, cyclophosphamide, vincristine, procarbazine, and prednisone) may be more effective than a regimen closely related to MOPP alternated with ABVD. If these promising findings hold up, Stanford V and BEACOPP may become standard treatments for Hodgkin lymphoma.

If you do not attain a complete remission with front-line treatment, your doctor may recommend a stem cell transplant. If you do attain a complete remission but then relapse, you may be treated with combination chemotherapy again or with a stem cell transplant. Radiation may sometimes be used instead of chemotherapy when the relapse is localized.

Regimens used in treating indolent (low-grade) NHL

Several distinct varieties of lymphoma are considered indolent, or slowly growing. In general, the same treatment approaches are used for all the indolent forms of disease. If your physician has told you that you have indolent, or low-grade, lymphoma, this discussion applies to you. Incidentally, if the term "low-grade" bothers you, remember that they're referring to the rapidity with which your lymphoma progresses—it's not intended as any sort of slur against *you*.

If you know how your lymphoma has been classified under either the Working Formulation classification system or the newer WHO classification system, you can find your specific category of lymphoma below. The discussion in the first part of the section on indolent lymphomas applies to the Working Formulation classifications of small lymphocytic lymphoma;

follicular small cleaved cell lymphoma (the most common form of indolent lymphoma);

follicular mixed small and large cell lymphoma;

and to the WHO classifications of

B cell chronic lymphocytic leukemia/small lymphocytic lymphoma;

lymphoplasmacytic lymphoma;

follicular lymphoma;

follicle center lymphoma, diffuse;

marginal zone lymphoma (MALT and nodal); and

splenic marginal zone lymphoma.

See Chapter 10 for a detailed description of the different forms of lymphoma and a discussion of the Working Formulation and WHO classification systems.

Some forms of lymphoma straddle the border between indolent and aggressive. These "borderline versions" are the Working Formulation categories of follicular large cell lymphoma (WHO classification: follicular lymphoma, grade III) and diffuse small cleaved cell lymphoma (several WHO classifications, including follicle center lymphoma, diffuse and mantle cell lymphoma).

The Working Formulation classifies both follicular large cell lymphoma and diffuse small cleaved cell lymphoma as "intermediate grade," which would fall into the aggressive category.

These forms progress more slowly than most of the aggressive lymphomas, and, unlike with the other aggressive lymphomas, it isn't clear that advanced cases are curable with current treatment regimens. Since some cases *may* be curable with the treatment regimens used against aggressive lymphomas, it makes sense to think of them as belonging therapeutically with this group. However, before you skip to the section on treating aggressive NHL (below), note that follicular large cell lymphoma, unlike most aggressive lymphomas, appears to be responsive to fludarabine, a drug commonly used to treat indolent lymphomas.

Mycosis fungoides, which generally behaves as an indolent lymphoma but has its own distinct set of treatment regimens, is discussed after the other indolent lymphomas. Mantle cell lymphoma, a "borderline" form, which has some features of indolent lymphomas but more features of aggressive lymphomas, is discussed separately.

At present, the approach to treating indolent NHL is fundamentally different from the approach to treating Hodgkin lymphoma or aggressive NHL.
That's because most advanced cases of indolent lymphoma are now considered
incurable. (*Localized* low-grade disease does seem to be curable and is often
treated with radiation, and it's possible that stem cell transplants can cure even
advanced cases.) Side effects that might be acceptable when curing an otherwise
rapidly fatal disease might not be acceptable in treating a disease that cannot be
cured and typically progresses very slowly.

Quality-of-life issues become more important. Most people would willingly
accept a few months of even the most unpleasant side effects of chemotherapy if
they know the treatment has a good chance of saving their life. On the other
hand, unpleasant side effects are less easy to tolerate if it isn't clear that the treatment will improve your chances of long-term disease-free survival.

A year or two before I was diagnosed with lymphoma, my father had a blood
test that suggested a possible diagnosis of indolent lymphoma. (As it turned out,
he didn't have cancer.) His doctor told him that he might be facing an incurable
disease, with a prognosis of about ten more years of life. A prognosis of ten years
didn't seem quite as terrible to my father—who was seventy-nine—as it might
have seemed to a twenty-nine-year-old (although being told you might have a
terminal illness is unwelcome news at *any* age). But he wasn't sure whether this
meant he would have to spend the next ten years undergoing chemotherapy for
an incurable disease. And:

"What kind of ten years will it be?" said my mother, with an expression of
fear and horror. It was clear that she was picturing him undergoing ten horrible
years of chemotherapy while growing ever more fragile and vulnerable. It was
clear that she wondered if they could bear ten years of such an existence.

Moreover, the pattern of response and relapse that characterizes indolent
lymphoma means that people with indolent disease are likely to undergo multiple rounds of therapy. Therefore, you and your doctor must carefully consider
the advantages and disadvantages of using drugs that are safe at low cumulative
doses but carry significant risks when they are administered for prolonged periods of time.

The trade-offs between the risks and benefits of long-term exposure to antineoplastic drugs need to be carefully balanced. If I—someone who was diagnosed with aggressive disease—develop heart disease in five years from the drugs
that saved my life eight years ago, I'm a lot better off than I would have been
without those drugs. (Although it would be nice if there were more antineo-

plastic drugs with no horrid short-or long-term side effects.) On the other hand, if I had indolent lymphoma and got heart disease five years after starting therapy for a disease that might have taken twenty years to kill me even if treatment had been *withheld* for a few years, I might be worse off than I would have been without that treatment.

The very slow progression of the indolent lymphomas also makes it difficult to determine whether a new therapy is curative; clinical trials need to run for many years before the long-term effectiveness of a given approach can be evaluated. It's easy to determine whether a new treatment can put the disease into remission; whether this translates into prolonged life—or possibly even cure—takes much longer to ascertain.

In general, more aggressive approaches to treating indolent disease seem to lead to longer remissions—and longer amounts of time without any apparent disease—but don't necessarily prolong life. Therefore, current treatment approaches to advanced cases of indolent NHL tend to be conservative. If stem cell transplants *do* turn out to cure indolent NHL (and there are some indications that this could be true), this approach to therapy may change. Current approaches to handling indolent lymphoma are also changing dramatically with the advent of the more highly directed "magic bullet" therapies involving monoclonal antibodies.

If indolent disease is asymptomatic, many oncologists practice a *watch-and-wait* (*or watchful waiting*) approach. You don't start treatment right away; the doctor simply checks up on you at intervals to see if the disease is progressing. Studies have indicated that people who are treated with a watch-and-wait approach, who begin therapy *only when treatment becomes necessary,* survive as long as people who start aggressive therapy as soon as their disease is uncovered.

Some people find it tremendously nerve-wracking to sit back and do nothing while waiting to see if (when) their cancer progresses. If you feel that way and your doctor has recommended a watch-and-wait approach, you may find it more appealing to think of this time as a reprieve, while you "watch and wait" for the discovery of an effective and nontoxic cure. A cure seems close enough that I have no doubt one will become available before some of us who are newly diagnosed with indolent disease are ready to start therapy.

If your disease is symptomatic (or undergoes significant progression), your doctor will likely recommend starting therapy. If your disease is threatening a vital organ (for instance, lymphoma has invaded your bone marrow and is choking out the cells that produce your white cells or platelets) or an enlarged lymph node is pressing on a nerve and causing pain, a watch-and-wait approach is no longer appropriate. It's time to start therapy.

Frustratingly, there is no clear consensus on the best approach to treating low-grade disease. Various regimens, using either single agents or combination chemotherapy, are used. (The good side to this is that if you relapse with disease that has become resistant to your initial regimen, there are a host of others to try.)

Traditionally, indolent lymphoma has been treated with single alkylating agents, such as cyclophosphamide or chlorambucil. Sometimes a steroid such as prednisone is given in combination with the alkylating agent (see descriptions of individual drugs under "Specific Drugs," below). Such single- (or double-) agent therapies are relatively mild—some people have no side effects at all from these treatments—and can sometimes keep indolent lymphoma under control for years. Moreover, both chlorambucil and cyclophosphamide can be taken as pills rather than as intravenous injections. While most people respond to single alkylating agents, the majority of people experience only a partial remission. Complete remissions to single alkylating agents (with or without a supplemental steroid) are less common, and these treatments do not appear to be curative.

Relatively mild drug combinations are also used to treat low-grade lymphomas. One combination is CVP: cyclophosphamide, vincristine, and prednisone. In this regimen, cyclophosphamide and prednisone are given by mouth on days 1–5 of a 21-day cycle, and vincristine is given by IV on day 1. Another combination is C-MOPP: cyclophosphamide, vincristine, procarbazine, and prednisone. Here, cyclophosphamide and vincristine are given by IV on days 1 and 8 of a 28-day cycle, and procarbazine and prednisone are given orally from day 1 through day 14. These combinations produce complete remissions more frequently than single alkylating agents do, but this doesn't seem to translate into increases in overall survival. While they're considered mild as far as combination chemo regimens go, side effects are not as mild as with cyclophosphamide or chlorambucil alone.

More recently, the antimetabolite drugs fludarabine and cladribine have proved to be effective in inducing remissions of indolent lymphoma. Fludarabine is frequently used as a single agent in initial therapy of low-grade disease. Clinical trials suggest that combination chemotherapies including fludarabine, such as fludarabine, mitoxantrone, and dexamethasone, may be even more effective. If the side effects turn out to be manageable, such combinations may become more common front-line treatments.

TREATING LYMPHOMA

Treatments aimed at recruiting your own immune system, like interferon-alpha or monoclonal antibodies, may be incorporated into the treatment regimen as well. Rituximab, a monoclonal antibody directed against the B cell marker protein CD20 that is sometimes used as single-agent therapy (see Chapter 5), is also frequently combined with various chemotherapy regimens. Interferon-alpha doesn't seem to do much when it's given with single agents but may improve the duration of remissions (and possibly overall survival) when it's given with the combination chemotherapy regimen CHOP (described under "Regimens used in treating aggressive NHL," below). This is surprising, since most studies have failed to find an advantage to treating indolent lymphoma with CHOP as compared with single agents or CVP. (See Chapter 5 for a discussion of monoclonal antibodies and the other "magic bullet" therapies used to treat lymphoma.)

There are a number of approaches to treating relapsed disease. Which one is best depends on individual circumstances, both in terms of response to the initial treatment and general overall health. Frequently, disease that responds to treatment with an alkylating agent, such as cyclophosphamide, and then relapses is still sensitive to the initial treatment. In this case, if the initial treatment was tolerable, it might make sense to re-treat with the same, relatively mild approach. If the disease no longer responds to the initial therapeutic regimen, it makes sense to switch to a new one: a monoclonal antibody (possibly labeled with a radioisotope; see Chapter 5), fludarabine or cladribine, or even a somewhat stronger regimen, such as CHOP.

Relapsed or nonresponsive disease may be treated with a stem cell transplant, although not everyone is a candidate for this form of therapy. If you have relapsed disease and are a good candidate for a stem cell transplant, the optimal timing can be difficult to determine. It's generally better to move on to a transplant sooner, rather than after many repeated courses of chemotherapy. This issue is discussed at greater length in Chapter 6.

Localized low-grade MALT lymphomas found in the stomach are a special case. As discussed in Chapter 11, there's evidence that these gastric lymphomas arise in response to chronic infection with the bacterium *Helicobacter pylori*. If they're caught early enough, they sometimes respond to treatments aimed at eradicating the bacterial infection. This consists of antibiotics given together with bismuth-containing compounds (like Pepto-Bismol). This sounds almost too good to be true: cancer treated with antibiotics! While it's not *certain* that antibiotic therapy is truly curative, so far the results of treating localized indolent gastric lymphomas with antibiotics are very encouraging. People whose gastric MALT lymphomas do not resolve after antibiotic therapy can be treated with more conventional chemotherapy or radiation. Gastric lymphomas, like other localized MALT lymphomas, are among the few forms of lymphoma frequently treated surgically.

Mycosis fungoides, a rare T cell lymphoma that involves the skin, is a special case as well. This disease, described in Chapter 10, is typically very indolent and shouldn't be confused with anaplastic T cell lymphomas of the skin (or with the occasional cutaneous B cell lymphoma). People whose mycosis fungoides involves *only* their skin (it hasn't spread to the blood or internal organs) are frequently treated with *topical agents*—substances applied directly to the affected areas rather than taken intravenously or by mouth—or localized treatments involving radiation. These treatments aren't necessarily curative, but they can control the disease for a long time.

Some approaches to localized therapy for mycosis fungoides use two of the antineoplastic drugs used systemically in treating other forms of lymphoma. For localized patches or plaques, mechlorethamine (nitrogen mustard) may be applied to the affected areas. The mechlorethamine can be dissolved in water or ointment and applied daily at home. Both mycosis fungoides and mechlorethamine treatment can cause severe itching and dry skin. Topical steroids (like cortisone cream), antihistamine pills, or over-the-counter skin creams and lotions may help. If dry skin is a problem, it's better to use mechlorethamine dissolved in ointment, since the ointment can act as a skin cream.

Some people become allergic to topical mechlorethamine. If that happens, you can undergo desensitization therapy or you can switch to another regimen. Sometimes BCNU (see "Specific drugs," below) is used topically. While fewer people develop allergic reactions to BCNU than to mechlorethamine, BCNU is more likely to be absorbed through the skin, and therefore systemic effects, like bone marrow suppression, are possible.

Localized mycosis fungoides can also be treated with various forms of radiation therapy: standard X-rays, electron beam therapy, and UV light. (All these treatments, as well as an unusual form of radiation therapy, *extracorporeal photopheresis*, are discussed in Chapter 4.) People with mycosis fungoides sometime receive injections of interferon-alpha or retinoids, drugs related to vitamin A that are beneficial in a variety of skin diseases. Both interferon-alpha and the retinoids are common components of combination regimens.

Mantle cell lymphoma

Mantle cell lymphoma progresses more rapidly than most indolent lymphomas. Indeed, most oncologists classify it with the aggressive diseases. However, the pattern of mantle cell lymphoma relapse and recurrence resembles that of most indolent lymphomas more than that of most aggressive lymphomas. Recent research suggests that very aggressive treatments involving stem cell transplants and/or several different treatment modalities (chemotherapy plus radiation plus one of the newer immunological therapies) may be more active against mantle cell lymphoma than standard chemotherapy regimens.

Regimens used in treating aggressive NHL

Aggressive NHL is somewhere between Hodgkin lymphoma and indolent NHL on the lymphoma curability spectrum. Even advanced cases are potentially curable with chemotherapy, but success rates aren't as high as those for Hodgkin lymphoma. With current treatment regimens, about half the people diagnosed with aggressive NHL can be cured.

For many years, the standard front-line therapy for most types of aggressive NHL was a combination chemotherapy regimen with the vaguely disturbing name of CHOP: *c*yclophosphamide, Adriamycin (also known as *h*ydroxydaunomycin), vincristine (also known as *O*ncovin), and *p*rednisone. (See descriptions of individual drugs under "Specific drugs," below.) It helps to think of the drugs as CHOPping the lymphoma, rather than CHOPping you. Cyclophosphamide, Adriamycin, and vincristine are given intravenously on day 1 of a 21-day cycle; prednisone is taken orally on days 1 through 5. As with many combination chemotherapy regimens, CHOP combines antineoplastic agents from different classes. Cyclophosphamide is an alkylating agent, Adriamycin is an anthracycline that attacks and cuts up DNA, vincristine is an antimitotic drug, and prednisone is a corticosteroid hormone. I participated in a clinical trial combining CHOP with the then experimental monoclonal antibody rituximab (R-CHOP; rituximab is described in Chapter 5). I was lucky to get into that trial. The preliminary results were amazing, and R-CHOP has now become the standard approach to therapy for aggressive B cell lymphomas. (Rituximab does not add any benefit to CHOP alone for people diagnosed with aggressive T cell lymphomas.)

The aggressive NHLs treated with CHOP (or R-CHOP) include the Working Formulation classifications diffuse mixed small and large cell lymphoma;

diffuse large cell lymphoma (the most common form of aggressive NHL); and

large cell, immunoblastic lymphoma.

Translated into the WHO system, these include

diffuse large cell lymphoma

and most of the aggressive T cell lymphomas, with the exceptions of T cell lymphoblastic lymphoma and adult T cell lymphoma/leukemia.

The aggressive lymphomas that are not usually treated with CHOP or R-CHOP (lymphoblastic lymphoma, Burkitt lymphoma, and adult T cell lymphoma/leukemia) are discussed separately. Mantle cell lymphoma has a relapse pattern similar to that of the indolent lymphomas but progresses more rapidly. It may be treated with CHOP or R-CHOP, but, unlike the more typical aggressive lymphomas, it isn't cured by either therapy. There is now some hope that mantle cell lymphoma may be curable with more aggressive regimens.

It's not clear whether it's most appropriate to classify the Working Formulation categories follicular large cell lymphoma (WHO classification: follicular lymphoma, grade III) and diffuse small cleaved cell lymphoma (several WHO classifications) as indolent or aggressive lymphomas in terms of the response to therapy. Since they may be curable with CHOP or R-CHOP, it makes sense to consider them as belonging with the aggressive lymphomas. Sometimes, follicular, mixed, small cleaved and large cell lymphoma and other indolent lymphomas may be treated with CHOP or R-CHOP as well.

While CHOP is a somewhat harsher regimen than the regimens commonly used in front-line therapy against indolent disease, many people discover that it isn't nearly as bad as they had expected. I took R-CHOP and was surprised to find that, for me, the worst effects were fatigue and weight gain (I also lost my hair). I considered R-CHOP pretty easy to tolerate. Others, however, have found the CHOP regimen much more difficult. Nonetheless, it's a pretty safe regimen, with only a 1 percent treatment-related fatality rate (mostly to do with infections). A 1 percent fatality rate is small comfort if you are in that 1 percent. And having lost a dear friend to infectious complications of chemotherapy, I don't take even a 1 percent risk lightly. But it's much better odds than you'll get from untreated aggressive lymphoma.

The major problem with CHOP (or R-CHOP) is that it doesn't cure everybody. Researchers have tried to identify those people who are likely to be cured by CHOP or R-CHOP and those who are likely to require additional treatment. If these groups of people can be identified, people who are likely to be cured by CHOP or R-CHOP can be treated with standard therapy, while those who are less likely to respond may be treated with a more experimental (possibly more toxic) approach. Evaluating the likelihood that a specific individual will respond successfully to CHOP or R-CHOP means taking into account age, general condition at the time of diagnosis, stage of disease, blood levels of the enzyme LDH (see Chapter 2, section on diagnostic tests), the size (bulk) of individual tumors, and the number of sites in your body where disease is found outside the lymphatic system.

If you look closely at these various factors, you'll see that they fall into two distinct groups. One group—stage of disease, size of tumors, serum LDH, number of extranodal sites—has to do with the extent of the disease. The other group—age and general condition—concerns the person's ability to withstand treatment. Both the severity of disease and the ability to withstand treatment play a role in determining a person's response to therapy.

The extent of the disease is important because the more cancer cells there are, the harder it is to eradicate them all. Lymphoma, like many other forms of cancer, is believed to arise from a single malignant cell. This means that, for you to be cured, *every single malignant cell* in your body must be wiped out. The more malignant cells present, the greater the likelihood (purely by chance) that *one* of those cells will manage to survive treatment. It may also be more difficult for antineoplastic agents to penetrate to the cells in the middle of a very large tumor, and this situation can help those cells to survive therapy. Even if all signs of disease have disappeared, that one resistant survivor can give birth to numerous daughter cells, leading to a relapse of the cancer.

The person's ability to withstand treatment is important, too. Someone in fragile health may not be able to withstand a full course of a regimen like CHOP. It does no good to cure cancer if the treatment further damages an already weakened heart. Similarly, someone with liver or kidney problems, or someone whose bone marrow is already working at suboptimal levels, might be unable to tolerate the full dose of CHOP. Under these circumstances, the physician may need to reduce the dosages of some of the drugs to avoid intolerable side effects of treatment.

The problem with taking reduced dosages of drugs, of course, is that although you're not hitting the person as hard with chemotherapy, you're not hitting the *cancer* as hard, either. So it's more likely that a few of the tougher malignant cells will survive the treatment. If these hardy cells do survive treatment, there's a good chance that their daughter cells will retain their chemo-resistant properties. In this case, the relapsed cancer may be even harder to eradicate than the lymphoma that was there in the first place.

Thus, both the extent of the disease and the general overall condition of the person can influence the likelihood that the person will be cured with a given regimen. Experimental therapies for people who are considered unlikely to be cured with conventional therapy address both of these issues.

Some experimental approaches to lymphoma therapy use new drugs, higher doses of conventional drugs, or different methods of drug delivery so that higher concentrations are applied to the tumor. These treatments are designed to make sure that no malignant cells escape therapy. Other experimental approaches involve finding ways to improve supportive care or designing dosage schedules that might be easier to handle. For instance, someone with fragile bone marrow and a weak heart who couldn't tolerate CHOP at the standard doses might be able to take CHOP if he or she took a drug that stimulates the bone marrow to produce new blood cells and a drug that protects the heart.

As someone who was diagnosed in poor physical shape, with a *very* large tumor and LDH levels through the roof, I didn't think I stood a very good chance of making it with the standard therapy. The only thing I had going for me was my youth. And, although I didn't know it at the time, my oncologist was concerned about my ability to withstand the treatment. I was weak and skinny and anemic. (In fact, I was able to tolerate the full-dose CHOP regimen; people can sometimes be surprisingly resilient.)

The current treatment of choice for people with aggressive disease that doesn't respond completely to (or relapses from) front-line therapy with CHOP or R-CHOP is high-dose chemotherapy followed by an autologous stem cell transplant (see Chapter 6). Sometimes, people at high risk of a relapse from CHOP move directly from CHOP or R-CHOP into a stem cell transplant during their first remission. People who are unable to tolerate a stem cell transplant (because of age or fragile health) may undergo an alphabet soup of salvage therapies. (Many people feel that the term "salvage" has depressing connotations, but it helps to remember that it stems from the same route as "save" and "salvation." Salvage therapy is therapy to try to save you, even if front-line treatment has failed.)

These salvage therapies use combinations of drugs that show activity against lymphoma but that aren't generally used in front-line treatment. They include DHAP (dexamethasone, cisplatin, high-dose cytarabine), ESHAP (etoposide, cytarabine, cisplatin, prednisone), MIME (mesna, ifosfamide, methotrexate, and etoposide), and MINE (mesna, ifosfamide, mitoxantrone, etoposide). Some of these same regimens are used to reduce the extent of disease prior to starting high-dose chemotherapy in preparation for a stem cell transplant.

Several forms of aggressive lymphoma have their own specific therapies. Most of these "special case" lymphomas involve "very aggressive" disease—disease that progresses more rapidly than disease that is simply aggressive. In the Working Formulation, these are the "high-grade" diseases.

Lymphoblastic lymphoma is a highly aggressive disease that is generally treated with its own distinct set of regimens. Lymphoblastic lymphoma, in which the malignant cell resembles a lymphocyte at an early stage of development (usually a developing T cell, less commonly a developing B cell), is very similar to but less common than acute lymphoblastic leukemia. Therefore, many of the regimens used to treat lymphoblastic lymphoma are similar to those used to treat acute lymphoblastic leukemia. These "leukemia-style" regimens are more complex than traditional "lymphoma-style" regimens. They may involve as many as ten different drugs, administered on various schedules. Moreover, these antileukemic "ten different ingredient soups" involve more extended treatment, in which the last phase of chemotherapy—known as the maintenance phase—can last for several years.

While the treatment plan will vary depending on the extent of disease, it's not uncommon for chemotherapy for lymphoblastic lymphoma to be divided into three phases. These are an *induction phase,* aimed at achieving a complete remission; a *consolidation phase,* to nail down the remission, catching any stray cells that might be lurking in hard-to-reach areas of the body; and a *maintenance phase,* which is frequently less intensive, to prevent late relapses.

Regimens for treating lymphoblastic lymphoma generally include vincristine, prednisone, an anthracycline (such as Adriamycin or daunorubicin), and methotrexate. Some of the other antineoplastic drugs used in treating lymphoblastic lymphoma are L-asparaginase, cyclophosphamide, cytarabine, 6-mercaptopurine, 6-thioguanine, hydroxyurea, and BCNU. Although studies indicate that the prolonged maintenance phase really does help prevent late relapses, it's not clear that complex induction regimens are essential for everyone with lymphoblastic lymphoma. For some people with localized disease, simpler regimens may be as effective as the more complex ones.

A major concern with lymphoblastic lymphoma is possible spread to the central nervous system (the brain and spinal cord). Therefore, one or more of several drugs, including methotrexate, cytarabine, or a corticosteroid, may be administered directly into the fluid surrounding the brain and spinal cord through a catheter (so as to bypass the blood-brain barrier). This introduces high doses of antineoplastic drugs into the cerebrospinal fluid—the fluid that surrounds and cushions the brain and spinal cord—in order to prevent spread of the disease to the central nervous system.

The process of delivering drugs into the cerebrospinal fluid is called intrathecal chemotherapy. In some cases, intrathecal chemotherapy involves delivering drugs into the spinal canal. Sometimes, methotrexate, steroids, or cytarabine are delivered directly into the fluid-filled cavities inside the brain known as *ventricles* through an Ommaya reservoir, which is implanted under the scalp. High-dose systemic methotrexate may be given intravenously into the circulatory system as well.

The small noncleaved cell lymphomas, Burkitt lymphoma and Burkitt-like lymphoma, are also highly aggressive. These lymphomas have their own special regimens. Most regimens used in treating the small noncleaved cell lymphomas incorporate the alkylating agent cyclophosphamide. Indeed, children with Burkitt lymphoma have reportedly been cured with cyclophosphamide alone. Most regimens for Burkitt and Burkitt-like lymphomas, however, also include vincristine, prednisone, and either methotrexate or Adriamycin. If your doctor is concerned about possible spread to the CNS (based on the location and size of the tumors), you may be given preventative doses of methotrexate delivered into the cerebrospinal fluid through a needle or an Ommaya reservoir.

Since the malignant cells in these very aggressive forms of lymphoma divide very rapidly (the tumor can double in size in just a few days), dosage schedule is very important. The goal is to prevent the tumor from growing back completely before the next dose of chemo, a situation that would put you in a perpetual chemical tug-of-war in which neither the patient nor the tumor ever quite wins. To avoid this scenario, it's common for the oncologist to tailor the chemotherapy schedule to the patient's individual response. White cell counts are carefully monitored, and the next dose is delivered as soon as the bone marrow has recovered enough to handle it (generally when neutrophil levels have reached 200–1,000 cells/mm³ of blood). This sort of dosage schedule can give the chemo an edge over the tumor, allowing the patient to win this battle.

The rapid rate of cell turnover found in the very aggressive lymphomas generally translates into extreme sensitivity to antineoplastic drugs. If you have extensive disease, this sensitivity to treatment can lead to large numbers of cells dying in synchrony and spilling their contents into your bloodstream. Such synchronized cell death can raise the levels of uric acid in your blood. If the uric acid concentration in your blood becomes too high, some of it may crystallize out. This can cause pain (if it crystallizes in your joints—this is what causes gout) or kidney damage (if it crystallizes in the tubules of your kidneys).

To prevent this, people with small noncleaved cell lymphomas may be given intravenous fluids and diuretics to help flush the excess uric acid out of their blood and into their urine, together with drugs like allopurinol or rasburicase, which respectively inhibit the synthesis of uric acid and increase the rate at which it is broken down. (It should be noted that this massive *tumor lysis syndrome*, leading to increased blood levels of uric acid, is more common with, but not unique to, very aggressive forms of lymphoma. I was given allopurinol before starting my own chemotherapy regimen.)

Adult T cell leukemia/lymphoma (ATLL) is one of the few forms of lymphoma that has been clearly linked to infection with a virus. As discussed in Chapter 11, ATLL is associated with the retrovirus HTLV-I, a relative of the virus that causes AIDS. Some studies have suggested that the antiviral drug AZT (zidovudine), more familiar for its role in treating AIDS, may be useful in treating ATLL, particularly in combination with interferon-alpha.

Specific drugs

Remember, you will *not* experience all the side effects of these drugs. Don't let the various alarming possibilities scare you.

Adriamycin

Adriamycin (doxorubicin, hydroxydaunomycin, "Big Red") is a member of a class of antineoplastic drugs (table 3.1) called the *anthracycline antibiotics*. (The others are daunorubicin, idarubicin, and mitoxantrone.) It is used in the ABVD regimen for Hodgkin lymphoma, as well as the CHOP and R-CHOP regimens for treating some forms of NHL. Adriamycin is a bright, fluorescent red drug that will turn your urine red for a day or so after it is administered. (Drink lots of water to flush it out of your kidneys and bladder; you'll know it's gone when your pee looks normal again.)

Like many antineoplastic drugs, Adriamycin causes bone marrow suppression and can cause mouth sores, moderate to severe nausea and vomiting, and hair

Table 3.1. Antineoplastic Drugs Used to Treat Lymphoma

Generic Name	Brand Name	General Class	Delivery
bleomycin	Blenoxane	similar to anthracycline	intravenous
carmustine	BCNU	alkylating	intravenous
chlorambucil	Leukeran	alkylating	oral
2-chlorodeoxyadenosine; 2-CDA; cladribine	Leustatin	antimetabolite	intravenous
cisplatin	Platinol	similar to alkylating	intravenous
cyclophosphamide	Cytoxan	alkylating	intravenous or oral
cytarabine; cytosine arabinoside; Ara-C	Cytosar-U	antimetabolite	intravenous
dacarbazine	DTIC-Dome	alkylating	intravenous
dexamethasone	Decadron	corticosteroid	intravenous or oral
doxorubicin; hydroxydaunomycin	Adriamycin; Doxil; Rubex	anthracycline	intravenous
etoposide; VP-16-213	VePesid	similar to anthracycline	intravenous or oral
fludarabine	Fludara	antimetabolite	intravenous
gemcitabine; difluorodeoxycytidine	Gemzar	antimetabolite	intravenous
ifosfamide	Ifex	alkylating	intravenous
lomustine	CeeNu	alkylating	oral
mechlorethamine	Mustargen	alkylating	intravenous
melphalan	Alkeran	alkylating	intravenous or oral
6-mercaptopurine	Purinethol	antimetabolite	oral
methotrexate		antimetabolite	intravenous or oral
methylprednisolone	Medrol	corticosteroid	oral
prednisone	Deltasone; Prednicot	corticosteroid	oral
procarbazine	Matulane	alkylating	oral
vinblastine	Velban	antimitotic	intravenous
vincristine	Oncovin	amtimitotic	intravenous

loss. It can also cause severe tissue damage if it leaks out of your veins during administration (if something seems to be going wrong during the intravenous drip, tell the nurse *at once!*). Of most concern, however, is that Adriamycin can sometimes cause heart damage. With Adriamycin, cardiac damage is the chronic dose-limiting toxicity. Therefore, people who are embarking on regimens that use Adriamycin frequently get baseline tests of cardiac function.

Heart damage generally occurs only after you've received cumulative doses of Adriamycin that are higher than those attained during standard treatment with ABVD, R-CHOP, or CHOP; it's most common in children and in the elderly. The potential for Adriamycin-induced damage to the heart is synergistic with the potential for radiation-induced damage. That is to say, doses of Adriamycin that wouldn't ordinarily cause cardiac toxicity might do so if you underwent radiation therapy to your heart as well. This drug/radiation synergy limits the amount of Adriamycin that can be given to people who are likely to require radiation to the chest (such as people who, like me, have mediastinal lymphoma).

It's possible that you might reach the safe limit for Adriamycin administration at a time when Adriamycin-sensitive cancer is still present in your body. Drugs that bind iron, like Zinecard, as well as antioxidant vitamins that inhibit the activity of free radicals, can protect your heart from Adriamycin-induced damage. Under certain circumstances, such protective agents can let you get away with higher-than-normal doses of Adriamycin. These protective agents aren't given routinely, however, since it's theoretically possible that they could protect the *cancer* cells from Adriamycin as well. Exercise may help protect against Adriamycin-induced damage to the heart by increasing the levels of certain cardiac enzymes that act to break down and detoxify free radicals.

BCNU

BCNU (carmustine) is a member of a subclass of alkylating agents known as the *nitrosureas*. Its major side effect is bone marrow suppression. With BCNU, bone marrow suppression takes longer to show up than with most antineoplastic drugs (with nadir occurring five weeks or so after treatment), and recovery may also be prolonged. This bone marrow suppression may be cumulative and is considered the dose-limiting toxicity for BCNU. BCNU has a moderate tendency to cause nausea and vomiting, and high doses may cause some lung damage. BCNU is given intravenously. If it is administered too rapidly, you may feel a localized burning sensation. Tell the nurse to *slow down.*

Bleomycin

Bleomycin binds to DNA and, in the presence of iron and oxygen, chops it up into pieces. It has an unusual spectrum of side effects, producing little bone marrow suppression (and therefore little effect on immune function) and only a moderate tendency to cause nausea and vomiting. It does tend to cause hair loss, frequently causes fever (especially the first few times you take it), and may cause mouth sores.

The most common adverse side effects of bleomycin, however, involve the skin and lungs. Skin effects range from the innocuous (darkening and thickening of the skin), to the more annoying (itching, hives, peeling skin, or rash), to the downright distressing (sores developing over pressure areas like elbows or knuckles). Bleomycin can also cause lung damage (oxygen, which is found at high levels inside the lungs, is involved in how this drug works). Lung damage can show up as a cough or as difficulty in breathing, or it may be seen on a chest X-ray before symptoms appear. While more people escape lung damage than develop it, it's important to let your doctor know at the first sign that you're developing a cough or difficulty breathing. If these symptoms are due to bleomycin, he or she may want to switch you to a different regimen before serious lung damage occurs. Damage to the lungs is more common with very high doses of the drug and is considered the dose-limiting toxicity for bleomycin. Lung damage occurs more commonly in smokers and in people over the age of seventy. It may be aggravated by radiation to the chest.

Rarely, people given bleomycin have an allergic reaction in which they develop high fever and chills, dizziness and confusion, and a drop in blood pressure. This occurs in about 1 percent of people given the drug. For reasons that are unclear but probably having to do with abnormal cytokine balance, this reaction is more common in people with lymphoma than in people with other sorts of cancer (we always knew we were special). Since this sort of severe allergic reaction can be dangerous if it isn't treated right away, many medical centers give a small test dose of bleomycin before starting therapy. After taking the test dose, you are carefully monitored for any signs of an allergic response. That way, any such reactions will be minimal and can be treated immediately.

2-chlorodeoxyadenosine

The drug 2-chlorodeoxyadenosine (cladribine, 2-CDA, Leustatin) is an antimetabolite. It is closely related to adenosine, which is a normal component of DNA (see Chapter 8), and is incorporated into newly synthesized DNA, leading to cell death. Adenosine is also part of the molecule ATP, which provides energy for the cell, and cladribine also acts to deplete cellular stores of ATP. This energy depletion also promotes cell death.

Cladribine is given intravenously, typically over the course of five to seven days, either through continuous drug infusion or through daily two-hour-long infusions. As with the related drug fludarabine, the immediate side effects of cladribine are generally mild. Cladribine causes bone marrow suppression, leading to reduction in the levels of both neutrophils and platelets. While this is generally fairly mild to begin with, it can become more pronounced with continued use.

Cladribine kills normal, as well as malignant, lymphocytes, and normal lymphocyte levels may remain suppressed for some time after therapy. Because lymphocytes play such an important role in the normal immune response, this suppression can cause increased susceptibility to infection. Therefore, antibiotics are frequently given along with cladribine-containing regimens in order to prevent the development of potentially serious infections. Cladribine may also cause anemia. Fever is a relatively common side effect, as is unusual fatigue.

Chlorambucil

Chlorambucil is an alkylating agent. Like the other alkylating agents, it binds to DNA. Unlike most antineoplastic drugs, it's effective when given by mouth. While chlorambucil causes some bone marrow suppression, affecting levels of both neutrophils and platelets, this suppression is often relatively mild. Persons with low grade lymphoma have taken chlorambucil for months, or even years, without experiencing severe suppression of bone marrow. Some people report *no* side effects from chlorambucil; others experience relatively mild nausea or fatigue or both. Like some of the other alkylating agents, chlorambucil may increase the chance of developing leukemia; this is more common with long-term use of the drug and must be considered if long-term use of chlorambucil is being contemplated.

Cisplatin

Cisplatin (Platinol) is a complex of platinum, ammonia, and chloride. That's right, platinum—you could be taking a drug that's literally worth more than its weight in gold. The antineoplastic activity of platinum-containing compounds was discovered accidentally, when researchers were investigating the effects of electricity on bacterial growth by passing electrical current from platinum electrodes through bacterial cultures. They discovered that the bacteria stopped dividing and grew long, strand-like processes. The researchers soon realized that these effects were due to platinum from the electrodes dissolving in the growth medium, rather than from the effects of the current itself. Since several antineoplastic agents were known to produce similar effects on bacteria, they tested the activity of cisplatin (the soluble complex formed by platinum under these conditions) against cancer.

Cisplatin probably works like the alkylating agents: it binds to multiple sites on DNA and links separate DNA strands together. It also interacts with various proteins, and this likely contributes to its side effects. Cisplatin, like many other antineoplastic drugs, can cause bone marrow suppression; not only neutrophil levels but platelet and red blood cell levels may be suppressed. Nadir is delayed compared with many other bone marrow-suppressing drugs, generally occurring two to three weeks after the drug is administered. Nausea and vomiting are frequent side effects of cisplatin; usually these can be controlled with Ondansetron and corticosteroids.

Cisplatin has some more unusual side effects as well. When it was first used in clinical trials, the dose-limiting toxicity involved kidney damage. Keeping the kidneys well flushed out can minimize the risk of kidney damage. *Be sure to drink a lot of fluids if you are on a cisplatin-containing regimen!* Generally, people are given an intravenous saline solution and diuretics with cisplatin to be absolutely certain the kidneys are well flushed. Drug effects on the kidneys can also disturb your blood levels of calcium and magnesium; your doctor will order blood tests to monitor levels of these and other serum electrolytes.

Cisplatin can also damage your inner ear. This side effect is more common in children than adults and can lead to hearing loss, vertigo, or ringing in the ears. With high concentrations or sustained use, cisplatin can cause a peripheral neuropathy that is characterized by numbness or tingling sensations in your fingers and toes. Rarely, cisplatin can trigger an allergic reaction. Like most allergic reactions, this can be controlled with corticosteroids, epinephrine, or antihistamines.

Cyclophosphamide and ifosfamide

Cyclophosphamide (Cytoxan) is an alkylating agent; like the other alkylating agents it binds to DNA and links different strands together. It was one of the drugs I took, and I have to admit that I was vaguely horrified to learn that I was going to be taking a drug whose trade name, Cytoxan, sounded suspiciously like it meant "cell poison." Fortunately, cyclophosphamide is very toxic to lymphoma cells but relatively easy on the rest of the body.

Cyclophosphamide is a key ingredient in several regimens used against NHL. These include CVP, CHOP, R-CHOP, and COMP. Indeed, it has been used as a single agent against Burkitt lymphoma. You can take cyclophosphamide either orally or intravenously (with CHOP, R-CHOP, and COMP it's given intravenously). Like most of the alkylating agents, cyclophosphamide suppresses the bone marrow (primarily affecting the neutrophils), causes hair loss, is likely to induce nausea and vomiting, and can lead to sterility in both men and women. It may also cause darkening of the skin, fingernail ridges, and mouth sores.

Cyclophosphamide can irritate your bladder (*cystitis*); this can lead to severe hemorrhaging from the bladder with significant blood loss. People who develop such hemorrhagic cystitis during treatment with cyclophosphamide are at increased risk of developing bladder cancer in the future. Since hemorrhaging is a potentially serious condition, if you see blood in your urine or experience painful urination while on a regimen including cyclophosphamide, be sure to alert your doctor right away.

Bladder damage is caused when toxic by-products of cyclophosphamide act directly on the cells lining the bladder walls. It may be avoided by drinking enough fluids to dilute the concentration of these toxic substances in your urine to low levels. *It is therefore very important to drink a lot of fluids—at least eight 8-ounce glasses a day—while you are on regimens that contain cyclophosphamide.*

People taking very high doses of cyclophosphamide, which are sometimes used in preparation for a bone marrow transplant, or those who take the closely related drug *ifosfamide*, are frequently given a drug called mesna. Mesna, which stands for 2-mercaptoethanesulfonate sodium, is not an organization for dyslexics with very high IQs. Rather, it is a drug that binds to the toxic by-products of cyclophosphamide and ifosfamide metabolism and prevents them from injuring the bladder wall. Mesna is not usually necessary at standard dosages of cyclophosphamide.

Very high doses of cyclophosphamide can have other toxic effects that are rarely seen at standard doses; these may include damage to the heart and lungs.

Sometimes cyclophosphamide may be given orally over extended periods of time. This may lead to a chronic low-grade upset stomach or persistent vague nausea, which can be difficult to control with antiemetic drugs. As with the other alkylating agents, long-term use of cyclophosphamide may lead to an increased chance of developing leukemia.

Cytarabine

Cytarabine (cytosine arabinoside, Ara-C) is an antimetabolite. Like cladribine, cytarabine is related to one of the components of DNA (but to cytosine, not adenosine) and is mistakenly incorporated into newly synthesized DNA. Although it is most commonly used to treat certain forms of leukemia, cytarabine is used in regimens against some types of lymphoma as well. It is given intravenously.

Cytarabine is given at different dosages; side effects depend on dose. The most common side effects are bone marrow suppression (affecting neutrophils, platelets, and red blood cells) and damage to the cells lining the gastrointestinal tract. This can lead to severe mouth sores, diarrhea, and abdominal pain. Cytarabine sometimes irritates the membranes lining the eyelids and covering the eye (conjunctivitis). It may also cause mild, reversible problems with liver function that can lead to jaundice (yellowing of the skin and eyes). At high doses it is likely to cause nausea and vomiting. Less commonly, high doses may lead to neurological damage involving the central nervous system; this shows up as slurred speech or *extreme* tiredness and is usually reversible. Cytarabine is one of the two drugs commonly used intrathecally to treat CNS lymphoma.

Dacarbazine

Dacarbazine is an alkylating agent used in the ABVD regimen to treat Hodgkin lymphoma. It is given intravenously. Dacarbazine is very likely to induce nausea and vomiting and should be accompanied by an appropriate antiemetic. It also causes some bone marrow suppression, which may affect neutrophils and platelets. It sometimes causes flu-like symptoms, including fever and associated aches and pains. It may cause increased sensitivity to sunlight; it's a good idea to cover up for several days after receiving dacarbazine therapy.

Dexamethasone

Dexamethasone, like prednisone, is a synthetic corticosteroid hormone. It is more potent than prednisone and longer lasting, but both its therapeutic actions and its side effects are similar (see "Prednisone," below, for discussion of the corticosteroid hormones). In addition to being an antilymphoma agent, dexamethasone acts as an antiemetic.

Etoposide

Etoposide is derived from a compound with the unwieldy name *podophyllotoxin*, which is extracted from the leaves and roots of a beautiful spring wildflower, the mayapple (or American mandrake, Latin name: *Podophyllum peltatum*). The roots and umbrellalike leaves of this plant are toxic; the lemon-colored fruit has been used to make jam. Extracts of this herb were used cautiously (large amounts were known to be poisonous) in American folk medicine to promote vomiting and purging and to expel worms. (Vomiting and purging were curiously popular remedies in traditional herbal medicine.) Podophyllotoxin is the chief component in podophyllin, a mixture of chemicals extracted from the mayapple that is applied locally to destroy warts.

Podophyllotoxin acts like the vinca alkaloids (described below), binding to the protein tubulin and inhibiting mitosis. Oddly, the two synthetic antineoplastic compounds derived from podophyllotoxin, etoposide (VP-16-213) and teniposide (VM-26), do not show significant antimitotic activity. Instead, they act like Adriamycin and the other anthracycline antibiotics, inhibiting the DNA repair enzyme topoisomerase II, which leads to cleavage of the DNA strands.

Etoposide at conventional doses causes mild bone marrow suppression (primarily of neutrophils) and has a mild to moderate tendency to promote nausea and vomiting. With higher dosage regimens it causes pronounced bone marrow suppression and is more likely to induce nausea as well as hair loss and mouth sores. Rarely, people who have been treated with high doses of etoposide develop leukemia.

Fludarabine

Fludarabine is an antimetabolite that is related to adenosine, a component of both DNA and RNA. It is given intravenously over a period of five days and is highly active against many indolent lymphomas. The side effects of fludarabine are generally rather mild. It does cause bone marrow suppression, which can be particularly significant following repeated use of the drug. Fludarabine can cause nausea and vomiting (usually mild), mouth sores, and sometimes fever. It is toxic to normal lymphocytes as well as malignant ones and may cause a prolonged reduction in the levels of circulating CD4 T cells. This can lead to enhanced susceptibility to infection. Therefore, antibiotics are frequently prescribed along with fludarabine-containing regimens to minimize the risk of contracting potentially severe infections.

Occasionally (particularly in older people given high doses) fludarabine may cause some nerve damage. This may appear either as peripheral neuropathy (see "Vinca alkaloids," below, for a description of peripheral neuropathy); effects on nerve cells in the brain that may lead to confusion or lethargy; or inflammation of the optic nerve, causing disturbances in vision. Very rarely, high doses of fludarabine may cause lung damage.

Gemcitabine

Gemcitabine (2′,2′-difluorodeoxycytidine, Gemzar) is an antimetabolite. Like cytarabine, gemcitabine is related to cytosine, one of the components of DNA, and is mistakenly incorporated into newly synthesized DNA. It also inhibits the production of some DNA components. Although rarely used in front-line therapy, it is often used to treat relapsed disease. It has been shown to be effective against Hodgkin lymphoma, aggressive NHL, and mycosis fungoides. Gemcitabine is given intravenously. It can suppress the bone marrow—affecting platelet production in particular—but its side effects are generally fairly mild.

Ifosfamide

See "Cyclophosphamide and ifosfamide," above.

Mechlorethamine

Mechlorethamine, or nitrogen mustard (related to mustard gas), was the first of the class of drugs known as alkylating agents used in clinical medicine and is the prototype of drugs in this class. It is very likely to induce nausea (more than 90 percent of patients given mechlorethamine experience some nausea) and should therefore always be taken with an appropriate antiemetic.

Like other alkylating agents, mechlorethamine causes bone marrow suppression, can cause hair loss and infertility, and should not be taken during the first trimester of pregnancy. It may also cause ringing in your ears or dizziness (usually only with high doses). It is administered intravenously; since it can irritate your veins, it is diluted by injection into an IV line of running saline. If mechlorethamine leaks out of a vein into the surrounding tissue, it can cause tissue damage (after all, mustards are known for their irritating properties). Therefore, if you notice *any* redness, pain, or swelling at the injection site, be sure to tell the oncology nurse right away so that he or she can treat it before any damage occurs.

Melphalan

Melphalan is related to nitrogen mustard. Although it is more commonly used to treat multiple myeloma, it is used in some lymphoma regimens, including BEAM, a high-dose therapy often used in preparation for bone marrow transplants, as well. Its major side effect is bone marrow suppression.

6-Mercaptopurine

6-Mercaptopurine and the closely related 6-thioguanine are both purine antimetabolites (like fludarabine and cladribine). That is to say, they resemble normal components of DNA. Unlike fludarabine and cladribine, which are derivatives of the purine base adenine, 6-mercaptopurine and 6-thioguanine are derivatives of guanine, another component of DNA. These two drugs are very active against leukemias but not most forms of lymphoma. However, they are used in some of the leukemia-style regimens used to treat lymphoblastic lymphoma.

Methotrexate

Methotrexate is also an antimetabolite; in fact, it was the first antimetabolite used in chemotherapy. It was the discovery of methotrexate's effectiveness against childhood leukemia that lead to the widespread development of this class of antineoplastic drugs. Methotrexate blocks the metabolism of folic acid. Folic acid, or folate, is one of the vitamins in the B complex and is required for the normal synthesis of DNA in dividing cells. In the absence of folic acid, chromosomes aren't replicated, and the cells aren't able to divide normally. Folic acid deficiencies can result from insufficient dietary folate, problems in folate absorption, or increased demand (high rates of cell turnover).

In the 1940s, researchers discovered that children with leukemia had low levels of folate in their blood. They tried to treat this deficiency by administering folic acid. To their horror, they found that folate treatment *worsened* the leukemia: the malignant cells were gobbling up the folate and using it to replicate themselves! The researchers reasoned that if folate made leukemia worse, a drug that interfered with folate metabolism might be beneficial. This led to trials of drugs like methotrexate that blocked the action of folic acid and the first dramatic remissions of childhood leukemia.

Since folic acid is important for rapidly dividing cells, methotrexate will target cells that are reproducing. Methotrexate has dramatic activity against various malignant cells but can also be toxic to rapidly dividing populations of normal cells. Therefore, high doses of methotrexate are frequently administered in combination with what's called a *leucovorin rescue.* Leucovorin is a compound that is closely related to folic acid. However, it feeds into the folate metabolic pathway *after* the point blocked by methotrexate. DNA synthesis can proceed as required; the cell is rescued from the toxic effects of folate inhibition.

Leucovorin rescue is like starting an airlift to an island that's critically dependent on supplies from the mainland after the bridge that forms the normal supply route falls down. Leucovorin rescues rapidly dividing cells in the bone marrow and the gut from the toxic effects of methotrexate after the malignant cells have already succumbed. Proper timing of leucovorin administration is critical to the success of the rescue mission: you need to time the airlift so that it takes place after the inhabitants of "Cancer Island" have starved to death, but while the inhabitants of "Bone Marrowland" are still hanging on.

Because inhibiting folate metabolism affects all rapidly dividing cells, methotrexate causes bone marrow suppression as well as mouth sores and other gastrointestinal problems (at the higher doses, where these effects are most pronounced, they will be minimized by the leucovorin rescue). High-dose regimens of methotrexate can sometimes cause kidney damage; administering intravenous fluids that contain sodium bicarbonate (which makes urine more alkaline) can minimize the potential for this side effect. Methotrexate has been associated with some risk of liver damage; this is generally a problem with high doses or very long term (years) use. Methotrexate is the main drug used intrathecally to treat CNS lymphoma (cytarabine and hydrocortisone may be given as well). This use exploits its targeting of rapidly dividing cells because mature nerve cells (neurons) in the brain do not continue to divide.

Methylprednisolone

See "Prednisone," below.

Prednisone

Prednisone is a synthetic glucocorticoid hormone that is used in many NHL regimens, including CVP and CHOP, as well as in MOPP for Hodgkin lymphoma. Its effects are similar to those of dexamethasone and methylprednisolone, two other glucocorticoids used in treating lymphoma, and it is discussed here as representative of the actions of glucocorticoid hormones in general.

Since our own glucocorticoids have so many different effects on metabolism and normal physiological function, it's not surprising that large doses of glucocorticoids given therapeutically should have a variety of secondary effects. Of all the drugs used in treating lymphoma, prednisone was most likely to trigger an avalanche of responses on the NHL mailing list.

I was a member of the minority of prednisone users who discovered that they *loved* prednisone. It gave me energy, helped me breathe more easily, and let me (literally) snap my fingers at the chronic joint pain that had plagued me for so long. Several chronic ailments (recurrent vertigo and hives) disappeared: prednisone made me feel better than I had for years.

The only thing I didn't like about prednisone was its effect on my appetite. It made me hungry. Constantly hungry. Unbelievably hungry. Paul watched in amazement as his dainty, 90-pound wife gobbled down three servings of dinner and then eyed his own not-yet-completed first serving with longing. I stopped eating because I knew I should, not because I felt full. It didn't even matter that everything tasted kind of funny—I was *hungry*.

This was probably a good thing at first, when I was underweight, but the 60 pounds I added during and after the eighteen weeks I was on chemotherapy was annoying. It seemed so unfair—the only *good* part about cancer had been my model-like appearance during the brief interim between "ideal weight" and "walking skeleton." I had always thought that people undergoing chemotherapy lost weight, becoming thin and frail. Instead, my body expanded like bread dough. This sort of weight gain on prednisone-containing regimens like CHOP is not uncommon. (People on some other lymphoma regimens, and even some people taking prednisone, *do* lose weight while undergoing chemotherapy.)

Prednisone can also give you the classic steroid "moon-faced" appearance and cause swelling of your feet and ankles. Long-term use can lead to a change in the distribution of body fat. People develop a characteristic "snowmanlike" appearance, with rounded faces, heavy abdomens, and thin, sticklike arms and legs. More serious effects of long-term prednisone use may include problems in carbohydrate handling that can make existing diabetes worse (or uncover a hidden tendency toward diabetes) and increased risk of ulcers, muscle weakness, and cataracts. Since people with diabetes appear to be at increased risk for developing NHL, this side effect of prednisone can be a serious problem.

Prednisone has multiple effects on how your body handles calcium, and long-term use can lead to osteoporosis, a serious condition in which calcium is lost from your bones, markedly decreasing their density. The loss in bone density can lead to increased susceptibility to hip fractures in response to a fall or to spontaneous fractures of your vertebrae (the bones in your spine), resulting in the development of a dowager's hump. If you need to be treated with prednisone or other steroids for extended periods of time, speak to your doctor about taking calcium supplements, and make sure that you get sufficient exercise and adequate supplies of vitamin D to combat the loss of calcium from your bones. Some oncologists prescribe alendronate (brand name: Fosamax), a drug that inhibits the loss of calcium from bone, for people undergoing therapy with steroids.

Osteoporosis is of particular concern to women who undergo early menopause as a consequence of chemotherapy, since early menopause, which leads to a premature decrease in the levels of the hormone estrogen (which acts to increase bone density), also increases your risk of developing osteoporosis. If you undergo early menopause as a result of chemotherapy and you need to take glucocorticoids for extended periods of time, you may want to discuss the advisability of taking hormone-replacement therapy with your doctor. Prednisone can also cause pain and damage to the joints of the hip and shoulder. In severe cases, joint replacement may become necessary.

The two complaints voiced most often, however, had to do with prednisone's effect on mood (which I never experienced) and its nasty taste (which I never noticed—I was too hungry to worry about taste). Many people experience intense effects on mood and behavior. These can include restlessness and insomnia (taking it first thing in the morning helps minimize problems with insomnia) and the kind of manic exuberance that leads people to buy everything in sight, drive into a lamppost, or quit their job and move to Paris on the spur of the moment. People on the NHL mailing list frequently referred to this as "flying Air Prednisone."

After prolonged treatment, people may experience the Air Prednisone crash: unpleasant withdrawal symptoms when they stop taking prednisone. Side effects of prednisone withdrawal may include fever, achiness, and general malaise, as well as tiredness and depression. It is sometimes possible to slowly taper off the dosage, rather than stopping abruptly, in order to avoid such withdrawal symptoms.

Procarbazine

Procarbazine is an alkylating agent that interferes with DNA, RNA, and protein synthesis. The drug as given is inactive: it must undergo metabolism in the liver before becoming active as an antineoplastic agent. Procarbazine causes bone marrow suppression, leading to neutropenia and thrombocytopenia, and can cause nausea and vomiting as well as mouth sores and skin rashes. Occasionally, procarbazine causes some neurotoxicity. This can cause drowsiness or agitation, as well as "pins and needles" sensations or dizziness upon standing up.

Procarbazine also has some adverse interactions with certain foods or drugs. It's a good idea to avoid alcohol while undergoing chemotherapy (to give your poor liver a break); this is particularly important with procarbazine-containing regimens. Procarbazine can have a nasty Antabuse-like effect, so that people who drink alcohol while on procarbazine can develop hot flashes and pounding headaches and become violently nauseated.

Procarbazine also inhibits the activity of the enzyme monoamine oxidase (MAO). Indeed, procarbazine was initially synthesized as an MAO inhibitor (a class of drugs sometimes used to treat depression) and was then discovered to have antineoplastic activity as well. MAO inactivates a class of compounds called monoamines. Some of these monoamines can increase your blood pressure. If a drug like procarbazine has inhibited MAO activity, circulating levels of these monoamines can rise, leading to dangerously high blood pressure.

People taking procarbazine or other MAO inhibitors should avoid foods high in the monoamine tyramine. These foods include red wine, fava beans, and liver (hmmm), smoked and pickled meats and fish, yeast extracts, avocados, aged cheese, and overripe fruit. Foods that are high in caffeine, such as coffee, tea, and chocolate, and various drugs including cocaine, the tricyclic antidepressants, and some antihistamines can also increase levels of circulating monoamines. Therefore, it can be dangerous to take them in combination with procarbazine as well.

Vinca alkaloids: vincristine and vinblastine

Vincristine (Oncovin) and vinblastine (Velban) act as antimitotic agents by binding to tubulin and interfering with the action of the mitotic spindles. This prevents cells from undergoing cell division and leads to apoptotic cell death. These drugs are derived from the leaves of a beautiful subtropical plant, the Madagascar periwinkle (Latin name: *Catharanthus roseus,* formerly *Vinca rosea. Note:* This is *not* the same plant as *Vinca minor,* the common periwinkle, which is grown as a ground cover). Tea made from the leaves of the Madagascar periwinkle was widely used in tropical folk medicine to treat diabetes. During the 1950s, researchers decided to see if it really was effective in controlling the disease. Although they were unable to observe any benefit of periwinkle tea on diabetes (it has some effect on blood sugar levels, but not enough to be useful), they discovered that diabetic rats injected with plant extracts died of massive infections. Since similar effects had been observed following injections of large amounts of cortisone, they wondered if they had discovered a natural source of corticosteroids. They discovered that the infections resulted from a tremendous suppression of the bone marrow that had nothing to do with corticosteroids.

This observation led to the isolation of several plant alkaloids from the periwinkle and trials of their efficacy in treating various forms of cancer. Two of these alkaloids, vincristine and vinblastine, are effective against both Hodgkin lymphoma and various forms of NHL.

Oddly enough, given the initial observation that *Vinca* extracts caused bone marrow suppression, vincristine actually has very little effect on the bone marrow. That means that it can be taken together with drugs that *do* suppress the bone marrow without worrying that the combination will reduce blood cell production to dangerously low levels. It also has very little tendency to induce nausea and vomiting: fewer than 10 percent of persons given vincristine alone experience nausea or vomiting as a side effect. Vincristine can—but doesn't always—cause hair loss. Vincristine that leaks out of your vein can damage the surrounding tissue, so let the nurse know right away if you notice any redness, pain, or swelling at the site of injection.

Not only are microtubules involved in forming mitotic spindles during cell division, but they also convey substances down the long processes found in many nerve cells. When vincristine binds to tubulin, it disrupts neuronal microtubules as well as those involved in cell division. This interrupts the delivery of substances down the nerve processes, which in turn can lead to neuronal damage. This neuronal damage (*neuropathy* or *neurotoxicity*) is responsible for most of vincristine's side effects. Since vincristine doesn't cross the blood-brain barrier, most of its neurotoxic effects involve the peripheral nervous system—those areas of the nervous system outside the brain and spinal cord. Damage to peripheral nerves is known as *peripheral neuropathy.*

Minor nerve damage is generally fully reversible, while more severe damage may not be. It is important to report any of the following side effects to your doctor so he or she can assess the extent of any neuropathy that may occur. Peripheral neuropathy may make itself known by either numbness or a "pins and needles" tingling. It shows up in the tips of your fingers and toes first, since they are innervated by the longest nerves. The peripheral neuropathy will usually start to clear up by the time you are given the next round of vincristine, but the effects of repeated doses tend to accumulate.

Peripheral neuropathy may be relatively mild—I experienced tingling, numbness, and deterioration of my handwriting and wouldn't have wanted to attempt sewing by hand or any delicate work in my laboratory—or fairly severe. A friend was so severely affected—she couldn't hold a pencil or feel her feet—that she needed to reduce her dosage. The full effects may be somewhat delayed. Several months after I completed chemotherapy I started experiencing numbness and a feeling of weakness in my lower legs after walking a block or two, and for several years I had trouble doing delicate manipulations in my lab. Both the numbness in my legs and the deterioration in my handwriting have mainly cleared up by now, and I've generally recovered from vincristine-induced neurological damage.

Less commonly, damage to the nerves that supply internal organs such as the gastrointestinal tract and the bladder may occur. The severe constipation known as "vincristine belly" is best treated prophylactically by eating lots of fruits and vegetables or other foods that are high in fiber. If you don't feel like eating very much, you can try drinking some of the high-fiber versions of liquid dietary supplements.

Disruption of the nerves to the bladder may cause problems with urination. Depending on the exact balance of affected nerves, this may show up either as difficulty in urinating or as an increase in frequency of urination. Occasionally people experience transient dizziness when they stand up, blurred vision, or difficulty in sweating. Even more rarely, vincristine may affect nerves in the brain, causing such symptoms as dizziness, confusion. or agitation. This is *very* rare at standard dosages.

Vinblastine, like vincristine, inhibits cell division. Although its chemical structure is very close to that of vincristine, its spectrum of activity against cancer is different, as are its possible side effects. It has a much more pronounced effect on the bone marrow, causing pronounced neutropenia with nadir occurring four to ten days after administration. It is more likely to cause mouth sores or a sore throat than vincristine and may cause jaw pain; perhaps in compensation, neurological side effects are less common. Hair loss may or may not occur.

Shortly after I started chemotherapy, my aunt gave me a book of poetry. I was startled to find the vinca alkaloids in Thomas Avena's beautiful poem "Cancer Garden":

> The cancer garden, protected by buildings, one unfinished. Still
> the wind will continue through the garden when these walls
> are sewn in. Everything known in the cancer garden devolves
> to breath. If we can, we open gray chambers and fingers
> of the lung. Such breath can sting. Here are vermilion
> snapdragons, mild blue agapanthus, poppy. Here in our
> veins is the blood of the Madagascar periwinkle: its sulfates
> vincristine, vinblastine, effective against neoplasm.

In the second verse, Avena refers to "neon colored serum," which I think must be "Big Red," Adriamycin.

If the drugs used in chemotherapy can be viewed as the blood of the plants growing in the cancer garden, the sunlight in the garden can be viewed as radiation therapy, a form of lymphoma treatment we'll consider in the next chapter.

The medical texts on lymphoma in the reference section for Chapter 1 all have chapters on treatment covering a broad range of topics, both traditional and more experimental. Additionally some of the following books and articles may be of interest.

This standard oncology text has excellent chapters pertaining to lymphoma:

DeVita VT Jr., Hellman S, Rosenberg SA, eds. (1997). *Cancer: Principles and Practice of Oncology.* 5th ed. Philadelphia: Lippincott-Raven.

Review articles that discuss various aspects of lymphoma therapy include:

Aisenberg A. (1999). "Problems in Hodgkin's disease management." *Blood* 93:761–769.

Bartlett NL. (1997). "Treatment of aggressive histology lymphoma." *Current Opinions in Oncology* 9:413–419.

Bendandi M, Pileri SA, Zinzani PL. (2004). "Challenging paradigms in lymphoma treatment." *Annals of Oncology* 15:703–711.

Fisher RI, Miller TP, O'Connor OA. (2004). "Diffuse aggressive lymphoma." *Hematology* 2004:221–236.

Fisher RI, Oken MM. (1995). "Clinical practice guidelines: Non-Hodgkin's lymphomas." *Cleveland Clinic Journal of Medicine* 62:S1–48.

Golomb HM. (1998). "Management of early-stage Hodgkin's disease: A continuing evolution." *Seminars in Oncology* 25:476–482.

Kasamon YL, Swinnen LJ. (2004). "Treatment advances in adult Burkitt lymphoma and leukemia." *Current Opinion in Oncology* 16:429–435.

Martelli M, De Sanctis V, Avvisati G, Mandelli F. (1997). "Current guidelines for management of aggressive non-Hodgkin's lymphoma." *Drugs* 53:957–972.

Vose JM. (1998). "Current approaches to the management of non-Hodgkin's lymphoma." *Seminars in Oncology* 25:483–491.

For a general overview of various drugs commonly used in cancer treatment:

Chabner BA, Allegra CJ, Curt GA, Calabresi P. (1996). "Antineoplastic agents." Chap. 51 in Hardman JG, Limbard LE, Molinoff PB, Ruddon RW, Gilman AG, eds., *Goodman & Gilman's Pharmacological Basis of Therapeutics.* 9th ed. New York: McGraw-Hill.

Hillman RS. (1996). "Hematopoietic agents: Growth factors, minerals and vitamins." Chap. 53 in Hardman JG, Limbard LE, Molinoff PB, Ruddon RW, Gilman AG, eds., *Goodman & Gilman's Pharmacological Basis of Therapeutics.* 9th ed. New York: McGraw-Hill.

And for a really comprehensive discussion of chemotherapy, which includes chapters on specific classes of drugs, complications of chemotherapy, drug delivery, and newer approaches (you will need some background in biology to read this book):

Chabner BA, Longo DL, eds. (1996). *Cancer Chemotherapy and Biotherapy: Principles and Practice.* 2d ed. Philadelphia: Lippincott-Raven.

For an exceptionally entertaining and enlightening account of the discovery of the anti neoplastic drugs vincristine and vinblastine by one of the major people involved:

Noble RL. (1990). "The discovery of the vinca alkaloids—chemotherapeutic agents against cancer." *Biochemistry and Cell Biology* 68:1344–1351.

Helpful information can also be found online:

The most up-to-date source of information on lymphoma therapy (and cancer therapy in general) is the National Cancer Institute's Physician's Database Query (PDQ), which gives treatment information summaries on many forms of cancer for both patients and physicians. PDQ is available from the National Cancer Institute site: cancernet.nci.nih.gov/cancertopics/pdq OR wwwicic.nci.nih.gov/cancertopics/pdq

Medscape is another outstanding source of up-to-date information (you need to sign up, but it's free): www.oncology.medscape.com/Home/Topics/oncology/oncology.html

CHAPTER 4

Radiation Therapy, Combined Modality Therapy, and Surgery

R adiation therapy, like chemotherapy, is intended to selectively kill malignant cells while sparing normal cells as much as possible. Like chemotherapy, radiation therapy (also called radiotherapy) is most active against rapidly dividing populations of cells. Unlike most forms of chemotherapy, radiation can be applied *locally*, to specific areas of the body, rather than spreading throughout the entire body via the bloodstream. Radiation therapy is sometimes used to treat localized disease. It may be used alone or in combination with chemotherapy (*combined modality treatment*).

Total body irradiation (TBI) is sometimes used to treat generalized disease in preparation for a bone marrow transplant. Chemotherapy is more common as a first line of therapy to treat widespread disease, however, and radiation is most often used for treating localized areas of involvement.

Several different kinds of radiation are used to treat lymphoma. High-energy X-rays and gamma rays are used to treat tumors deep within the body. These high-energy forms of radiation penetrate some distance into the body before they interact with tissue. Electron beam therapy, which doesn't penetrate as deeply, may be used to treat more superficial tumors. Ultraviolet light may be used to treat lymphomas like mycosis fungoides that involve the skin.

All these forms of radiation therapy are known as external radiation therapy, or external beam therapy, because you're exposed to a beam of radiation emitted by a piece of equipment outside your body. Radiation can also be delivered internally by means of radioisotopes attached to monoclonal antibodies (see Chapter 5).

Radiation fields

External beam therapy may involve greater or lesser portions of your body. *Involved field radiation* is delivered only to sites of known disease. Involved field radiation may be given as palliative treatment to people with widespread indolent NHL. In this case, the radiation is intended not to be curative but to reduce the size of a particularly troublesome region of disease. *Extended field radiation* includes not only the sites of known disease but also lymph node chains that are adjacent to them, to kill off microscopic cancers that may have spread beyond the regions where disease is apparent. Involved or extended field radiation therapy may be given with curative intent to people with localized low-grade disease.

Involved or extended field radiation therapy may also be used in combination with chemotherapy for people with Hodgkin lymphoma or some presentations of aggressive NHL. For example, people with very large (very large or "bulky" tumors are generally defined as greater than 10 cm—about 4 inches—in diameter) mediastinal tumors are frequently treated with combined modality therapy. Chemotherapy is given first, to reduce the size of the mass, followed by extended or involved field radiation to any remaining abnormal areas. This reduces the exposure to radiation. Localized involvement of certain sites, including the stomach, the testes, the thyroid, the socket of the eye, and the brain, is frequently treated with localized radiation as well (sometimes in combination with chemotherapy).

The amount of tissue that should be irradiated in treating localized disease remains controversial and is an area of ongoing research. With Hodgkin lymphoma, which typically spreads directly from one node to the next, fewer relapses occur when the radiation field is extended beyond sites known to be involved with lymphoma. Presumably, that's because the adjacent lymph nodes contain microscopic disease that can't be visualized.

It *isn't* clear, however, that increasing the irradiated area improves your chances of long-term survival. In part, this is because Hodgkin lymphoma that relapses from front-line treatment with radiation usually responds well to further treatment with chemotherapy. It may also have to do with a greater likelihood of long-term toxic side effects of the treatment if a larger area of normal tissue is exposed to radiation.

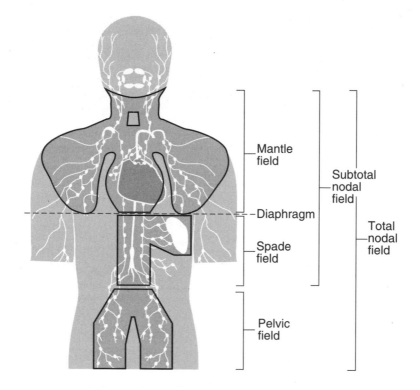

Figure 4.1. *Standard radiation fields.* Localized Hodgkin lymphoma without "B" symptoms (Stage I and II A) is sometimes treated with one of several standard radiation fields. The *mantle field* covers the region of the body containing the lymph node regions below the jaw and above the diaphragm. These include the lymph nodes in your neck, above your collarbone, in your armpits, and deep within your chest. *Subtotal nodal irradiation* includes the mantle field plus the abdominal *spade field,* which consists of the spleen and paraaortic lymph nodes. The *pelvic field* includes the femoral and inguinal lymph nodes. Radiation delivered to the pelvic and the abdominal spade regions is sometimes called the *inverted Y field.* *Total nodal radiation* includes all the lymph node regions in the mantle, spade, and pelvic fields.

Localized Hodgkin lymphoma without "B" symptoms (Stage I and II A) may be treated with one of several standard radiation fields (fig. 4.1). The *mantle field* covers the lymph node regions below the jaw and above the diaphragm. These include the lymph nodes in the the neck, above the collarbone, in the armpits, and deep within the chest. *Subtotal nodal irradiation* includes the mantle field plus the abdominal *spade field,* consisting of the spleen and paraaortic lymph nodes.

Localized Hodgkin lymphoma that occurs only above the diaphragm is sometimes treated with a mantle field alone but may also be treated with subtotal nodal irradiation. *Total nodal irradiation* includes the mantle field, the spade field, and the lymph nodes in the groin and pelvis. The spade field plus the pelvic lymph nodes make up the *inverted-Y field*, used to treat people whose disease is present only below the diaphragm. Sometimes total nodal radiation is used to treat Stage III A disease, although treatment for Stage III disease more commonly involves chemotherapy.

With NHL, which doesn't necessarily spread from one node to the next but may jump from one lymph node region to another one far away (possibly circulating to distant sites through the blood), the value of irradiating lymph node regions adjacent to sites of known disease is even less clear except possibly in the case of bulky mediastinal disease. It is common to deliver high levels of radiation to sites of known disease and to irradiate surrounding regions with a reduced dose.

Total body irradiation (radiation delivered to your whole body) may be given in preparation for a bone marrow transplant. Electron beam therapy to all of your *skin* is sometimes used for mycosis fungoides. Since the electron beam doesn't penetrate as deeply as X-rays or gamma rays, this type of radiation will not have as many systemic effects as the total body irradiation given before a bone marrow transplant.

Treatment planning

Before undergoing radiation therapy, you'll undergo a *treatment simulation.* In this planning session, the radiation oncologist and radiation technicians take X-rays to determine exactly where the disease is located and where the treatment will be directed. The simulation ensures that all the diseased tissue is included in the treatment area (*radiation port* or *radiation field*) but as little healthy tissue as possible is irradiated. You will have to lie very still on a table while these X-rays are being taken, to make sure that an accurate image of the sites of disease is obtained.

The radiologist will mark your skin in the region of the treatment area with semipermanent ink or a tiny tattooed dot (smaller than a freckle). When you come in for treatment, these marks are used to line up a beam of light that's delivered through the same piece of equipment used to deliver the X-rays, to be certain that the X-rays will be delivered to exactly the right place. The ink marks are easier to line up but messier for you. (A nonchlorine bleach will help get ink off your clothes.) Usually, the technician will measure the contours of your body with a lead wire or some other such flexible device so the radiation can be directed to the appropriate *depth* inside your body.

After you undergo the radiation simulation planning session, special shields, or *blocks,* may need to be constructed—these are placed inside the machine that will deliver the radiation. The blocks, which are made of a very dense metal alloy, are opaque to radiation and will direct the radiation to the appropriate areas of your body. Uninvolved areas, and sensitive tissues like your heart and lungs, are shielded. Your blocks will be constructed especially for you, like a pair of custom-made shoes. This may take a few days, so plan on having a few days off between the simulation and starting radiation therapy.

Radiation used to treat lymphoma is given in *fractionated doses.* That is, rather than receiving all the radiation at once, treatment is spread out over an extended period. Generally, radiation is given five times a week (you get the weekends off). Palliative therapy may be delivered for only a few weeks; curative therapy may extend over four to six weeks. Research has shown that radiation given in divided doses is less damaging to normal tissue, which has time to recover between treatment sessions, but is still deadly to the cancer.

In some cases, particularly if you're undergoing total body irradiation in preparation for a stem cell transplant, you may be given *hyperfractionated doses* of radiation. In this case, you will undergo more than one treatment a day, over a period of several days.

If your treatment plan involves delivering a smaller dose of radiation to an extended field and a larger dose to the tumor itself, the size of your shields will be progressively increased, so that the radiation field gradually becomes smaller and smaller. Less and less tissue will be exposed to radiation as the therapy becomes more focused on the sites most affected by the disease. Periodically, the radiation oncologist will take X-rays to track any changes in the size and shape of the malignant tissue, and these changes can be used to direct modifications in the size and shape of your radiation shields.

Undergoing radiation therapy

You'll be asked to change into a hospital gown before undergoing irradiation, so wear clothes you can change in and out of quickly. Getting irradiated takes only a few minutes. You'll be very precisely placed, either on a table or in a chair (depending on the sites to be irradiated), and you will need to remain very still while the radiation is being administered. Sometimes it is necessary to use plaster or plastic forms, put a cage over your head, or have you bite onto something to make sure you remain *absolutely* still during treatment. That's to ensure that the correct areas—and only the correct areas—are irradiated.

After a technician helps you get positioned and lines up a beam of light with your ink marks or tattoos, everyone else will leave the room for a few minutes while you get irradiated. You'll hear the machine go on but generally won't feel anything (people receiving total body irradiation sometimes feel some warmth and tingling of their skin). The machine may be moved around so that you are irradiated from different angles. This minimizes the amount of radiation absorbed by any normal tissue in "line of sight" of the tumor (fig. 4.2). In this case, different shields may be inserted between shots.

External beam radiation is essentially like getting a superdose of X-rays, so you don't need to worry about being made radioactive. You're not, and it's therefore impossible for you to irradiate other people.

Side effects

Like chemotherapy, radiation damages normal tissue as well as cancer cells; this tissue damage can have both short-term and long-term side effects. Side effects will depend on the site to which radiation was delivered, the total amount of radiation you receive, the form of radiation given, and whether radiation is given in combination with chemotherapy.

The most common side effect of radiation therapy is fatigue. This is partly because of the energy required to rebuild normal tissue that's been damaged and may also have to do with substances released by the dying malignant cells. Radiation-induced fatigue usually develops after a few weeks of treatment and may last some time. Some people feel better within a few weeks of ending treatment; others take months or even years to regain their energy. During this time, you may need to get more rest and take naps during the day. As with chemotherapy-related fatigue, getting regular, moderate exercise and eating a well-balanced diet may help.

You may become nauseated and lose your appetite. This is most common if large areas of your body are contained within the radiation port or if the field encompasses part of your gastrointestinal tract. The antiemetics used to control nausea with chemotherapy are also helpful in combating radiation-induced nausea. Small meals may be easier to cope with than large meals, and avoiding fried foods, or other foods that are high in fat, and eating bland food may help. Even if you don't feel much like eating, it's important to try. Maintaining adequate nutrition really seems to make a difference in your ability to cope with the treatment.

Radiation may also affect your skin. This can range from mild (faint pink or lightly tanned skin) to severe (like a very bad sunburn). Dry, itchy skin or a mild rash is fairly common. The intensity of your skin reaction will depend on the

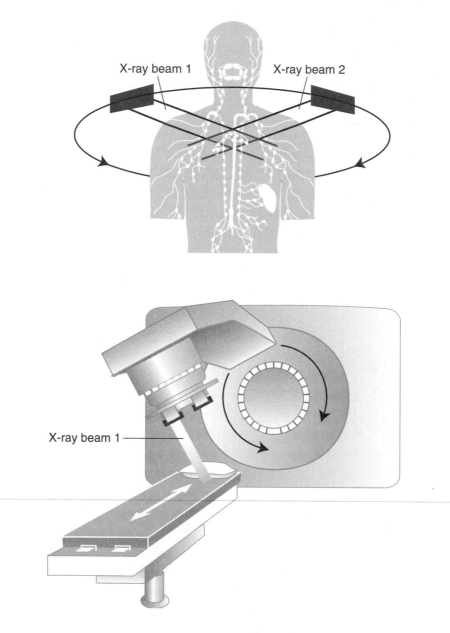

amount of radiation you receive per dose, the total cumulative dose, whether the beam is directed at superficial lymph nodes close to your skin or lymph nodes deep within your body, whether you've undergone chemotherapy, and your individual sensitivity. I was lucky in this respect; my radiation was delivered deep within my chest, and I escaped with faint reddening and itchy skin. A friend of mine, who had radiation to superficial lymph nodes close to the surface of her body, developed second- and third-degree burns that had to be treated to prevent infection.

Be careful to avoid irritating your skin any further while you're undergoing radiation therapy. Wear loose clothing and wash with lukewarm water and mild, unscented soaps (and don't scrub the area). Don't use *any* lotions or creams on the irradiated skin without first OKing them with your doctor: they can increase the radiation absorbed by your skin, leading to burns. Similarly, avoid deodorants if your underarms are in the radiation field. (Some facilities permit special deodorants that don't contain any metals during the first weeks of treatment.)

Once radiation therapy is complete, you can use nonperfumed lotions, like petroleum jelly, cold cream, or aloe vera gel, to help heal damaged skin. Your skin will remain sensitive for some time, and you'll need to protect it from excess exposure to the sun for *at least* a year. Even though I had only a very mild skin reaction, my skin is still sensitive to the sun years after having completed radiation therapy. I need to wear a hat or turtleneck if I expect to be in the sun for any extended amount of time. My friend who got second- and third-degree burns still has to cover up more than five years after completing radiation. Hats, scarves, or other clothing provide the best protection from the sun. Check with your doctor about using sun-blocking lotions with SPF greater than 30.

Figure 4.2. *Overlapping radiation fields.* Radiation may be delivered from different angles so that the dose of radiation delivered to the cancerous tissue (where the individual irradiated regions overlap) is greater than that delivered to any healthy tissue through which an individual beam must pass. For instance, as shown in the upper part of the figure, radiation beams delivered from "ten o'clock" and "two o'clock" meet in this person's mediastinal region. Thus, the mediastinal lymph nodes will receive more radiation than any other part of the body that the radiation beam passes through. The machine shown in the bottom is set to deliver X-ray beam 1 shown above as coming from "ten o'clock." After this beam has been delivered, the apparatus can be swung around to deliver X-ray beam 2 (shown as coming from "two o'clock" in the upper part of the figure).

Since bone marrow is very sensitive to radiation, bone marrow suppression, accompanied by reduced levels of white cells or platelets (or both), may occur. You'll need to get frequent blood tests to monitor this. Lymphocytes, particularly helper T cells, are extremely sensitive to radiation, and it may take a very long time (years) for your lymphocyte levels to return to normal.

Other effects of radiation depend on the location of the radiation fields. Radiation frequently causes hair loss, or *alopecia*. Radiation-induced alopecia is restricted to the areas directly in (or close to) the radiation field. The lost hair may not return.

Radiation to your head and neck may affect your salivary glands, leading to a seriously dry mouth. Your mouth and throat may feel sore, and you may find it difficult to swallow. You may experience changes in how things taste and become more susceptible to cavities. If you wear dentures, radiation-induced swelling of your gums may affect how dentures fit. Drinking cool fluids throughout the day may help with dry mouth. Some people find that carbonated beverages are particularly helpful. You'll probably want to put sauces or gravy on your food to moisten it. Your doctor can prescribe swish-and-swallow products to coat and numb your mouth and throat. If necessary, he or she can also prescribe artificial saliva or pilocarpine (brand name: Salagen), a drug that stimulates the salivary glands, to help make it easier to swallow.

It's important to observe good oral hygiene while undergoing radiation to your head and neck, and it's a good idea to see a dentist before you get started (to make sure you have no dental problems). Brush your teeth frequently, using a soft toothbrush. Salt and baking soda rinses may help (irrigating devices like a Water-Pik are also a good idea), but avoid commercial mouthwashes that contain alcohol, since alcohol will dry out the irritated tissues of your mouth even more. (Because of this drying effect, you should also avoid alcoholic drinks while you're undergoing radiation to the head, neck, or chest.) It's also a good idea to keep up with your dental visits after undergoing radiation to the head and neck. Radiation can weaken your jawbone, and it's better to have your dentist spot this *before* your teeth start to fall out.

Radiation to the chest can irritate the *esophagus*, the tube that carries food from your mouth to your stomach. This can make it feel like you have a lump in your throat. You may also develop a sore throat, unrelenting hiccups, a dry mouth, or a cough. Esophageal irritation following radiation to the chest can make it very difficult to eat. It can be painful to swallow food that presses on the inflamed tissues of your esophagus (it's like having an internal sunburn), and you may experience nausea and vomiting. You may also develop heartburn; medications that suppress acid production may help with this.

Again, your doctor can prescribe thick, numbing medications to help alleviate the pain and medications to help heal ulcerated tissues. You may find it easier to eat very soft, pureed food (in a pinch, you can always resort to baby food). If necessary, you can take liquid nutritional supplements.

Abdominal radiation can also irritate your gastrointestinal tract. In this case, you may experience severe intestinal cramps and diarrhea. Again, eating small amounts of soft, easily digested food, like rice and bananas, may help. In severe cases, you may need to go on a clear liquid diet (water, weak teas, clear juices, broth, sherbet, gelatin) to avoid triggering diarrhea. If you do get diarrhea, drink a lot of fluids so you don't become dehydrated.

Radiation to the gonads can cause temporary or permanent sterility in both men and women (and this isn't a good time to even *think* about getting pregnant). You may also experience bladder irritation. Drinking lots of fluids may help, and your doctor may be able to prescribe medication that will reduce the symptoms. Women may go through menopause after receiving radiation to the pelvis. People who need to undergo gonadal irradiation and are interested in maintaining the option of having children may wish to look at the discussion on preservation of sperm or fertilized ova in the "Reproduction and infertility" section of Chapter 3.

Some women who need to undergo radiation to the pelvis have avoided menopause, and preserved their fertility, by undergoing a surgical procedure called an *oophoropexy*. With an oophoropexy, the ovaries are moved closer to the uterus. This shields them from the radiation, and women have been able to become pregnant after undergoing this procedure.

Radiation is generally considered easier to tolerate than chemotherapy. Someone who had undergone a treatment regimen similar to mine told me that, compared with chemo, radiation was a walk around the park. Having breezed through R-CHOP, which is considered a fairly rough chemo regimen, I was anticipating an easy time with radiation.

I was to receive fractionated radiation five days a week for five weeks, so it was impossible to make a daily commute from home to the hospital for treatment. We rented a tiny furnished studio apartment in Boston, a mile or so from the hospital. While I couldn't bring the NordicTrack I'd so faithfully worked out on while undergoing chemo, I figured I'd get in my daily exercise walking to and from the hospital. I was looking forward to spending spring in Boston: visiting the Public Gardens, eating out, and enjoying life in the city.

As it turned out, my expectations couldn't have been further off base. A freak April Fool's Day blizzard took care of the stroll to and from the hospital for the first week or so of treatment, and after that I was too sick to care. And every day, something went wrong with the elegant, overpriced apartment we'd rented. The phone didn't work properly, and we couldn't turn off the hot water faucet in the bathroom. The bathroom turned into our own private sauna, and the paper began to peel from the walls.

Although slow to come on, showing up only after the second week of treatment, the anticipated "esophageal irritation" was severe. In addition to the worst sore throat I could possibly imagine, I developed some sort of spasm: it felt as though my esophagus were tied in a knot, and what food made it past my throat stayed there for an hour or so before returning whence it came, rather than passing docilely into my stomach. The numbing rinse of Maalox, lidocaine, and Benadryl that my radiation oncologist had given me helped with pain but had no effect on the spasms.

I had to laugh, thinking about the earnest instructions I'd received from the hospital dietitians to avoid eating anything hard or crunchy that might damage my throat. Trying to get a feel for what they meant by "hard," I had asked about eating bread. They had thought things over seriously and told me that bread was OK, but not bagels. Once the effects of radiation hit in full force, there was no way I could possibly have choked down a piece of bread or anything harder than oatmeal!

For about a week, I subsisted on very soft mushy foods, thick soups, and supplements like Ensure and Sustacal. But eventually the sore throat and difficulty in swallowing developed into intractable hiccups and uncontrollable nausea and vomiting. As I leaned out of bed to vomit into the bowl Paul had brought over for me, I heard a retching noise from the corner. The dog, feeling neglected, had decided that she wanted to get in on the action! We had to go to the emergency room in the middle of the night so I could get intravenous antiemetics and sedatives to knock me out. (Friends took care of the dog for the rest of the radiation experience.)

I spent four days in the hospital, receiving intravenous fluids, before I was able to continue with treatment. I continued taking the numbing rinses, as well as a medication that suppressed the production of stomach acid and one that pro-

TREATING LYMPHOMA

moted healing of the esophagus, and was able to complete radiation with no further horrific episodes. (Radiation *isn't* always this tough. Four years later, when I underwent radiation therapy for breast cancer, the experience was the expected walk in the park.)

While most of the immediate effects of radiation clear up within a few weeks of stopping therapy, a few may linger, and some may show up only after a delay. As I've indicated, fatigue, reduced levels of circulating lymphocytes, and sensitivity to the sun can all persist for some time after you complete treatment. Radiation-induced hair loss is generally permanent, as is radiation-induced infertility and some radiation-induced tissue damage. I developed a permanent susceptibility to severe heartburn and can no longer eat sweet or acidic food—so much for the morning glass of orange or grapefruit juice. As for the occasional glass of wine that I gave up when I was trying to become pregnant, and then during chemo, and then during radiation . . . well . . . I was never much of a drinker, anyway.

Wearing turtlenecks and avoiding orange juice is no big deal. However, some delayed complications of radiation therapy can be serious. Many of these potentially serious delayed side effects depend on the site to which you have received radiation.

People who've received radiation to their throat frequently become *hypothyroid.* Their thyroid gland produces less thyroid hormone, or *thyroxine,* than necessary. Hypothyroidism can lead to fatigue, weight gain, difficulty tolerating the cold, depression, thinning eyebrows, and dry hair and skin. I developed hypothyroidism about a year after completing radiation therapy; for some people it takes several years before this side effect of treatment shows up. Hypothyroidism can be detected with a blood test and is treated with synthetic thyroxine pills.

There's some evidence that taking thyroxine, which suppresses thyroid activity, *while* you're undergoing radiation therapy can reduce the risk of subsequently becoming hypothyroid and of developing thyroid cancer. This is worth discussing with your doctor if you need to undergo radiation to your neck.

Lhermitte syndrome, in which you develop a tingling or "electric" sensation in your legs and feet after bending your neck, sometimes shows up several months after you receive radiation to the mantle field. This condition, which results from temporary damage to the sheath covering the nerves in your spinal cord, usually clears up spontaneously in time. Other delayed complications of radiation therapy include cataracts if your eyes were exposed to the radiation field and damage to your heart or lungs. Both lung and heart damage may be acute (appearing at the time of treatment) or chronic (showing up after therapy is over). Heart and lung damage is more common when radiation has been given in combination with certain chemotherapy regimens, and careful shielding during delivery of the radiation can minimize both.

As with chemotherapy, the most serious potential long-term side effect of radiation therapy is development of a second malignancy. Radiation, however, is more commonly associated with solid tumors, while leukemias are the malignancies that most commonly appear after chemotherapy. These solid tumors almost always show up within the area of the radiation port.

Depending on the site where you were irradiated, you may be at increased risk for cancers of the head and neck, salivary glands, thyroid, lungs, bone, stomach, and breast; melanoma of the skin; and soft-tissue (tendons, ligaments, and muscle) sarcomas. Don't be overwhelmed by this list of possible cancers: you certainly won't get them all, and you *probably* won't get any. While the incidence of chemotherapy-induced leukemias peaks and then falls off with time, so that ten years or so after therapy is completed your risk of getting leukemia returns to normal, that doesn't happen with tumors induced by radiation. You remain at increased risk for these solid tumors for the rest of your life. Therefore, it's *very* important to be conscientious about post-treatment follow-up visits with your doctor.

While the risk of developing some radiation-induced tumors increases with age, radiation-induced breast cancer is more common following irradiation in girls and young women. The effects of radiation on lung cancer are synergistic with those of smoking. If you smoke and you receive thoracic irradiation, it's even more important to quit smoking, and to avoid smoke-filled rooms, than it is for the general population. Having smoked when I was younger and then quit years before I was diagnosed with lymphoma, I didn't think that this would be a problem. But I found all my latent cigarette-longing violently reactivated by undergoing radiation therapy. Somehow the knowledge that I *couldn't* smoke any more made me long to take it up again. I even dreamed about cigarettes for close to a year after undergoing radiation therapy.

Mycosis fungoides

Just as mycosis fungoides, a slowly growing lymphoma of the skin, has its own particular set of chemotherapy protocols, it also has its own particular set of radiation regimens. Mycosis fungoides is sometimes treated with electron beam therapy. Since the electron beam doesn't penetrate as deeply into the tissues of your body as X-rays or gamma rays do, larger doses can be applied to more extensive areas of your body. It's not uncommon to treat mycosis fungoides with total skin electron beam therapy.

Total skin electron beam therapy is generally given while you're standing. It's like trying to get an allover suntan—you need to figure out how to expose all of your skin to the treatment. You may need to move around to expose different areas of your body to the electron beam, or you may receive therapy while you're standing on a rotating platform. Areas of your body that aren't exposed to the radiation beam when you're standing—like the soles of your feet, the top of your head, or under your breasts (if you're a woman) will need to be treated separately. Total skin electron beam therapy may be delivered daily for as long as ten weeks.

Mycosis fungoides is sometimes treated with an unusual form of radiation therapy called *PUVA*, which stands for psoralens plus ultraviolet A (UVA). *Psoralens* are naturally occurring compounds that are found in various plants, including limes, lemons, and parsnips. Ultraviolet A is the longest wavelength, most deeply penetrating form of ultraviolet light. (Ultraviolet B, which has a shorter wavelength, plays a more prominent role in tanning and sunburn.) PUVA is frequently given in combination with *retinoids*, compounds closely related to vitamin A. It may also be given in combination with interferon-alpha.

The psoralens act as *photosensitizers*. That is to say, they sensitize your skin to the effects of ultraviolet radiation. They bind to DNA and, when acted on by UVA, act to cross-link it. This DNA cross-linking is similar to the action of alkylating agents. Strands of DNA attach to each other in abnormal ways and can't function properly. However, unlike alkylating agents, psoralens act predominantly on your skin, since UV light can't penetrate throughout your body. PUVA therapy is used to treat benign skin conditions, such as psoriasis and vitiligo (a loss of skin pigmentation), as well as mycosis fungoides. In addition to cross-linking DNA, PUVA may induce the production of cytokines that contribute to the therapeutic response.

Psoralens can be applied topically or taken as pills. When they are taken orally, they may cause nausea. Nausea is decreased if the pills are taken with a meal. You can also take antiemetics. You'll need to wear goggles when you're undergoing PUVA to protect your eyes from the ultraviolet radiation. Since you've received a photosensitizing drug, it's important to avoid exposure to the sun. Cover up when you're not undergoing treatment. Long-term treatment with PUVA may increase the likelihood of certain forms of skin cancer as well as cataracts.

A variation of PUVA therapy is sometimes used to treat mycosis fungoides that has spread to the blood. This treatment is called *extracorporeal photopheresis.* In extracorporeal photopheresis, blood is withdrawn from your body. Psoralens are added to the blood, which is exposed to UVA and then returned to your body. Typically, six photopheresis cycles, in which your blood is withdrawn and irradiated, are performed in a day. The procedure is continued for two days, and the two-day treatment is repeated once a month.

Combined modality treatment

In the early days of chemotherapy, people often experienced dramatic responses to therapy with a single drug, only to relapse when a small population of resistant cells continued to grow and multiply. Combination chemotherapy addresses this problem by simultaneously hitting the cancer with several drugs, each of which interferes with a different aspect of cellular function.

The idea is that, while individual cells may be resistant to any one drug, or even any *class* of drugs, it's less likely that the same cell would be resistant to them all. This tends to be true: in the curable lymphomas, combination chemotherapy is much more successful than single-agent chemotherapy. Unfortunately, though, it's not always the case. Some cancer cells can resist different classes of antineoplastic drugs. They may develop mechanisms, for instance, that allow them to get rid of all unwanted chemicals, dumping them back out into the extracellular fluid before they can do any harm.

Combined modality treatment, combining chemotherapy and radiation, starts with the same basic idea of hitting the cancer cells in different ways at the same time but takes things a step further. Ionizing radiation kills cancer cells by creating free radicals, highly reactive substances that damage DNA and other cellular constituents. While this is similar to the mechanism by which many antineoplastic drugs work, there is a fundamental difference between using radiation and using drugs. Radiation is a completely different *modality* of treatment.

The fact that radiation and chemotherapy represented two distinct modalities led to the idea that combining radiation with chemotherapy might be more effective at destroying malignant cells than either modality alone. And, indeed, combined modality therapy does a better job of destroying cancer cells than either chemotherapy or radiation used alone. However, the two modalities used together are frequently more toxic to *healthy* tissue as well as to cancer. Therefore, in deciding whether to use a combined modality approach, your physician must carefully weigh the advantages (improved chance of curing the cancer) against the disadvantages (increased likelihood of a serious side effect somewhere down the line).

At present, there's controversy about exactly when combined modality therapy should be used. In this book, I report general trends concerning the situations in which doctors are more or less likely to use combined modality treatment. These general trends may or may not be applicable to your situation. Remember, only a physician who knows your case can make the most appropriate treatment decisions.

Combined modality therapy is most frequently used to treat localized disease or to treat generalized disease in which there is a specific bulky component. With Hodgkin lymphoma, combined modality treatment is frequently used to treat people with massive mediastinal tumors. That's because, in this particular presentation, neither radiation nor chemotherapy alone provides sufficient likelihood of a cure.

In other localized presentations of Hodgkin lymphoma, the risk of relapse following initial treatment with either radiation *or* chemotherapy is smaller. While combined modality therapy may reduce the risk of relapse even further, it's not clear that, under these circumstances, the benefits of combined modality treatment outweigh the risks. In this case, people who *do* relapse can be treated with the alternate modality (if it's appropriate), and people who *don't* relapse will be spared the additional toxicities of combined treatment. At this point, the balance seems to be tilted against heavy-duty combined modality treatment—with full-length courses of chemotherapy—for Hodgkin lymphoma, although combined modality treatment in which a reduced number of cycles of chemotherapy are given in combination with radiation therapy is sometimes used.

With NHL, the decision to use combined modality treatment is influenced by your age and the subtype of disease. For children and young adults (under twenty-one) with localized aggressive disease (lymphoblastic, small noncleaved cell, diffuse large cell), chemotherapy alone appears to be as effective as combined modality treatment.

Two recent large-scale studies have investigated the efficacy of combined modality therapy compared with chemotherapy alone in adults. One study of adults with *localized* aggressive disease (*mostly* diffuse large cell, but also follicular large cell, diffuse small cleaved cell, diffuse mixed small and large cell, and diffuse small cleaved cell) found that three cycles of CHOP plus involved field radiation was preferable to eight cycles of CHOP alone. Fewer people relapsed with combined modality treatment during the first seven years after treatment, and overall survival (with and without relapse) through the first nine years was better in the combined modality group as well. However, more late relapses occurred years after therapy was completed in the group of people treated with combined modality therapy, suggesting that for some individuals, a short course of chemotherapy combined with radiation is not sufficient to cure the disease.

Similarly, a large-scale study of people with bulky Stage I or Stage II disease suggested that eight cycles of CHOP plus irradiation to previous sites of disease was preferable to eight cycles of CHOP alone when people were evaluated within six years of treatment. However, by ten years after treatment, there was no difference in overall survival between people treated with combined modality therapy and people treated with CHOP alone. Since some of the more serious complications associated with radiation therapy—such as secondary cancers—may show up only after many years, it will be important to see what happens as the participants live longer and longer past the time they underwent treatment. At present, it seems likely that the best treatment for a given individual will vary depending on the specific details of his or her illness.

At this point it isn't clear whether it's desirable to use combined modality treatment for people with localized indolent disease or to treat this relatively rare presentation of low-grade disease with radiation therapy alone.

Combined modality therapy is frequently used to treat people with CNS lymphoma—both people with primary CNS lymphoma (which arises in the CNS and is generally confined there) and people whose disease has arisen outside the CNS and spread there. Although the optimal treatment for CNS lymphoma is not yet clear, treatment often includes chemotherapy regimens incorporating high-dose methotrexate (which can penetrate the blood-brain barrier) and radiation to the whole brain. Intrathecal chemotherapy may be given as well. Whole brain irradiation may also be given as *prophylactic* (preventative) therapy as a component of the treatment of people who are considered at risk of their disease spreading to the CNS. People with highly aggressive lymphoma such as Burkitt lymphoma, Burkitt-like lymphoma, or lymphoblastic lymphoma (or diffuse large cell lymphoma in the testes or sinuses) may receive such prophylactic treatment.

Surgery

Because most forms of lymphoma spread throughout your body rather than remaining localized, surgery is only rarely used as a form of treatment. That's something I found surprising. Since the odds of developing a cell that's resistant to therapy increase with the total number of malignant cells, I thought that people like me who are diagnosed with a single, very large tumor would benefit by having the tumor removed surgically prior to undergoing chemotherapy. Get rid of most of the cells, and you'd reduce the risk that one would be resistant to treatment. This is the approach taken to treat many other forms of cancer.

Having undergone several successful surgeries to remove fibroids and endometriosis, I had a pronounced bias in favor of surgical approaches to treatment. I wanted the damn thing cut out of me, and out of me *now*, rather then going through the long and uncertain processes of chemotherapy and radiation. However, for most people with aggressive disease, surgery really doesn't seem to be beneficial, and my oncologist convinced me that, for me, chemo and radiation were the way to go.

Surgery is mostly used to treat people with a form of low-grade lymphoma called a MALT lymphoma (see Chapter 10) when it is found localized to an area like the stomach or thyroid. MALT lymphomas tend to remain localized for long periods of time; therefore, there's a good chance that surgery will remove all the cancer and either cure the disease or permit less aggressive adjunctive treatment. Surgery is also used to treat intestinal lymphomas, some low-grade lymphomas that primarily involve the spleen, and some Burkitt lymphomas that involve the abdomen in children. Intestinal lymphomas and abdominal Burkitt's in children require chemotherapy in addition to the surgery. Localized MALT lymphomas removed surgically may or may not require adjunctive chemotherapy or radiation.

SUGGESTIONS FOR FURTHER READING

Diehl V. (2004). "Chemotherapy or combined modality treatment: The optimal treatment for Hodgkin's disease." *Journal of Clinical Oncology* 22:15–18.

Diehl V, Stein H, Hummel M, Zollinger R, Connors JM. (2003). "Hodgkin's lymphoma: Biology and treatment strategies for primary, refractory, and relapsed disease." *Hematology* 2003:225–247.

Fisher RI, Miller TP, O'Connor OA. (2004). "Diffuse aggressive lymphoma." *Hematology* 2004:221–236.

Golomb HM. (1998). "Management of early-stage Hodgkin's disease: A continuing evolution." *Seminars in Oncology* 25:476–482.

Horning SJ et al. (2002). "Final report of E1484: CHOP v CHOP + radiotherapy for limited stage diffuse aggressive lymphoma." *Proceedings of the 43rd Annual Meeting of the American Society of Hematology.*

Lister A, Abrey LE, Sandlund JT. (2002). "Central nervous system lymphoma." *Hematology* 2002:283–296.

Loeffler M et al. (1998). "Meta-analysis of chemotherapy versus combined modality treatment trials in Hodgkin's disease." *Journal of Clinical Oncology* 16:818–829.

Meyer RM, Ambinder RF, Stroobants S. (2004). "Hodgkin's lymphoma: Evolving concepts with implications for practice." *Hematology* 2004:184–202.

Miller TP, Dahlberg S, Cassady JR, Adelstein DJ. (1998). "Chemotherapy alone compared with chemotherapy plus radiotherapy for localized intermediate- and high-grade non-Hodgkin's lymphoma." *New England Journal of Medicine* 339:21–26. *Follow-up:* Miller TP et al. (2001). "CHOP alone compared to CHOP plus radiotherapy for early stage aggressive non-Hodgkin's lymphomas: Update of the SWOG randomized trial." *Blood* 98:724a.

Specht L, Gray RG, Clarke MJ, Peto R. (1998). "Influence of more extensive radiotherapy and adjuvant chemotherapy on long-term outcome of early-stage Hodgkin's disease: A meta-analysis of 23 randomized trials involving 3,888 patients." *Journal of Clinical Oncology* 16:830–843.

CHAPTER 5

Monoclonal Antibodies and
Other Magic Bullet Therapies

Wе've come a long way in lymphoma treatment over the past forty years. The majority of people with Hodgkin lymphoma can now be cured, and they will move on from their brush with death to have normal, healthy lives. Many people with aggressive NHL and some with indolent NHL can now be cured as well.

But we still have a long way to go. A substantial minority of people with Hodgkin lymphoma will *not* be cured; and a substantial minority of those who *are* cured will experience serious long-term side effects from the therapy. Similarly, about half of those diagnosed with aggressive NHL will be cured, but half *won't*. Many of us will experience dangerous, debilitating, or distressing long-term side effects from the therapy that saved our lives. And the majority of people with low-grade lymphoma are still incurable.

Until *all* lymphomas can be reliably cured, with little danger of long-term toxicity from the treatment, we cannot afford to be complacent. Fortunately, cancer research continues to push forward the range of available therapies, and right now we're poised on the brink of some dramatic breakthroughs. Lymphoma therapy is already distinctly different from when I was diagnosed. We can hope that advances in the treatment of NHL over the next few years will be as dramatic as the advances in treating Hodgkin lymphoma some thirty years ago. We can also hope that therapies for those forms of lymphoma that are now curable continue to evolve in the direction of becoming less and less dangerous and unpleasant.

This chapter describes some of the newer approaches to treating lymphoma. While new antineoplastic drugs are continually being developed, and though some of them may well be dynamite against lymphoma, the treatments I discuss in this chapter are based on new *types* of anticancer therapy. These are *directed therapies* based on advances in our understanding of cancer or of the means our bodies use to fight disease. They differ from the older forms of cancer therapies (chemotherapy and radiation) in their selectivity against cancer cells. Many of these newer therapies promise to act as the long-sought "magic bullets" that shoot down cancer cells but leave the rest of the body untouched.

These directed therapies include *immunological therapies* (or *immunotherapies*), which involve the immune system; *biological therapies*, defined here as therapies using living cells to create an anticancer response; and therapies that depend on a detailed understanding of biological mechanisms underlying cancer. I discuss some directed therapies that are now in common use against lymphoma, such as monoclonal antibodies, as well as some that are still experimental.

Over the past twenty years, our understanding of *immunology*, the branch of biology concerned with the function of the immune system, has really exploded. Several of the new approaches to cancer therapy in general (and lymphoma in particular) make use of this knowledge. And it somehow seems appropriate that the power of the immune system itself should be harnessed to fight these immunological cancers.

Immunotherapies
Monoclonal antibodies

As discussed in more depth in Chapter 9, B cells and plasma cells, which are the completely differentiated form of the B cell, are considered part of the *humoral immune system.* Their immunological actions are mediated by *antibodies*, proteins secreted into the blood that recognize and bind to *antigens.* Antigens are defined as substances that can stimulate the production of antibodies. In general, they are substances that the immune system recognizes as foreign (and therefore potentially dangerous). Antibody/antigen interactions are very specific: an antibody that recognizes a particular antigen (say, a protein on a poliovirus) won't recognize any other.

When a secreted antibody recognizes and binds to its antigen, it sets a series of events into play. These are designed to neutralize and get rid of the antigen.

When antigens are part of a foreign cell, antibodies can flag that cell as a target for other components of the immune system to destroy. There are various ways in which the immune system can act against cells that have been targeted by an antibody.

In some cases, the bound antibodies trigger a direct attack by other cells in the immune system. Macrophages, neutrophils, and natural killer cells can all recognize bound antibodies. When an antibody signals these cells that a given cell is dangerous, they come over and deliver the "kiss of death," discharging toxic substances at the antibody-coated cell. These toxic substances include highly reactive chemicals, like peroxide, and proteins that can punch holes in the cell membrane or enter the cell and trigger *apoptosis*—a process in which cells essentially commit suicide. In any case, the cell under siege is destroyed.

Bound antibodies can also trigger *complement*, a collection of proteins found in your blood that helps eliminate pathogens. The activated complement proteins can either destroy the targeted cell directly or help recruit monocytes, macrophages, and neutrophils into the fight, thus *complementing* the recruiting efforts of the antibody itself.

Many years ago, researchers came up with the idea of using antibodies to target *tumor* cells for destruction. This is a terrific idea. In contrast to conventional chemotherapy and radiation, which are more or less active against *all* rapidly dividing cells, a targeted antibody can be highly specific. Ideally, you could target the antibody to some antigen that was found *only* on the tumor cells. In that case, the antibody would ignore all your healthy tissue and zero in on the tumor cells, marking them for destruction by your own immune system. Because of this specificity, this sort of therapy would have far fewer side effects than conventional forms of cancer therapy. However, developing antibody-based therapy has been far more difficult in practice than it sounds in theory.

In order for antibody-based cancer therapy to work, three basic conditions must be fulfilled. First, you need to have an antibody that specifically recognizes tumor cells and ignores healthy cells. Second, you need an antibody that can effectively recruit immune cells—particularly natural killer cells—and/or activate complement to help destroy the tumor cells that it flags. Finally, you need to be able to produce your specific and effective antibody in quantities that are sufficient to destroy all of someone's lymphoma cells. Ideally, you'd want a single antibody that would work for *everybody* with lymphoma (or at least everyone with a certain type of the disease), since it could be very time consuming, and prohibitively expensive, to custom-build a different antibody for each individual.

How could someone create an antibody that recognized lymphoma cells but not the other cells in the body? As discussed in Chapter 9, each new B cell that develops in bone marrow carries immunoglobulin. This immunoglobulin is unique to each developing B cell and is specialized to recognize a single antigen. Most B cell lymphomas continue to manufacture immunoglobulin. And since each cell in the tumor is descended from the same initial malignant B cell, all the cancer cells will carry the same identical immunoglobulin. So one approach to developing a tumor-specific antibody is to make an antibody that recognizes the *specific* region of the *tumor cells'* immunoglobulin that makes that immunoglobulin unique. Similarly, for T cell lymphomas, antibodies could be generated against the unique portion of their T cell receptors that allows *them* to specifically recognize antigens.

Such an approach would be incredibly selective and is therefore tremendously appealing. With our present technologies, however, it is impractical to synthesize specific antibodies against each lymphomaniac's own unique tumor immunoglobulin (unless you happen to be a Gates or a Rockefeller). Moreover, in clinical trials, when people with lymphoma were treated with antibodies directed against their own tumor immunoglobulin, their tumors escaped destruction by developing slightly different versions of immunoglobulin that were no longer recognized by the antibody.

The next best approach is to use antibodies that recognize only the general *type* of cells that your tumor arose from. Different classes of cells can be characterized according to their *immunophenotype*, the specific repertoire of proteins found on their surfaces. Like most cancer cells, lymphoma cells resemble the normal cells that gave rise to them. Therefore, it's not too surprising that most lymphomas display certain characteristic proteins that are found on normal lymphocytes as well.

For instance, most B cell lymphomas make the proteins CD19, CD20, and CD22. (You can remember them as the "young adult" cell markers.) These three proteins are found on mature B lymphocytes but not on early stem cells or fully mature plasma cells. Similarly, many T cell lymphomas carry the proteins CD2, CD3, CD5, and CD7 (the "childhood" markers), which are characteristic of normal T lymphocytes. The Reed-Sternberg cells found in Hodgkin lymphoma carry CD25 and CD30, which are typically found on lymphocytes that have been activated to proliferate. While these proteins aren't quite as specific as an antibody directed against tumor immunoglobulin, they *are* specific for lymphocytes. Thus antibodies directed against lymphocyte marker proteins would act against both your normal and malignant B cells or T cells (depending on whether you were given an anti–B cell antibody or an anti–T cell antibody), but not against the other cells in your body.

Since most lymphomas carry these marker proteins, one wouldn't need to custom-develop a new antibody for each individual but could mass-produce an antibody in quantities sufficient for everybody. Therefore, researchers have tried treating lymphoma with antibodies directed against B cell–specific marker proteins, T cell–specific marker proteins, and proteins found on both B and T lymphocytes.

These antibodies are generated by injecting purified target proteins into mice. Since the mouse's immune system will recognize human lymphocyte proteins as foreign, the mouse's plasma cells will oblige by making antibodies against the human proteins. Individual mouse plasma cells, descended from different mouse B cells, will produce slightly different antibodies that recognize and bind antigen more or less effectively. In order to obtain unlimited supplies of a good antibody (one that recognizes the target protein very specifically and binds to it very tightly), researchers have devised a method for churning out indefinite quantities of a given antibody.

After the mouse is immunized against the human lymphocyte protein (let's say we're interested in the B cell antigen CD20), its antibody-producing plasma cells are harvested. Some of these plasma cells will manufacture antibody directed against human CD20. Supplies of these antibodies would ordinarily be limited by the lifetime of the isolated mouse plasma cells. Around thirty years ago, Georges Köhler and Cesar Milstein developed a technique for growing specific strains of antibody-producing cells indefinitely. They *fused* the mouse plasma cells with human myeloma cells that didn't produce antibody themselves but retained the capacity to do so. The resulting hybrid cells can be grown indefinitely because the myeloma cells are immortal.

This means that a mouse plasma cell that produces a particularly effective antibody can be *immortalized* so that its descendants can be grown forever. These immortal cells will continue to produce the effective strain of mouse anti-CD20 antibody. This takes care of antibody supply and specificity. Since the whole line of immortal antibody-producing cells is descended from a single mouse plasma cell fused with a single human myeloma cell, it is called a *clonal* cell line. The strains of identical antibodies produced by the clonal cell line are called *mono-*

clonal antibodies. Köhler and Milstein were awarded a Nobel Prize for developing this technique of producing monoclonal antibodies, which are used in immunophenotyping cells during diagnosis as well as in cancer therapy.

Surprisingly, clinical trials using monoclonal antibody therapy to treat cancer have historically met with relatively little success. Recently, researchers realized that a major flaw in the approach was that *mouse* antibodies were unable to interact effectively with the *human* immune system. They bound to their target cells all right, but they didn't do a very good job of stimulating an effective immune response.

Researchers therefore devised ways to *humanize* the mouse antibodies. That is to say, the portions of the mouse immunoglobulin involved in recruiting complement and macrophages and natural killer cells into the fight are replaced with the corresponding regions from human immunoglobulins. Only the mouse variable portions that recognize and bind to the antigen are retained. Antibodies that mix mouse and human immunoglobulin are sometimes called *chimeric* antibodies, after the mythological Chimera, which was a mixture of goat, lion, and serpent.

Humanized monoclonal antibodies promise to revolutionize cancer therapy, and they are *already* revolutionizing the fight against lymphoma. The first monoclonal antibody approved by the Food and Drug Administration (FDA; in 1997) for treating cancer (indolent B cell lymphoma) was a humanized monoclonal antibody directed against the B cell protein CD20. Called Rituxan or rituximab, it recognizes and binds to most B cell lymphoma cells, as well as normal B lymphocytes, but not early B cell precursors or mature plasma cells. It's able to recruit both complement and natural killer cells into the fight against lymphoma and thereby stimulate an effective immune response. Additionally, rituximab appears to inhibit lymphoma cell growth and proliferation, and promote a cell suicide process, simply by binding to CD20, which plays a role in the process of B cell growth and activation.

About half of the people with indolent B cell lymphomas who are treated with rituximab respond with at least a partial remission. Typically, these partial remissions involve about a 75 percent shrinkage of the tumor mass. Since the side effects of rituximab are very mild compared with those of conventional chemotherapy or radiation, it can be given to people who would ordinarily be considered too fragile to withstand treatment, such as the very elderly, or people who have relapsed soon after a bone marrow transplant.

Rituximab can also be given as maintenance therapy, or repeatedly, in case of a relapse. It usually remains effective for multiple cycles of retreatment—sometimes even more effective the second time around—although doctors are now beginning to see people who relapse with mutated lymphoma cells that no longer express CD20 and are therefore no longer a target for rituximab.

In studies using antibodies directed against marker proteins found on animal tumors, scientists have found that relapses resulting from this sort of *escape mutation* (by which the tumor cell escapes detection by the antibody) are very common. Treating animal tumors with two different antibodies directed at two different cell markers is far more effective than treating with one alone, since it is much less likely that a cancer cell will undergo simultaneous mutations leading to the deletion of *both* target proteins. It therefore seems possible that combining rituximab with a similar antibody directed against another B cell marker protein, such as CD19 or CD22, could be more effective in eradicating human tumors than using rituximab alone. Indeed, recent studies have been initiated investigating the effects of combining rituximab with epratuzumab, an antibody directed against CD22, or galiximab, an antibody directed against CD80.

About half of the people who are treated with rituximab experience side effects. Most commonly, side effects include flu-like symptoms such as fever, aches, and shaking chills. For most people, this reaction is mild and shows up only during the first treatment. Giving rituximab with very slow rates of infusion can minimize these flu-like symptoms, so it can take five or six hours to get your first dose.

Since rituximab destroys healthy B lymphocytes as well as malignant ones, you might expect that people undergoing rituximab therapy would be very susceptible to infection. However, this doesn't seem to be the case. Another humanized antibody, CAMPATH1H (also known as alemtuzumab), which is directed against an antigen found on both T cells *and* B cells, is active against some lymphocytic leukemias and against some T cell lymphomas, including mycosis fungoides. However, unlike rituximab, clinical trials suggest that CAMPATH1H can significantly increase susceptibility to infection, so that people undergoing therapy with CAMPATH1H need to take antibiotics and antiviral agents while they are undergoing therapy.

People with large tumor masses sometimes experience *tumor lysis syndrome* in response to therapy with rituximab. As noted in Chapter 2, tumor lysis syndrome, which can also occur following chemotherapy in someone with a very large, rapidly growing tumor, is the result of too many tumor cells dying at once and spilling metabolic products like uric acid into the bloodstream. It produces symptoms like gout and can be avoided by taking medications like allopurinol that suppress the production of uric acid.

Rituximab is even more effective when given in combination with chemotherapy than it is alone. The first clinical trial combining rituximab with CHOP for people with indolent B cell NHL showed a *100 percent response rate* for people who received the combined treatment. While many of those people eventually relapsed, 60 percent remained in remission an average of five years after completing therapy. At last report sixteen of thirty-eight patients from this trial remain in remission six to nine years after receiving this therapy! Although it is too early to be certain, it is possible that some people may actually have been cured of their disease. Combining rituximab therapy with chemical messengers that promote the expression of CD20 on lymphocytes (see "Cytokines," below) promises to enhance effectiveness as well.

Rituximab alone is not very effective against aggressive forms of lymphoma. However, preliminary studies suggest that it has a chemosensitizing effect: it helps chemotherapy be more effective against aggressive disease. Clinical trials have investigated the effectiveness of rituximab plus CHOP against newly diagnosed aggressive lymphoma and of rituximab plus different salvage therapies against relapsed disease or against lymphoma that does not respond well to chemotherapy in the first place. The results have been very encouraging, and combination antibody-chemo regimens are rapidly becoming the standard approach to therapy for many aggressive B cell lymphomas.

I participated in the first clinical trial to test the efficacy of rituximab plus CHOP (R-CHOP) against aggressive B cell lymphomas. This trial took place prior to the FDA approval of rituximab to treat indolent lymphoma, and I was lucky enough to have stumbled into it. Not long ago, a woman who was interested in cancer clinical trials asked me if my background as a biologist had involved the use of monoclonal antibodies and if this had influenced me during my research of possible therapeutic approaches to lymphoma.

I had to laugh at the idea of my calmly sitting down to research the best approach to the treatment of my lymphoma and deciding to go with monoclonal antibodies because I'd used them in my own research. Nothing could have been further from the reality of my diagnosis and decision to participate in the antibody trial.

By the time I was diagnosed, I was in pretty bad shape. Shortly after my diagnosis, in a frantic search for information, I discovered a Web site that gave truly horrible survival statistics for lymphoma. As far as I could tell, I had just about run out of luck.

I spent the next few weeks in a state of numb horror, going through the various tests and procedures that were required before I could start treatment. It was clear that my oncologist was worried about lost time and thought we had no more time to lose. She scheduled my biopsy, and the preliminary tests, as soon as possible. The only time I have ever seen her stern was when I asked if I could delay therapy for a few weeks to try to harvest some ova before beginning the chemotherapy that would destroy them and leave me unable to bear children.

"You've got to get your priorities straight here," she said; "we have *one chance* to save your life."

It was clear she didn't think it was very much of a chance, but she was determined to help me put up a good fight. She started me on allopurinol, to avoid tumor lysis syndrome when I started chemotherapy, and sent me home for a week. She told me to eat as much as I could to try to put on some weight. She mentioned that there was an ongoing clinical trial involving monoclonal antibodies. She said she didn't know all that much about it, but she gave me the protocol to read over, just in case it looked like the right therapy for me.

It was a rough week. I had an unusual response to allopurinol, becoming violently ill, and spent the week lying down and throwing up. I couldn't eat anything, and I grew weaker and weaker as the week wore on. I lost even more weight. Death seemed to be looming very close. I found myself breaking down and crying a lot.

I cried seeing a documentary about Janis Joplin, remembering growing up carefree in the sixties. Janis had died young, and most likely I would, too. I cried seeing a documentary about a space probe that had been launched to discover if there was water on one of the moons of Jupiter. I wouldn't be alive to find out.

I read the antibody protocol and was not impressed by the efficacy of the antibody as a solo agent against aggressive disease. The antibody seemed highly effective against indolent disease, but I didn't have indolent disease. It occurred to me that I wouldn't make it to the millennium. For some reason, it seemed particularly dreadful that I wouldn't make it to that milestone. I thought about the research I would never do, after all those years of training, living on a graduate student stipend below the national poverty line. I thought about Paul, who had uprooted his life to be with me, left a widower less than two years after getting married. I pictured my parents grieving as they buried their youngest child. Somehow, that seemed the saddest part of all.

The day I was to start chemotherapy was gray and wintry and stormy. I was expecting to start a form of chemotherapy called CHOP. Even the acronym sounded ominous, as though I would be CHOPped up by the treatment. I knew the names of the four drugs I was to take and that one of them sounded like "cell poison" and another could cause heart damage, but that was about it.

Paul drove us to the hospital in Boston. I had lost another ten pounds over the past week, from the reaction to allopurinol, and was even weaker than before. I held a kidney-shaped pink plastic basin in my lap as I heaved up the chocolate Ensure Paul had forced into me for breakfast. Brownish, slightly used Ensure sloshed onto my jeans and the car upholstery whenever we took a curve too fast, but I was too weak and miserable to really care.

During the whole three-hour drive to Boston, all I could think about was a poem called "The Erl King." This poem, set to ominous music, describes a father desperately riding on horseback through the night during a violent storm with his sick child. The child, feverish and delirious, insists that the Erl King, who represents death, is pursuing them. The father tries to be reassuring; it's only the wind—not the Erl King. But the child, hysterical, insists that the Erl King is following and is trying to entice the child to join him. The poem ends with the father arriving at his destination. But it's too late; the child is dead in his arms.

All through that cold, gray ride, Paul tried to be cheerful and reassuring. But all I could hear were the ominous opening chords: "Ba-da-da-da-da-da-*da*-bom-bom" of the Erl King. All I could do was hope that we were driving fast enough to elude him.

We arrived at the hospital. Too weak to sit up, I lay down on the examining table. Ba-da-da-da-da-da-*da*-bom-bom. My oncologist came into the room. She leaned over me. Her voice seemed to be coming from very far away.

"I've learned some more about that antibody trial," she said. "I think it looks promising. I think it might be worth trying. But you'll need to read and sign a consent form. Have you looked over the protocol?"

I had read the protocol. I wasn't terribly impressed with the data on the efficacy of the antibodies as solo therapy against aggressive disease. But I thought they were unlikely to do me any harm, and I didn't think I had much chance with conventional therapy alone. I had a massive tumor and looked like a stick and couldn't even tie my shoes without collapsing in exhaustion. I had gone a long way down a bad road, and the odds were stacked against me. Why not do my best to tilt the odds in my favor? I thought about growing up in the sixties and about Janis singing "Freedom's just another word for nothin' left to lose."

I didn't have much left to lose, and I was free to do whatever I wanted. In some ways, freer than I'd ever been before. What the hell, I thought. I was a scientist;

I might as well do my bit to add to the sum of human knowledge about lymphoma therapy.

"OK," I said, "let's do it."

"Are you sure you understand?" she said. "We think the antibodies could help, but they're experimental. We don't really know what they'll do; they might even harm you."

"I understand," I said; "let's do it." I signed the consent form lying flat on my back, too weak to sit up. A little while later, I went upstairs to receive my first infusion of rituximab.

Because of the concern about a possible allergic reaction, a nurse set up an IV line to drip the antibodies very slowly into a vein in my arm. A nurse checked my temperature and blood pressure every fifteen minutes for the first hour and then every half hour. That first infusion seemed to take forever. I wasn't used to IV lines yet, and I was afraid to move my arm. The hospital personnel kept me an additional hour to make sure that my blood pressure was OK, and then Paul and I joined my parents, who had driven up from New York. The four of us spent the next day in a hotel room. The following day (two days after the rituximab) I would receive my first infusion of CHOP, and then the whole sequence would be repeated (with a slightly faster antibody drip rate) in three weeks' time.

I experienced no adverse side effects from the rituximab—no difficulty breathing, no fever, chills, nausea, aches, or low blood pressure. In fact, I noticed only two side effects following antibody administration. The first was that breathing became easier the day after I received the antibodies. The second, which occurred only during the first three cycles, was that my urine became very cloudy and foul smelling for the two days after antibody administration. I suspect this had to do with the excretion of breakdown products of dead tumor cells.

After I went into remission, it occurred to me that rituximab might have wiped out my *memory* B cells and destroyed my humoral immunity. Since memory B cells, like other mature B cells, carry CD20, this seemed like a real possibility. In that case, I could be susceptible to diseases to which I was supposed to be immune. This would include both diseases I'd weathered as a child, like measles, and diseases I'd been vaccinated against, like smallpox, diphtheria, and polio. My doctor checked to see if I had antibodies against these viruses. We discovered that I had normal levels of antibodies, so somehow or other my memory B cells survived.

Rituximab is designed to recruit your own immune system into the fight against lymphoma. And other humanized antibodies like it are now available or in the drug development pipeline. However, antibodies can also be used independently of your immune system, as guided missiles that carry toxic substances to the tumor. In this situation, in which antibodies are simply the guidance system used to deliver some explosive substance to the tumor cell's doorstep, it isn't necessary to use humanized antibodies, since ordinary mouse antibodies do a great job of recognizing antigens on human lymphocytes. Right now, monoclonal antibodies against CD20 tagged with either radioactive iodine (Bexxar, tositumomab) or radioactive yttrium (Zevalin, ibritumomab tiuxetan) are being used against lymphoma.

Radioactively tagged antibodies such as Bexxar and Zevalin allow radiation to be delivered precisely to the right location. Since X-rays don't need to pass through normal tissue between the radiation source and your lymphoma, you can use antibodies to deliver higher doses of radiation to the tumor itself.

Moreover, since antibodies are microscopic, they can circulate through your bloodstream to seek out and destroy even small clusters of cancer cells that are undetectable by conventional imaging techniques (and thus wouldn't be targeted with conventional means of radiation therapy).

The radiation emitted from the radioactively tagged antibodies travels for several cell lengths within your body. In some situations, this provides an advantage to using radiolabeled antibodies rather than untagged antibodies. In a tumor in which some cells bear the marker protein and some don't, radiation scatter can kill unmarked cells that would escape the surveillance of the "naked" antibodies.

On the other hand, radiation scatter limits the use of radioactively tagged antibodies in other situations. If your bone marrow is heavily infiltrated with lymphoma cells, it could be dangerous to use radioactively tagged antibodies, since the radiation could destroy healthy stem cells along with the lymphoma.

Since the thyroid gland uses iodine to produce thyroid hormone, it accumulates iodine from the blood. The thyroid is very sensitive to radiation and is unable to distinguish radioactive iodine from ordinary nonradioactive iodine. Consequently, thyroid damage is a possible side effect of treatment with monoclonal antibodies labeled with radioactive iodine. While the thyroid can't take up radioactive iodine that's attached to the antibodies, it's possible that a little radioactive iodine could become detached from the antibodies. If that happens, the free radioiodine becomes fair game for your unsuspecting thyroid.

People taking radioiodine-labeled antibodies are therefore given nonradioactive iodine as a pretreatment in the hope that the thyroid will satisfy all its iodine needs before any radioactive iodine comes along. In spite of this, some people absorb some radioactive iodine into their thyroid. If your thyroid is damaged by radioiodine, you may need to take supplemental thyroid hormone. This isn't really a big deal. I sustained some thyroid damage after undergoing (external) radiation therapy to my neck. Except for realizing that I can't permanently flee civilization to live in some tropical paradise, since I'm dependent on a daily dose of thyroid hormone, this hasn't affected my life.

Radioiodine emits γ-rays, which pass through the body and can pose a danger to others nearby. Therefore, people given radioiodine-labeled antibodies as lymphoma therapy may be hospitalized during therapy so that they can be kept isolated from other people until most of the radioisotope has decayed. This is not a problem with yttrium-labeled antibodies, since yttrium emits very few γ-rays.

At this point, it has become apparent that radioisotopically labeled antibodies produce higher overall response rates and more complete remissions than do the same antibodies given without attached radioisotope. However, it is not yet clear whether this increased response rate ultimately leads to longer survival.

Similar to antibodies tagged with radioisotopes, antibodies carrying toxic substances can deliver ultrahigh doses of antineoplastic drugs directly to the tumor. This avoids the dose-limiting toxicities that appear when your whole body is exposed to high levels of these drugs. Some cell membrane proteins—like CD19 and CD22—are engulfed by the cell that carries them whenever something binds to them. Toxin-bearing antibodies directed against such proteins will be carried into the cell along with the internalized target protein. This provides a neat way of delivering into malignant lymphocytes toxins that are active only when they get *inside* a cell.

A recent study found that eleven of sixteen people with an indolent lymphoid malignancy (hairy cell leukemia) who had become resistant to standard chemotherapy had complete remissions when treated with an immunotoxin consisting of the antigen-binding portion of an antibody to CD22 fused with part of a bacterial toxin, and two had partial remissions.

Antibodies tagged with very low doses of radioisotopes can also be used together with sensitive detection techniques to determine the location of any cancer cells. Antibodies can also be used to purge bone marrow before using it in a transplant. Antibodies tagged with radioisotopes or toxins can target and destroy any contaminating cancer cells in autologous transplants (see Chapter 6), while untagged antibodies can act as tiny, molecular fish hooks to seek out and capture stem cells from the mix of cells found in any bone marrow specimen.

Although rituximab and the other monoclonal antibodies are by no means the ultimate lymphoma treatment, they represent a major leap forward. Immunotherapy with monoclonal antibodies now represents a standard component of lymphoma therapy. And the combination of antibodies with radiation or with classical chemotherapy has produced even more encouraging results than the results seen with antibodies alone. The development of humanized monoclonal antibodies directed against tumor cell markers has ushered in a brave new world of more effective, less toxic approaches to cancer treatment.

Cytokines

Cytokines are chemical messengers that are secreted by many different types of cells in our body. These chemical messengers bind to, and influence the behavior of, other cells. The recipient cells—whose behavior is influenced by cytokines—are often called *target cells,* since they're the targets of cytokine action.

There are many different cytokines, and each of them has distinctive effects. Different cytokines can act on different types of target cells. Moreover, different cytokines can stimulate a particular type of target cell to divide, differentiate along one pathway or another, or stop proliferating. All the cells in the immune system—including normal lymphocytes—are subject to regulation by different cytokines, and some lymphoma cells have retained this sensitivity.

Cytokines are used in various approaches to lymphoma therapy. One use is in *supportive* therapy, to minimize undesirable side effects of other treatments, like chemotherapy and radiation. The cytokines known as *granulocyte colony-stimulating factor,* which stimulates the growth and differentiation of all the granulocytes, and *granulocyte and macrophage colony-stimulating factor,* which stimulates the growth of macrophages as well (I bet you guessed that), are used to treat people whose neutrophils have dropped to levels that leave them vulnerable to infection.

Similarly, *erythropoietin,* a cytokine made by cells in the kidneys that stimulates the production of red blood cells, can be used to treat anemia. This avoids the need for a blood transfusion. Another cytokine, *interleukin-11,* may be used to stimulate platelet production.

The colony-stimulating factors are frequently used as supportive therapy for people who are undergoing stem cell transplants (see Chapter 6). They are used before the harvest to stimulate the production of peripheral blood stem cells and after infusion of the donor stem cells to shorten the length of time to engraftment. This decrease in the amount of time it takes for the new stem cells to kick in and start producing white blood cells has decreased the risk of post-transplant complications and has made transplants much safer and easier to tolerate than they used to be.

Some tumor cells are believed to escape immunological surveillance by T cells because of their very low levels of certain cell surface molecules, called the MHC complex (see Chapter 9 for a discussion of the role of MHC molecules in T cell activation). The *interferons* act to increase the number of MHC molecules on the cell surface and also activate natural killer cells. Therefore, administering interferons to increase the density of MHC molecules may make such tumor cells easier for the immune system to detect and destroy. Some interferons are used in combination with certain chemotherapy regimens to try to prolong remissions in follicular lymphomas, as well as to try to stimulate a graft versus lymphoma effect following a stem cell transplant.

In addition to their role in *treating* lymphoma, cytokines are involved in various aspects of the disease process. The tumors in Hodgkin lymphoma typically contain a very small percentage of malignant cells amid a whole host of normal reactive lymphocytes. These normal lymphocytes aggregate in the vicinity of the cancer cells in response to cytokines secreted by the malignant cells. And the Ann Arbor "B" symptoms of weight loss, fever, and night sweats are probably caused by cytokines secreted by the lymphoma (as well as by the other cells of the immune system responding to the disease). The suppression of the immune response that occurs with Hodgkin lymphoma and some forms of NHL is likely related to secretion of inhibitory cytokines by tumor cells that trick your body into thinking that it's producing too many of the normal lymphocytes that would ordinarily produce those same cytokines.

And while one generally thinks of cancer cells as being autonomous, growing merrily away on their own, independent of external signals, at least some forms of lymphoma *do* seem to be sensitive to external cytokine cues. These lymphoma cells retain sensitivity to the same cytokines that signal normal lymphocytes to divide. This means that, for people with lymphoma, cytokines can be a very powerful but potentially double-edged sword.

Thus, some low-grade B cell lymphomas found in the stomach are stimulated by cytokines secreted by T cells that proliferate in response to infection with the bacterium *Helicobacter pylori.* When the underlying bacterial infection is treated with antibiotics, the number of T cells drops and the cytokine-dependent B cell tumor regresses (and may disappear entirely)! It's likely that other forms of lymphoma are stimulated by abnormal cytokine production as well and that the spontaneous growth and regression of low-grade lymphomas that people sometimes see are responses to a changing cytokine balance.

For instance, interleukin-3, which is produced by activated T cells, normally stimulates the proliferation of bone marrow stem cells. Follicular lymphoma cells appear to be sensitive to stimulation by interleukin-3 as well. Thus, anything that increases the number of activated T cells in the vicinity of a nest of follicular lymphoma cells could potentially lead to growth of the tumor, while decreases in interleukin-3 production could allow tumor regression.

Abnormal production of cytokines in response to certain viral infections almost certainly plays a role in the development of some forms of lymphoma. Interleukin-2 is a cytokine produced by activated T cells that stimulates other T cells to grow and divide (its other name is "T cell growth factor"). The virus HTLV-I, which is associated with adult T cell leukemia/lymphoma, forces infected T cells to increase their production and secretion of interleukin-2. HTLV-I also stimulates the production of interleukin-2 *receptors*—the cell surface proteins that allow T cells to recognize and respond to interleukin-2. Since interleukin-2 stimulates T cell production, these viral effects are almost certainly involved in adult T cell leukemia/lymphoma.

For those forms of lymphoma that are sensitive to cytokines, a better understanding of their dependence on cytokines could lead to novel forms of treatment. A new drug used to treat mycosis fungoides, a low-grade T cell lymphoma that involves the skin, makes use of the selectivity with which cytokines bind to their target cells. This drug, denileukin diftitox (brand name: Ontak), consists of interleukin-2 fused to a portion of the toxin produced by the bacterium that causes diphtheria. The interleukin-2 part of the drug binds to its receptors, delivering the toxin to the malignant T cells and bypassing cells that don't bear the interleukin-2 receptor. (Ontak will also bind to normal T cells and other forms of lymphoma that carry the interleukin-2 receptor.) Alternatively, if you had a form of lymphoma that was dependent on a certain cytokine, you could treat it with a molecule that interfered with the actions of that cytokine. An "anticytokine" molecule that interfered with the synthesis or binding of the cytokine, or with the downstream signaling pathways that cytokine turned on, could be synthesized and targeted to the malignant cells to keep the lymphoma under control.

On the other hand, you'd want to think very carefully about the possible implications of undergoing any form of therapy that increased production of the cells that *produce* the specific cytokines that your lymphoma responded to. As we continue to learn more about the immune system and the molecular signals that govern the growth of both normal and malignant cells, therapies that involve cytokines will likely become more and more commonplace and more and more effective.

Vaccines

Giving someone with lymphoma a monoclonal antibody directed against his or her tumor cells is known as *passive immunization*. While these antibodies can recruit your immune system into the battle against the tumor, they don't confer a permanent immunity against cancer. If any cancer cells escape detection while you're undergoing antibody therapy, the tumor may reappear once the antibodies have been eliminated from your body.

Cancer vaccines are designed to "immunize" you against your lymphoma by eliciting an immune response from your own T cells and B cells. It's the same idea as exposing you to a dead or inactive virus to immunize you against smallpox or polio. This form of therapy is known as *active immunization*, since the cells of your own immune system produce the response (as well as participating in it). Once an active immune response has been elicited, it should be permanent, since you'll have made memory B cells and memory T cells that recognize the cancer. In this situation, it's critical that the immune response be directed against a protein that's completely unique to the lymphoma. While you can get along without your normal B lymphocytes for a few months while you're undergoing rituximab therapy, you wouldn't want to develop a permanent immune response against your own lymphocytes.

For this reason, research on antilymphoma vaccines has been aimed at lymphomas that produce immunoglobulin. As discussed in the section on monoclonal antibodies, each B cell lymphoma cell in your body is descended from one original malignant B cell and manufactures an identical version of immunoglobulin. Therefore, an immunological response mounted against the variable region—the specific part of the protein that makes that immunoglobulin unique—will be completely specific to the cells that make up the lymphoma.

Cancer vaccines directed against the lymphoma's immunoglobulin avoid the two drawbacks of using monoclonal antibodies against tumor immunoglobulin. In inducing an active immune response, you'll activate a number of different lymphocytes, each of which produces a slightly different immunoglobulin. Each activated lymphocyte will give rise to a clonal population of daughter cells, producing the same antibody as the parent cell. Each clonal population of lymphocytes recognizes a slightly different portion of the tumor immunoglobulin's variable region, so minor mutations in the tumor immunoglobulin won't make it unrecognizable. It may become unrecognizable to antibodies produced by *one* clone of lymphocytes, but not to all of them. And even though lymphoma vaccines need to be custom-manufactured for each patient, this is much easier than producing individually tailored monoclonal antibodies. Therefore you (or your insurance company) can actually afford the therapy.

Lymphoma vaccines show tremendous potential in treating lymphoma; however, they haven't yet been perfected. Therefore, different variations on this approach are being tested. The simplest approach is to remove some lymphoma cells from your body, grow them in a sterile environment, and get them to produce large quantities of immunoglobulin. The tumor immunoglobulin is harvested, and its unique variable regions are attached to some protein that elicits a very strong immune response. Meanwhile, you undergo conventional chemotherapy to induce a complete remission.

Once you have attained a complete remission (or as good a partial remission as you can), you're vaccinated with the combination of tumor immunoglobulin variable region attached to the strongly antigenic protein. In a recent study, people who developed a lymphoma-specific immune response (about half of the people in the study) sustained remissions averaging about eight years (*much* longer than would normally be expected).

Considering the current pace of cancer research, the emergence of a treatment that produces an average remission of eight years is tremendously encouraging. However, modifications of the vaccine approach are being tested to try to increase the success rate (and perhaps prolong the eight-year remission into a cure).

The vaccine, as described, is most effective at recruiting B cells, since B cells can recognize antigenic substances found outside cells. An interesting variation, the *dendritic cell vaccine*, is aimed at recruiting the other class of lymphocytes, the T cells, which recognize antigens found on other cells.

Dendritic cells are one of the classes of cells that activate T cells. Dendritic cells roam the body in search of antigens. If they find an interesting antigen, they take it up, process it, hustle back to the lymph nodes, and present it to T cells along with a co-stimulatory signal. If a T cell recognizes that antigen, then the antigen-presenting dendritic cell activates it. The activated T cell proliferates and differentiates into a tribe of functional daughter cells. Dendritic cells do a better job of activating T cells than any other form of stimulation.

Therefore, one approach to lymphoma vaccines has involved not only isolating your tumor immunoglobulin but also harvesting some of your dendritic cells. The dendritic cells are grown—or cultured—outside your body in the presence of a nutrient medium containing cytokines that allow them to grow and proliferate. These cultured dendritic cells are then exposed to the variable regions from your tumor-specific immunoglobulin. The idea is that they will take up the tumor-specific antigen and process it for presentation to T cells, just as they would any other antigen.

Once you've attained a complete remission with chemotherapy, you're reinoculated with your own antigen-primed dendritic cells so that they can activate a population of antigen-specific T cells. Then, the activated T cells roam your body searching for tumor antigen and destroying any remaining lymphoma cells. The dendritic cell vaccine can be given either on its own or in combination with injections of your immunoglobulin variable region coupled to the antigenic protein.

I was so excited about the possibilities of this approach that I resolved that, if R-CHOP didn't work, I'd try to get into a clinical trial using antilymphoma vaccines. I was disappointed to learn that, so far, vaccines were used only with indolent disease and that my form of lymphoma—primary mediastinal large cell lymphoma—was not only aggressive but one of the few B cell lymphomas that didn't produce surface immunoglobulin, so these particular vaccines would be useless against my form of the disease.

While R-CHOP seems to have worked for me, I certainly hope that progress continues in the exciting realm of antilymphoma vaccines, so that this approach can be extended to those of us with more aggressive disease, and that new lymphoma-specific proteins will be discovered, making this form of therapy potentially available to us all.

Other forms of directed therapy
Antisense

Another form of directed therapy utilizes genetic techniques to inhibit the activity of certain genes. Genes are the blueprints that tell cells how to manufacture specific proteins; specific genes are active only where and when the protein they code for is required. For instance, red blood cells *express* the genes that encode hemoglobin—allowing them to manufacture this protein—whereas skin cells (which don't need hemoglobin) do not. The basic idea behind *antisense gene therapy* is that lymphoma—like other forms of cancer—results from dysfunctions in gene expression.

Dysfunctions of gene expression can lead to cancer in several ways (as discussed in Chapter 8). Sometimes, a critical gene becomes disabled, so the protein it specifies no longer works properly. Forms of lymphoma that are characterized by mutations in a gene called *p53*, which prevents cells with a severely damaged genome from proliferating and which can trigger apoptosis (programmed cell suicide), fall into this category. In other cases, a given protein can work perfectly—but because gene regulation has gone awry, the protein is manufactured in the wrong type of cell, or it turns up at the wrong time, with disastrous consequences.

For many people with lymphoma, problems in gene regulation involve a gene called *bcl-2*. *Bcl-2*, which stands for B cell lymphoma-2 (it was discovered in B cell lymphomas, although it's associated with some other forms of cancer as well), codes for a protein that inhibits apoptosis. In addition to its role in eliminating damaged cells, apoptosis is the process through which ineffective lymphocytes are eliminated during normal lymphocyte development (see Chapter 9).

A cell suicide mechanism is important. It ensures that unnecessary cells are eliminated and only those that are necessary and useful survive. Otherwise we'd be overrun with nonfunctional and superfluous cells. It's also desirable to have a gene that can keep certain cells from committing suicide when their counterparts do. For instance, *bcl-2* plays an important role in the development of memory cells—the long-lived lymphocytes that confer permanent immunity to diseases you've previously encountered.

However, *abnormal* activity of *bcl-2*—whereby those cells that are *supposed* to die are rescued—can lead to problems. Most follicular lymphoma cells carry a mutation that leads to permanent activation of *bcl-2* (see Chapter 10). In follicular lymphomas, part of a gene that is concerned with regulating where and when immunoglobulin is manufactured (which is permanently turned on in B cells, since their job is to make antibodies) becomes attached to the gene that tells the cell how to make the Bcl-2 protein. Therefore the cell will continuously, and inappropriately, churn out Bcl-2 protein (as though it were immunoglobulin). For reasons that are unclear, the cells in some other forms of indolent lymphoma make high levels of Bcl-2 protein, even without this mutation.

The cells with permanently activated *bcl-2* continue to divide and proliferate as they normally would at this stage in development (unlike the memory B cells, which don't proliferate except in response to an activating signal). However, the high levels of Bcl-2 protein prevent them from undergoing apoptosis when it would be appropriate for them to do so. This leads to a buildup of follicular lymphoma cells. This may be critically important in the response to treatment. Some antineoplastic drugs damage the genetic material, thereby triggering apoptosis. Since *bcl-2* inhibits apoptosis, it helps make these cells resistant to chemotherapy. One approach to gene therapy involves inhibiting *bcl-2*. This should keep cells with abnormally turned on *bcl-2* from accumulating and make them more sensitive to chemotherapy.

How could you inhibit the activity of a gene? One way involves giving *antisense* to the gene. As discussed in Chapter 8, DNA, the primary genetic material, is essentially a molecular blueprint of the instructions required to make an organism. The DNA for a given gene is used as a template to manufacture the messenger molecule RNA for that gene, and then RNA is used to make that gene's protein. DNA is organized into two complementary strands, only one of which is used as the RNA template. The message that RNA carries encodes for a protein: it makes molecular sense. The DNA strand that corresponds to the messenger RNA sequence is sometimes called the *sense strand*. The other DNA strand is the *antisense strand*, and it is this strand that serves as the template for messenger RNA synthesis. *Antisense nucleotides* correspond to the antisense DNA strand: they bind to the RNA that encodes a particular protein and *inhibit* production of the protein. Antisense RNA refers to the nucleotide sequence you would get if you copied the *wrong strand* of DNA.

By giving people with follicular lymphoma small strands of nucleotides that correspond to the antisense strand of the *bcl-2* gene, you can inhibit production of Bcl-2 protein. This should allow apoptosis to take place in follicular lymphoma cells and make them more susceptible to chemotherapy. Clinical trials in which people were given *bcl-2* antisense (called augmerosen, Genasense, G3139, or oblimersen) have shown promising results.

As predicted, antisense to *bcl-2* seems to increase the lymphoma's susceptibility to chemotherapy. And as far as we can tell, this particular antisense compound is without harmful side effects. If future trials bear out the promise of this approach, we can expect not only a new weapon in our armamentarium against follicular lymphoma but also an expansion of the antisense technique to target other abnormally regulated genes.

Inhibitors of angiogenesis

A few years ago, an article appeared in the *New York Times* that electrified cancer patients all over the country. The article had to do with a technique called *antiangiogenesis* that promised to revolutionize cancer therapy. Antiangiogenesis, pioneered by Dr. Judah Folkman, is based on a very simple (but in many ways novel) idea. This is that tumor cells, like all the other cells in your body, require a constant blood supply. A good blood supply is necessary to bring oxygen and glucose (food) to your cells and to carry away waste products.

Folkman's idea was that, in order for tumors to grow to a size where they became dangerous, they needed to develop a blood supply. And this could take place only if the tumor cells sent out signals that caused new blood vessels to develop, grow toward them, and supply them with blood—a process called *angiogenesis.* This meant that if you could find compounds that inhibited angiogenesis—called *antiangiogenic* compounds—you could starve the tumors to death.

Antiangiogenic compounds would act against the cells making up the new blood vessels that supply the tumor, rather than against the cancer cells in the tumor itself. Antiangiogenesis is an appealing approach to cancer therapy for several reasons. One is that since antiangiogenesis therapy doesn't act directly against the cancer cells, which are genetically unstable, but against the normal, healthy cells making the blood vessels that supply them, it is far less likely that drug resistance will develop. Moreover, antiangiogenesis should, in theory, be active against all sorts of tumors (since all require a blood supply).

A host of compounds with antiangiogenic activity have recently been identified. Some of these occur naturally in our bodies, and some are synthetic. These antiangiogenic compounds have shown tremendous activity against cancer in mice. Unfortunately, oncology research is littered with promising drugs that cured cancer in mice but not in people. As one oncologist put it: "We've been able to cure cancer in *mice* for twenty years."

Early trials of antiangiogenic agents indicate that they may be active against some forms of cancer in people, although they are probably not as effective as initially hoped. Whether antiangiogenic therapy works against lymphoma remains to be determined.

Czuczman MS, Weaver R, Alkuzweny B, Berlfein J, Grillo-Lopez AJ. (2004). "Prolonged clinical and molecular remission in patients with low-grade or follicular non-Hodgkin's lymphoma treated with rituximab plus CHOP chemotherapy: 9-year follow-up." *Journal of Clinical Oncology* 22:4659–4664.

Three excellent articles in a special issue of *Scientific American, What You Need to Know about Cancer,* from September 1996 on directed therapies:

Folkman J. (1996). "Fighting cancer by attacking its blood supply." *Scientific American* 275:150–154.

Old LJ. (1996). "Immunotherapy for cancer." *Scientific American* 275:136–143.

Oliff A, Gibbs JB, McCormick F. (1996). "New molecular targets for cancer therapy." *Scientific American* 275:144–149.

Some other interesting reviews include:

Blattman JN, Greenberg PD. (2004). "Cancer immunotherapy: A treatment for the masses." *Science* 305:200–205.

Cotter FE. (1997). "Antisense therapy for B cell lymphomas." *Cancer Surveys* 30:311–325.

Fielding AK, Russell SJ. (1997). "Gene therapy for B cell lymphomas." *Cancer Surveys* 30:327–342.

Greten TF, Jaffee EM. (1999). "Cancer vaccines." *Journal of Clinical Oncology* 17:1047–1060.

Press OW. (1998). "Prospects for the management of non-Hodgkin's lymphoma with monoclonal antibodies and immunoconjugates." *Cancer Journal from Scientific American* 4:S19–26.

Press OW, Leonard JP, Coiffier B, Levy R, Timmerman J. (2001). "Immunotherapy of non-Hodgkin's lymphomas." *Hematology* 2001:221–240.

Waldmann TA. (2003). "Immunotherapy: past, present and future." *Nature Medicine* 9:269–277.

Winter JN, Gascoyne RD, Van Besien K. (2004). "Low-grade lymphoma." *Hematology* 2004:203–220.

Information can also be found online:

Many oncologists believe that anyone diagnosed with low-grade lymphoma should consider participating in a clinical trial. Information about clinical trials is available at the National Cancer Institute: *www.cancernet.nci.nih.gov/clinicaltrials* and CenterWatch: www.CenterWatch.com/patient/studies/area12.html.

The online journal for which I am now an editor, *Science's STKE,* has recently published several articles concerning different forms of directed therapy:

Adler EM. (2004). "Tailoring the immune response." *Science's STKE* 2004:eg9.

Engleman EG, Brody J, Soares L. (2004). "Using signaling pathways to overcome immune tolerance to tumors." *Science's STKE* 2004:pe28.

Olszewski AJ, Grossbard ML. (2004). "Empowering targeted therapy: Lessons from rituximab." *Science's STKE* 2004:pe30.

Opalinska JB, Gewirtz AM. (2003). "Therapeutic potential of antisense nucleic acid molecules." *Science's STKE* 2003:pe47.

CHAPTER 6

Stem Cell Transplants

The first time I met my oncologist, she told me about *stem cell transplants*. She didn't know whether I would be cured with front-line therapy, and she wanted to reassure me that we had backup options. A stem cell transplant is a procedure that uses high doses of antineoplastic drugs, or of radiation, that would ordinarily be toxic to wipe out any cancer cells that have proved resistant to more gentle methods of therapy. There are three basic types of stem cell transplant: *autologous* transplants, *syngeneic* transplants, and *allogeneic* transplants. They are distinguished from each other by the source of the stem cells that will repopulate your bone marrow after you receive this treatment. I found the idea of a stem cell transplant frightening, and the prospect of getting one loomed threateningly over me until I had passed the "unlikely to relapse" mark, two years after completing chemo and radiation.

However, a stem cell transplant is essentially just an extension of chemotherapy (and sometimes radiation therapy and immunotherapy). While the regimens involved are usually harsher than those involved in standard chemotherapy, making them harder to tolerate, transplant methodologies continue to be improved and extended. As the techniques involved in transplantation technology have been refined, the population eligible for a transplant has increased—so that people who wouldn't have been eligible for a transplant ten years ago can have them today—and the procedure has become much less difficult to undergo. This isn't your father's stem cell transplant.

In discussing chemotherapy, I talked about the idea of dose-limiting drug toxicity. The dose-limiting toxicity occurs at drug doses at which the side effects are so severe that you cannot risk taking any more of that drug. If the dose-limiting toxicity of the drug occurs at a higher concentration than the therapeutic concentration—the dose of drug required to wipe out the cancer—then everything's fine. The drug gets rid of the cancer; you put up with the side effects, and then move on. Treatment becomes problematic, however, when the dose-limiting toxicity is close to, or below, the therapeutic dose. In this case, you can't take enough of the drug to wipe out the cancer without incurring the risk of life-threatening complications.

Combination chemotherapy takes one approach to this problem. Different antineoplastic drugs with distinct dose-limiting toxicities are given together. The cancer cells are hit simultaneously from several different angles, but no healthy organ or system is excessively stressed. Stem cell transplants take a slightly different approach. In a stem cell transplant, you are given one or more antineoplastic drugs (sometimes combined with total body irradiation) whose dose-limiting toxicities are due to bone marrow suppression. You take very high doses of these drugs—enough to wipe out the cells in your bone marrow (as well as destroy the cancer).

As discussed in more depth in Chapter 9, your lymphocytes, and all the other blood cell types, are derived from *hematopoietic*—or blood-producing—stem cells found in your bone marrow. These stem cells, which are also found circulating in the blood, essentially function as the "seeds" of the bone marrow, giving rise to all the different types of blood cells. Therefore, eliminating the stem cells in your bone marrow would ordinarily wipe out your immune system, your platelets, and your red blood cells, leaving you subject to the first pathogen that comes along, as well as terribly anemic and vulnerable to massive bleeding in response to the most minor injuries. A truly fragile state of existence! With a stem cell transplant, however, you are saved from this dire fate by an infusion of hematopoietic stem cells, which magically find their way to the proper sites inside your bones to reproduce and reconstitute all your different blood cells.

The ability to perform a stem cell transplant—sometimes called a *stem cell rescue*—allows antineoplastic drugs to be given at much higher doses than normal: up to the point where other dose-limiting toxicities (that don't show up at normal therapeutic doses) start to emerge. The hope is that such high levels of drugs will eradicate even those populations of cancer cells tough enough to survive normal levels of antineoplastic agents. You're essentially hitting the cancer with the biggest guns in the therapeutic arsenal, and your stem cells are innocent bystanders shot down in the process. The use of these intensive therapies that obliterate your bone marrow is called *conditioning*.

In an *autologous* transplant, you supply the stem cells yourself. You are both *donor*, the person who supplies (or donates) the stem cells, and *recipient*, the person who receives the stem cells. Some of your own stem cells are harvested (usually from those circulating in the blood, but sometimes directly from the bone marrow) before you undergo the conditioning regimen, to be returned to your body after you complete the high-dose chemotherapy. Your returned stem cells can then repopulate your bone marrow. Autologous transplants are the most common form of transplant for people with lymphoma.

If you have an identical twin, you can get a *syngeneic* transplant. In this type of transplant, your twin is the donor, and you are the recipient. Since identical twins are identical all the way down to their genes, having started out as a single fertilized egg, the stem cells you receive in a syngeneic transplant are genetically equivalent to your own. This means that any lymphocytes included with the donor stem cells will recognize the cells in your body as "self." With a syngeneic transplant, like an autologous transplant, you avoid any problems of immunological incompatibility between the donor cells and the cells of your body. You don't need to worry that immune system cells in the donated marrow will consider the rest of you foreign. In a syngeneic transplant, moreover, you'll escape the possibility that some of your own malignant cells could be reintroduced along with the stem cells in the transplant (see below).

Finally, you can receive stem cells from someone who is not genetically identical to you but whose blood cells are similar enough to yours that receiving their stem cells will not lead to severe immunological complications. This is called an *allogeneic* transplant. Most commonly, the donor in an allogeneic transplant is a brother or sister, since your siblings are most likely to have cells that match yours immunologically. If you are a candidate for an allogeneic transplant but don't have a brother or sister whose cells match yours, other relatives may be tested. The closer the relationship, the more likely they are to match up. Sometimes, someone who is completely unrelated to you will have cells that match yours well enough to be used in a transplant. This is called a *matched, unrelated donor* (or MUD) transplant.

If you are going to have a stem cell transplant, whether you have an autologous, syngeneic, or allogeneic transplant will depend on the type of lymphoma you have, your age and general condition, whether the lymphoma has invaded your bone marrow, and whether a suitable donor can be located. Autologous stem cell transplants, using your own stem cells, are the most common form of stem cell transplant used to treat lymphoma. In fact, autologous transplants are performed more frequently for NHL than for any other condition. Syngeneic transplants, of course, are restricted to the 0.3 percent of people who have identical twins. People with extensive lymphoma in their bone marrow are more likely to receive an allogeneic transplant.

For people who do not have lymphoma in their bone marrow, autologous transplants are much more frequently performed than are allogeneic transplants. They appear to be curative for many people with aggressive NHL or Hodgkin lymphoma. They can produce long-term remissions in people with low-grade NHL, and some individuals with low-grade lymphomas may have been cured by autologous stem cell transplants, but, at present, it's hard to be sure.

Autologous transplants are easier to tolerate than allogeneic transplants. You don't need to worry that the lymphocytes derived from the donor marrow will perceive your body as foreign and attack it or that any remaining lymphocytes of your own will attack the transplanted cells. People given autologous transplants have fewer problems with the transplanted cells "taking" (a process called *engraftment*) and are less likely to develop severe infections than people undergoing allogeneic transplants. Therefore, autologous transplants are generally considered safer than allogeneic transplants, and mortality rates from treatment-related complications are low (less than 5 percent of transplantees at experienced centers).

On the other hand, allogeneic transplants may be more likely than autologous transplants to cure certain forms of lymphoma. Although the initial treatment-related mortality is higher with allogeneic transplants, relapses of the lymphoma appear to be less common. There are two reasons for this. If the lymphoma has massively infiltrated your bone marrow, some malignant cells may be harvested along with the healthy stem cells in preparation for an autologous transplant, and it may be impossible to eliminate all of them. This would lead to reintroducing cancerous cells with the transplanted stem cells, defeating the whole purpose of the transplant.

And while a lymphocytic attack on your body from cells in the transplanted marrow is one of the major concerns with an allogeneic transplant, this effect, called *graft-versus-host disease,* has a positive side as well. The donor lymphocytes in an allogeneic transplant may recognize any malignant cells remaining in your body as harmful and seek them out to destroy them. This is called the *graft-versus-lymphoma* or *graft-versus-tumor* effect, and it doesn't occur with autologous or syngeneic transplants.

TREATING LYMPHOMA

Syngeneic transplants fall somewhere between the other two forms in terms of curative potential. It is very unlikely that your identical twin would also have lymphoma (although, rarely, this is the case, so he or she will have to be tested). Therefore, it is also very unlikely that any malignant cells would be infused together with the healthy stem cells. On the other hand, the graft-versus-lymphoma effect seen in allogeneic transplants is absent. For this reason, relapses from syngeneic transplants are more common than relapses from allogeneic transplants.

Because stem cell transplants typically involve very high doses of chemotherapy, not everyone is a good candidate to undergo one. This depends on your age and your general health (aside from the lymphoma, of course). For example, someone with significant preexisting heart or lung disease might not be able to tolerate a stem cell transplant and would therefore not be a candidate for one. This needs to be determined for each individual on a case-by-case basis. Younger people generally have an easier time with transplants than the elderly, and there are upper limits to the age at which you are considered eligible for a transplant. (There are no lower limits, and very young children have successfully undergone stem cell transplants.) These age limits vary from one center to the next and have been revised upward as transplant procedures became more sophisticated. At present, you would be unlikely to be a candidate for an autologous transplant if you are over seventy and unlikely to be a candidate for an allogeneic transplant if you are over sixty.

Finding a donor for allogeneic transplants

The first step in undergoing an allogeneic transplant is finding a donor. The donor must be immunologically compatible with the recipient. This means that the cells of the donor's immune system must not consider the recipient's cells "foreign." This depends on a group of proteins found on the surfaces of cells known as the *human leukocyte antigens* (HLA; antigens are substances that can cause an immunological response). The HLAs, which are proteins involved in the normal immunological response (see Chapter 9), differ slightly from one individual to another. Certain T cells, members of a class of white blood cells that is important in the immunological response, distinguish "self" cells from "foreign" cells by detecting slight differences in their HLAs. They attack and destroy the foreign cells as part of their job of protecting the body from potentially harmful foreign invaders.

If the donor is not immunologically compatible with the recipient, these donated T cells will attack the cells in the recipient's body. It is this "friendly fire" that causes graft-versus-host disease.

Six HLA antigens between the potential stem cell donor and the recipient must be compared in order to determine whether the donor and recipient are immunologically compatible. The better the match between donor and recipient HLAs, the less likely you are to develop severe graft-versus-host disease. A six-out-of-six match is ideal; most transplant centers will accept five out of six, and sometimes a match of four out of six can be accepted. Your best chance for a six-out-of-six match is with your siblings. That's because the different HLA proteins are usually inherited together as a set. As with any other gene, everyone inherits two sets of genes coding for the HLA proteins: one set inherited from each parent. Since each parent has two sets of HLA genes inherited from *his or her* parents, the chances that a given sibling will match with you are one out of four (fig. 6.1).

If you have siblings, an easy test to determine whether they are HLA compatible with you is to see whether *your* lymphocytes cause *their* lymphocytes to proliferate. A sample of your white blood cells is killed (by radiation) and put in a dish with some of your sibling's lymphocytes. If his or her lymphocytes start to divide (yours can't divide any more, of course, being dead), it means that they recognize some protein on your cells as foreign and are preparing for the assault. Lymphocytes from your sibling's marrow would probably respond the same way to the cells in your body—in other words, you're HLA incompatible. On the other hand, if your sibling's lymphocytes accept yours and just sit there quietly, it's likely that they'll accept the rest of you as "self."

Since people who are not related to you are likely to have inherited different *sets* of HLAs from *their* parents, you may have difficulty finding a matching donor. It's been estimated that there's about a 1 in 20,000 chance that your HLAs will match perfectly with those of someone who is unrelated to you (the exact figure varies depending on your genetic heritage). Nonetheless, there are about 5 million volunteer donors, so that compatible unrelated donors *have* been identified, and matched unrelated donor (MUD) transplants are performed when no related donor is available. To identify an unrelated donor you must be *tissue-typed*. This means that the set of HLA antigens that you carry is characterized so that it can be compared with that of any potential donors.

The National Marrow Donor Program maintains lists of people who have been tissue-typed and are willing to donate marrow. If you belong to a racial minority or are descended from an unusual ethnic group, your chances of finding

TREATING LYMPHOMA

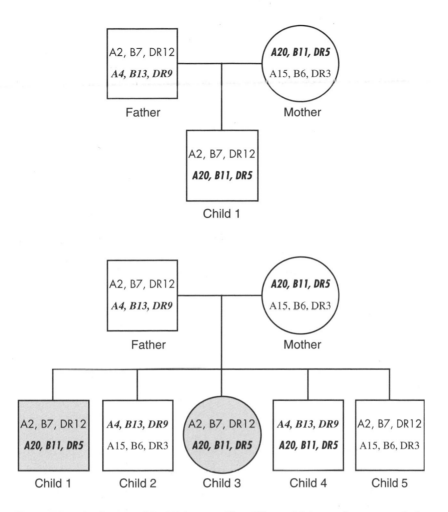

Figure 6.1. *Inheritance of the HLA genes.* The different HLA proteins are usually inherited together as a set. As with all genes, every person inherits two sets of genes coding for the HLA proteins: one set from each parent. In the "family tree" of HLA inheritance shown in this figure, the father and mother each have two sets of the HLA "A," "D," and "DR" genes. The father's sets are A2, B7, and DR12 and A4, B13, and DR9, while the mother's are A20, B11, and DR5 and A15, B6, and DR3. In this figure, their first child inherited the "top set" of genes from both parents, ending up with A2, B7, and DR12 from his father and A20, B11, and DR5 from his mother. However, he could also have inherited the "top set" from one parent and the "bottom set" from the other or the "bottom set" from both. Therefore, the chances that a given sibling will match with another are no more than one out of four. In the bottom row, which shows the different possible combinations of HLA genes for offspring of this couple, only Child 1 and Child 3 have a six out of six HLA match.

a matched unrelated donor are poorer than those of someone who belongs to a more common ethnic group (because of genetic diversity). Therefore, marrow donation programs have been particularly interested in enlisting healthy members of racial minorities and underrepresented ethnic groups.

With a MUD transplant you are somewhat more likely to develop graft-versus-host disease even with a perfect six-out-of-six HLA match. This is likely due to mismatches in other cellular proteins that are recognized as antigens by the donated T cells.

Obtaining stem cells

When stem cell transplants were first developed, stem cells were harvested directly from the bone marrow, and the procedure was frequently called a *bone marrow transplant*. More recently, a less invasive procedure called a *peripheral blood stem cell harvest* (PBSCH) has been developed; in this procedure, circulating stem cells are isolated from the bloodstream rather than extracted directly from the marrow. Today, PBSCHs are performed much more frequently than bone marrow transplants, particularly for autologous transplants (about 90 percent of the time). However, bone marrow transplants are still performed in some cases, and both procedures are described here.

Bone marrow harvest

The bone marrow harvest is similar to a scaled-up bone marrow biopsy. It's usually performed under a general anesthetic, so the donor will probably need to stay in the hospital overnight. The marrow is withdrawn from the large hipbones of the pelvis (and occasionally from the breastbone). The physician makes several small incisions and then withdraws twenty or thirty syringes full of marrow. About a pint or two of marrow is taken altogether. This sounds like a lot of bone marrow, but it's equal to only about 3 to 5 percent of the donor's developing blood cells. The procedure takes an hour or so and is considered extremely safe (if not a lot of fun).

Occasionally, there may be significant blood loss during the bone marrow harvest. Therefore, many donors store a unit or two of their own blood in advance of the donation, just in case. (If the donor doesn't need the stored blood, this blood can be given to the recipient during the time the new marrow is starting to become established, as long as the red cell types also match.) There will be some residual soreness around the site of the incision, and the donor may feel tired. This tiredness usually resolves within about a week (or less), and the donor will replace his or her harvested marrow and cells within a few weeks. Rarely, as with any wound, the incision may become infected, and the donor will need to be treated with antibiotics.

The harvested marrow is filtered to remove tiny fragments of bone and to break up any clumps of cells. It may or may not undergo further treatment to remove or modify the T cells as a means of avoiding problems with graft-versus-host disease. The HLA antigens used in tissue-typing bone marrow are different from the more familiar A, B, and O red cell blood types. If your donor has a red cell blood type that is incompatible with yours, the red cells will be removed from the marrow before it is given to you to prevent antibodies in your blood from attacking the donated red cells. Once the new stem cells have taken hold and have started producing blood cells, your blood type will change to that of your donor.

The processed marrow can be transplanted immediately or frozen for long-term storage. Frozen marrow is treated with dimethyl sulfoxide (DMSO), which is a *cryoprotectant:* it protects the cells in the marrow from being killed during the process of being frozen. DMSO prevents the formation of ice crystals, which would otherwise rupture various cell membranes and destroy the cellular structure.

Unfortunately, in addition to being a great cryoprotectant, DMSO has a really nasty smell. It's sort of like rotten garlic. The first time I smelled it, I thought that something had died and rotted in the room. The stored cells in the harvested marrow smell like DMSO, and, for a day or so after the transplant, so will you. (Most people who receive bone marrow preserved with DMSO don't notice the smell themselves, but people around them do. Ah, well, a small enough price to pay.)

Frozen and stored, the harvested bone marrow will last for at least several years. Therefore, people who expect to undergo an allogeneic bone marrow transplant in the future and have an HLA-matched sibling who may not be readily available some years hence (for instance, if he or she travels to exotic locales) may choose to have the marrow harvested and stored safely in advance as a sort of cellular insurance policy.

Peripheral blood stem cell harvest

Although the highest concentration of stem cells is found in the bone marrow, some stem cells are also found circulating in the bloodstream, which makes peripheral blood stem cell harvest another option. PBSC transplants are easier on the donor than traditional bone marrow transplants and are now much more commonly performed than bone marrow transplants, particularly with autologous transplants.

In a PBSC harvest, blood is withdrawn from a vein in your arm (or from an implanted catheter, if you have one) in a process called *apheresis*. During apheresis, stem cells found circulating in the blood are collected and saved for the transplant, and the rest of your blood is returned to you. Apheresis takes a few hours (the process may be repeated several times in order to obtain enough cells) and doesn't require anesthesia. You may experience some feelings of lightheadedness, coldness, or cramping in your hands.

Since the number of peripheral stem cells in blood is lower than the number in bone marrow, people are often treated to *mobilize* their stem cells, or increase the number circulating in the blood. People who have recently undergone chemotherapy frequently have increased levels of circulating stem cells. This is probably associated with increased levels of cytokines as your body recognizes the need to repopulate your blood with the types of cells that have been destroyed by the treatment. Therefore, PBSC harvests for autologous transplants are often performed when you are in remission following standard chemotherapy, before you receive high-dose chemotherapy or total body irradiation to destroy any remaining malignant cells in your body.

Another means of mobilizing stem cells is to give cytokines that increase the production of blood cells, such as granulocyte colony-stimulating factor. If you are getting an allogeneic transplant, your donor will not be expected to undergo chemotherapy (I suspect you'd have an *awfully* hard time finding willing donors) but may be given colony-stimulating factors.

People given PBSC transplants tend to engraft more rapidly than those given bone marrow transplants. That is to say, the newly transplanted stem cells take hold and start producing new blood cells more rapidly. This reduces the amount of time you are most vulnerable to infection and minimizes the number of transfusions you will need to replace red blood cells and platelets. While the more rapid engraftment seen with PBSC transplants may reflect differences between the stem cells likely to be found circulating in the blood and those who stay home in the marrow, it may be related to the growth-promoting factors that are given to mobilize the stem cells. If the latter proves to be the case, it may become standard practice to administer colony-stimulating factors before bone marrow harvests as well.

Umbilical cord blood transplants

A newer form of allogeneic transplant utilizes stem cells found in blood from the umbilical cords and placentas of newborn babies! After the baby is born and the umbilical cord is tied off, blood from the cord and placenta can be withdrawn with a needle and syringe. This *cord blood* is very high in stem cells, and it has been used successfully in allogeneic bone marrow transplants.

Cord blood transplants have certain advantages compared with traditional allogeneic transplants. The T cells in newborns and in cord blood are immature (probably so the baby's T cells won't attack any maternal proteins they might encounter) and less able to mount an effective immunological attack than adult T cells. This T cell immaturity minimizes the chances of severe graft-versus-host disease in cord blood transplants. This is a major advantage for people who don't have an HLA-matched relative and might not otherwise be able to find a compatible donor. While the best results have been seen with matched transplants from the cord blood of relatives, cord blood transplants that are incompletely matched in terms of HLA compatibility have been successful as well.

Cord blood is also less likely to contain certain viruses that may lurk in the stem cells of adults, which could pose a danger to immunocompromised marrow recipients. Finally, harvesting cord blood poses really minimal inconvenience to the donor. Once the baby is born, the umbilical cord and placenta become unnecessary and superfluous. While blood from a single umbilical cord contains enough stem cells to repopulate the bone marrow of most children, it may not contain enough for an adult. However, recent techniques have enabled researchers to propagate stem cells in vitro, making it likely that this former throwaway item will prove a major resource for adults requiring MUD transplants.

Autologous transplant

Autologous stem cell transplants are frequently performed on people whose lymphoma has not invaded their bone marrow. The great majority of autologous transplants involve PBSC. While you cannot undergo an autologous transplant if you have massive involvement of your bone marrow with lymphoma, some centers will perform autologous transplants on people whose marrow shows only a small amount of lymphoma.

For instance, you can have a bone marrow biopsy that shows some infiltration with lymphoma cells before you undergo chemotherapy. In this case, after you undergo chemotherapy your bone marrow biopsy may appear perfectly normal under a microscope, but sensitive tests such as the *polymerase chain reaction* (PCR), which are capable of detecting the presence of DNA from a single malignant cell in a sample of bone marrow, may show evidence of minimal residual disease.

Some transplant centers may go ahead with the autologous transplant as though there were no evidence of lymphoma in your marrow, believing that such low numbers of lymphoma cells will be destroyed by your immune system (once it has become reconstituted) and therefore pose little threat to your well-being. Other physicians are concerned that reinfusing *any* malignant cells may contribute to your chances of experiencing a relapse. Therefore, some transplant centers *purge* stem cells that show any sign at all of lymphoma in an attempt to remove every single malignant cell from your stem cells before they are returned to your body. If you have some bone marrow involvement and are preparing for an autologous transplant, you will want to discuss purging with your doctor.

There are several different approaches to purging. These include treating the harvested stem cells with antineoplastic drugs and using monoclonal antibodies that recognize specific proteins on the cell surface. Monoclonal antibodies can be used in either *negative selection* or *positive selection.* In negative selection, monoclonal antibodies that recognize antigens found on lymphoma cells are used to destroy those cells or to remove them from your stem cells. In positive selection, antibodies to specific proteins found on early stem cells, but not on lymphoma cells, are used to fish the stem cells out.

In theory, purging sounds like a great idea. There's something distinctly unappealing about the idea of going through a stem cell transplant only to have even a small number of malignant cells returned to your body. And some research centers have obtained results that suggest that purging your stem cells reduces your chances of experiencing a relapse.

Other centers, however, have found little difference in how well people who have received purged stem cells do, compared with those who've received unpurged stem cells. Moreover, some forms of purging may prolong the amount of time required for the transplanted stem cells to settle in and start producing new blood cells. This delay in engraftment increases the time that you are anemic and highly susceptible to infection. Thus, whether or not purging autologous stem cells is the "best practice" remains controversial.

If purging seems to be the best option for you, additional stem cells will be removed during the harvest in order to make up for those cells removed in the purge.

Conditioning

The high-dose chemotherapy with or without total body irradiation that is given in preparation for the stem cell transplant is known as the *conditioning regimen*. The conditioning regimen is intended to destroy any cancer cells that have proved resistant to more conventional, lower-dose chemotherapy treatments. With allogeneic transplants, the conditioning regimen is also intended to destroy the recipient's immune system, to keep any remaining immune cells from attacking and destroying the donated stem cells. Generally, the conditioning regimen is given after you have already attained the best possible response to conventional therapy.

Different conditioning regimens are used for different kinds of lymphoma, and even the same type of lymphoma may be treated with different regimens at different facilities. At this point, it's very difficult to say which regimen(s) is (are) best. One thing that *is* important, though, is finding a facility that performs stem cell transplants on a regular basis and has an experienced staff. The differences in outcome between centers that perform many transplants and those that perform very few are substantial enough to make even travel to a distant city for the transplant, if necessary, worthwhile. (The Corporate Angel Network, 914-328-1313, helps arrange free air transportation for cancer patients and stem cell donors to distant treatment centers.)

The conditioning regimen is frequently administered as a countdown (Day −10, Day −9, Day −8, . . . Day −1, transplant!), with the transplant itself performed on Day 0. The pretransplant preparative stage, whether it involves chemotherapy alone or chemotherapy plus total body irradiation, is brief (several days to a few weeks) but very intense. You are likely to experience nausea and vomiting (although, thankfully, modern antiemetics can alleviate much of this), as well as mouth sores, hair loss, diarrhea, and disturbances in how things taste. All the usual chemo side effects, but more intense (varying, depending on what drug you are given). On Day −1, you get to rest.

Because the conditioning regimen is designed to obliterate your bone marrow, you will become extremely susceptible to infection—even more so than with conventional chemo regimens. The early part of the regimen may be performed on an outpatient basis, with you coming in to the clinic only to receive intravenous drugs and to get your blood monitored. Once your blood counts drop, however, you will be admitted to the hospital or other transplant facility to protect you from infection.

While the greatest risk of infection comes from pathogens already present in the body, the facility will take precautions designed to protect you from further exposure to infection. The specific procedures vary somewhat among different facilities. You may be isolated in your own room. The air that supplies the room may be filtered to screen out any bacteria or fungi. You may have a laminar flow room, in which the filtered air moves in regulated layers, like a series of curtains. This prevents air in different portions of the room from mixing and helps keep you even more isolated from any pathogens that might get into the room.

The nursing staff must always wash their hands before coming to see you and may scrub as though they were preparing for an operation and put on clean clothes, masks, and gloves. If your center allows visitors, they will not be permitted to see you if they are ill, and they should not bring plants or flowers. You will eat an "immunosuppressed diet," similar to that described in the chemotherapy section, and will be instructed in "stem cell transplant personal hygiene." Again, this is similar to that described in the section on chemotherapy but even more rigorous.

Day 0

Day 0 is the transplant itself. After going through the conditioning regimen (not to mention all the events that led up to the transplant), many people find the transplant itself anticlimactic. The bag containing your precious stem cells is connected to your central line, and the marrow is slowly dripped into your blood, just like a blood transfusion. This takes several hours and is usually uneventful, although you may have some mild allergic reactions such as chills, fever, or hives. If the marrow has been frozen, you get to experience the unforgettable scent of DMSO.

Engraftment and recovery

After the transplant, you sit back and wait for the new stem cells to find their way to the proper sites inside your bones and start repopulating your body with blood cells. This process of engraftment usually takes several weeks but can take as long as a month. Many transplant centers will give you cytokines, such as granulocyte and macrophage colony-stimulating factor and erythropoietin, to help speed up the production of your new blood cells. You may experience bone and joint pain as the new marrow takes hold and starts manufacturing new blood cells.

During this time you are very vulnerable to infection. You will continue to observe all the precautions described above and will be carefully monitored for any signs of infection. In spite of all this care, most people undergoing transplants develop at least one infection. These infections can be treated with antibiotics. Some centers will start antibiotics prophylactically; others may wait until signs of infection—such as a high fever—occur. The antibiotics will be continued until your new white cells reach levels high enough to control infections on their own. You may also be given gamma globulin (the antibody-containing fraction of human blood). This may consist of general immunoglobulin or immunoglobulin targeted against specific pathogens.

Levels of blood cells, as well as your kidney and liver function, will be monitored with frequent blood tests. (You can see why getting a central line is so desirable.) Since your own marrow was obliterated prior to the transplant, levels of all your blood cells will drop, not just the white cells. Therefore, not only are you at risk for infection, but you will be anemic (low red cells) and at risk for bleeding problems (low platelets).

Because red cells and platelets develop more slowly than white cells, you'll need transfusions of both during the time your new marrow is engrafting. You may get whole blood transfusions or simply transfusions of packed platelets or red cells. Platelets may be needed daily, while red cells are usually given less often (once or twice a week). Whole blood and other blood products given post-transplant are irradiated to destroy any lymphocytes, since they could cause a graft-versus-host-like reaction, or otherwise depleted of white cells.

The first newly minted white cells generally start to appear in your blood two to four weeks after the transplant (even sooner, if you're getting cytokines). However, they may take some time to become fully functional. Neutrophils, for instance, start to appear between two and six weeks after the transplant but may not be fully functional for up to four months. While some cell types—such as natural killer cells—show up and are ready to go very soon after the transplant, other cell types—such as T cells and B cells—may take much longer.

Frequently, the balance of the different *types* of T lymphocytes is disturbed long after the transplant. You'll need to stay in the hospital until your blood cell levels have reached a point where you are reasonably safe from infection. While it may take months—or even years—for the levels of all your blood cells to return *completely* to normal, you can leave the hospital after they've reached certain minimal levels.

Usually, neutrophil levels need to reach 500 to 1,000 for two consecutive days before you can be released from the hospital. Ideally, you should no longer require platelet or red cell transfusions, with minimum platelet counts of 30,000 and a hematocrit of at least 30. This can take a month or two. You'll also need to be off antibiotics for at least two days without showing signs of infection; to have any nausea and vomiting under control; and to be able to eat.

You still need to check in frequently for blood work, bone marrow biopsies, and so forth. If you are at a transplant center that's far from home, you will need to stay somewhere local, so you can come in for checkups. Day 100 post-transplant is considered a big landmark. If everything has gone well and there have been no serious complications, you can cut down on your blood work, bone marrow biopsies, CT scans, and so forth. You may be able to get rid of your central line (yay!). If you live far from the transplant center, you will finally be able to return to your own home.

Even after being discharged from the hospital and passing Day 100, you will need to come in periodically for checkups. You will need to maintain strict rules about hygiene, avoiding crowds, eating only appropriate food, and so forth for the first six months. Gradually, as your new marrow takes hold and you begin to feel healthier and stronger, you will be able to return to the normal routines of your daily life.

Complications

There's no denying that undergoing a stem cell transplant is a rough experience, and various complications may arise. The likelihood and severity of these complications are greater in allogeneic than autologous (or syngeneic) transplants. These complications include graft-versus-host disease, graft failure, infections, and organ damage.

It can be scary to learn about things that might go wrong. In this discussion, it's important to remember that transplant methodologies (including supportive care) are improving all the time. Although complications still occur, the short-term treatment-related mortality for people undergoing autologous transplants at experienced centers is now less than 5 percent. In other words, 95 percent of people make it through.

Graft-versus-host disease

As discussed in more depth in Chapter 9, lymphocytes recognize foreign antigens and destroy cells carrying them. That's their job, and it's critical for normal immune function, but it poses a problem if the lymphocytes infused with the donor stem cells recognize *you* as foreign and start attacking the cells in your body. Since your own reinfused lymphocytes will still recognize you, graft-versus-host disease is a problem only with allogeneic transplants.

Graft-versus-host disease occurs in about 50 percent of allogeneic transplants. It's more likely to occur with an HLA mismatch and is more common with MUD transplants than with allogeneic transplants from close relatives. It is also more common (and more severe) in older individuals. This is a major reason for the age limits imposed on candidates for allogeneic transplants.

There are two forms of graft-versus-host disease: acute graft-versus-host disease, which develops within three months of the transplant, and chronic graft-versus-host disease, which can develop as long as three years after the transplant. Acute graft-versus-host disease is mediated by donor T cells. The skin, gastrointestinal tract, and liver are the sites most commonly attacked. Symptoms can be relatively mild or very severe.

Acute graft-versus-host disease of the skin may start out as reddening and burning of the palms of your hands and the soles of your feet. It can develop into a relatively innocuous rash that covers most of your body, or into severe blisters and skin ulcers, or even into large areas of your skin peeling and flaking off. Similarly, graft-versus-host disease affecting the gastrointestinal tract can be mild or can lead to severe nausea, vomiting and diarrhea, loss of the cells lining the intestine, bleeding from the intestinal tract, and a totally understandable inability to eat.

With liver involvement, increased levels of liver enzymes circulate in your blood, together with increased levels of metabolic products that are normally broken down by the liver. Liver graft-versus-host disease can be accompanied by swelling of your liver and *jaundice*, a yellowing of your skin and of the whites of your eyes that is caused by the buildup of these substances.

Chronic graft-versus-host disease develops more than three months after the transplant. It has been known to show up as long as two or three years post-transplant. You are more likely to get chronic graft-versus-host disease if you've had acute graft-versus-host disease, and it may be more common in people who have received PBSC transplants than those who have received marrow transplants.

Since most of the T cells present three months (or longer) post-transplant will have developed in your own body, they should no longer recognize you as foreign. Therefore, the causes of chronic graft-versus-host disease are less clearly understood than are those of acute graft-versus-host disease. The mechanism is probably similar to that underlying certain forms of autoimmune disease (also poorly understood) and may involve problems in T cell development. In fact, chronic graft-versus-host disease resembles such autoimmune diseases as scleroderma (which means scarring of the skin), rheumatoid arthritis, and lupus. A chronic inflammatory condition may develop in which thick, hard, scarlike tissue forms in your skin, joints, liver, or gastrointestinal tract. The mucous membranes lining your mouth and eyes may become dry and irritated. Your skin may become itchy and scaly, or darkened and very hard. You may develop jaundice or problems with bile flow because of liver involvement. Rarely, scar tissue may develop in your lungs, making breathing difficult.

People generally recover completely from mild attacks of graft-versus-host disease, but severe attacks can be fatal. Therefore, severe graft-versus-host disease is considered one of the most serious potential complications of allogeneic transplants. Since graft-versus-host disease is mediated by donor lymphocytes, it's generally treated with immunosuppressant drugs. These include high doses of corticosteroid hormones, like prednisone, and drugs that suppress T cells, like cyclosporine or tacrolimus.

These drugs inhibit the synthesis of a cytokine, IL-2, that stimulates T cell production (see Chapter 9) and therefore suppress the T cell proliferation that takes place in response to an antigenic stimulus. Methotrexate may be given as well. Cyclosporine also inhibits any of your own remaining T cells from attacking the donor marrow as foreign (which could lead to graft rejection).

Usually, some combination of these agents is given to *prevent* graft-versus-host disease in people who have received allogeneic transplants, and higher doses (or different combinations of drugs) are given to people who *develop* graft-versus-host disease in spite of this prophylactic therapy. Antibodies directed against T cells may be given as well. Chronic graft-versus-host disease of the skin is sometimes treated with PUVA therapy (see section on treatment of mycosis fungoides in Chapter 4), and photopheresis is used to treat more generalized forms of chronic graft-versus-host disease.

While immunosuppressive therapies like high-dose steroids or cyclosporine may be effective in controlling graft-versus-host disease, they increase the risk of infection. This can be problematic for someone who is already in an immunologically fragile state. Moreover, damage to your skin and gastrointestinal tract (as a result of either the conditioning regimen or the graft-versus-host reaction) gives pathogens easier access to your body. Therefore, the risk of serious infection is higher for people undergoing allogeneic transplants, and you and your doctors will need to walk a narrow tightrope between suppressing the negative aspects of the immune response and losing the beneficial ones.

Since donor T cells play a role in mediating graft-versus-host disease, researchers have tried depleting the donor stem cells of T cells prior to the transplant. Although T cell depletion *does* reduce the incidence of graft-versus-host disease, it has several unwanted side effects. The chances of a relapse are increased because T cells are also involved in the graft-versus-lymphoma effect. The process of T cell depletion also increases the likelihood that the new marrow will fail to engraft (see "Graft failure," below). Finally, T cell depletion increases the risk (usually *quite* low in people getting stem cell transplants) of developing an Epstein-Barr-virus (EBV)-related donor B cell lymphoma (see "Viruses and the pathogenesis of lymphoma" in Chapter 11), as sometimes occurs in people who are severely immunosuppressed. Therefore, T cell depletion isn't generally performed.

Allogeneic transplants hold great potential for cure for people whose own bone marrow is severely affected and who therefore can't undergo autologous transplants—but also the potential for frightening side effects. When graft-versus-host disease is conquered, it's likely that many more of us will be cured of lymphoma by allogeneic transplants, particularly those of us without HLA-matched siblings. Therefore, much research is aimed at developing strategies to preserve the beneficial effects of graft-versus-lymphoma effect while minimizing the risks of graft-versus-host disease.

Some of these strategies involve making sure that T cells are present—but only in the right place at the right time. Researchers have isolated donor T cells and used genetic engineering to insert a *suicide gene* into them. This gene allows the researchers to trigger the donor T cells into killing themselves without disturbing your other cells. For example, they have inserted a gene that causes cells to make a protein that converts certain antibiotics into a toxic substance. That way, the T cells can be included with the rest of the marrow, so they can suppress any EBV-related abnormal B cell proliferation, create a graft-versus-lymphoma effect, and promote engraftment. But if you started getting severe graft-versus-host disease, you could take an antibiotic and kill them off. You'd eventually go on to develop your own new T cells (missing the suicide gene) from the stem cells in the transplant.

Other research suggests that the *timing* of the T cell donation may be important, so that if you simply delay giving the T cells, you'll get the beneficial effects without the harmful ones. Still other research has suggested that the specific populations of T cells (and perhaps natural killer cells) that mediate graft-versus-host disease are distinct from those involved in the graft-versus-lymphoma effect. If this is true, cytokines could be used to enhance the action of the good T cells and suppress the activity of the bad ones.

Transplanters play various immunological tricks to try to induce the graft-versus-lymphoma effect. One approach has been to administer cytokines (including interferon, interleukin-2, interleukin-12, and interleukin-15) to increase the chance that the donor lymphocytes will recognize the tumor as a target and stimulate them into action. Another approach has been to administer cytokines that increase the production or function of other immune system cells that activate T cells (see Chapter 10). Paradoxically, low doses of the immunosuppressant drug cyclosporine work as well.

Researchers also hope that cytokines can be used to stimulate a graft-versus-tumor effect in people undergoing autologous transplants—without putting them at risk of graft-versus-host disease.

Graft failure

Graft failure, in which the donor stem cells fail to take hold and start producing new blood cells, is an equally serious complication (although less common). In this case, you are left without an immune system and without the ability to produce new red cells or platelets. This can occur in allogeneic transplants if you have any remaining T cells that recognize the donor stem cells as foreign and mount an attack. This type of graft rejection is more likely to occur in transplants with HLA mismatches. The immune suppressant drug cyclosporine can help prevent this sort of rejection. (It's used for this purpose in people with normal immune systems who get organ transplants.) As mentioned above, failure to engraft is also a problem with T cell-depleted stem cells.

If you undergo an autologous transplant after previously undergoing extensive chemotherapy, your stem cells may simply be too worn out to rally. If the surrounding cells in the marrow to which the stem cells must home are severely damaged (either from extensive chemotherapy or from the disease itself), engraftment may be a problem as well. Active infections, and certain drugs, including both some immunosuppressive drugs and some antibiotics, can also affect engraftment.

If you fail to engraft on the first try, don't give up hope. It's worth remembering the old maxim: "If at first you don't succeed, try, try again." Sometimes failure on the first attempt is followed by success on the second (or later) tries.

Infection

Stem cell transplants make people very susceptible to infection, particularly while engraftment is taking place. Transplant associated infections are very common. Though they aren't any fun, they *are* usually treatable. Since it's usually easier to prevent infections than to treat them once they become well established, many centers use prophylactic (preventive) antibiotics, and all centers are extremely vigilant about spotting the very first signs of infection.

Using colony-stimulating factors to speed neutrophil regrowth along with the superobsessive regimens designed to isolate a person from pathogens has minimized the incidence (and danger) of bacterial infections. These are now less common and less serious than they were in the early days of bone marrow transplants. Bacterial infections, if they do occur, can be treated with antibiotics. These infections may cause high fevers and often develop around your central line. The area may be sore to the touch and reddened. (But it won't have any pus, which requires the white cells you don't have—an unexpected benefit of being immunosuppressed.)

Fungal infections, parasitic infections, and viral infections may also arise. Fungal infections (such as *Aspergillus* and *Candida*) can be treated with their own classes of antibiotics, but they tend to be more resistant to treatment than bacterial infections. And the antifungal antibiotics tend to have more side effects than the antibacterial ones.

I took the antifungal drug fluconazole (generally used against *Candida*) for the chronic yeast infection I developed around the time I was diagnosed with lymphoma. I found fluconazole to be pretty innocuous, although some people develop nausea and vomiting with high doses. Amphotericin, though, which is the antibiotic of choice for *Aspergillus* infections, has been nicknamed "amphoterrible." It may cause fever and chills and will likely cause some red cell suppression (just what you need at this point!). Anyone taking amphotericin must be carefully monitored for possible kidney damage.

Pneumocystis carinii is generally considered a protozoal parasite, although recent research suggests that it's more like a fungus. Most familiar as causing an unusual form of pneumonia in people with AIDS, it's also a potential hazard when you are undergoing a stem cell transplant. It is frequently treated prophylactically with the antibiotic combination of sulfamethoxazole-trimethoprim and inhaled pentamidine. If, like me, you are allergic to sulfa drugs, an antibiotic called atovaquone can be substituted for the sulfamethoxazole-trimethoprim combination.

If you have had chicken pox (they can test your blood for antibodies to the chicken pox virus prior to the transplant), recurrence of the virus as shingles (herpes zoster) may occur. Shingles is associated with terribly uncomfortable (or even painful) blisters on your trunk or face. Latent herpes simplex virus may become activated to produce cold sores. Both shingles and cold sores can be controlled by the antiviral drugs acyclovir or valacyclovir; shingles can also be controlled with immunoglobulin directed against the virus that causes it. Acyclovir and valacyclovir are among those very rare drugs to be deeply cherished because they are not only very effective but essentially without side effects.

Cytomegalovirus infections, although less common now than previously, are sometimes a problem (primarily with allogeneic transplants). These are usually treated with another antiviral drug, ganciclovir, in combination with anti-cytomegalovirus immunoglobulin. Ganciclovir has the unwanted side effect of inhibiting white cell production; colony-stimulating factors can help combat this.

Organ damage

The conditioning regimen, which, after all, consists of powerful antineoplastic agents given at dosages beyond the usual dose-limiting toxicity, can cause organ damage. Usually this damage is temporary; sometimes it is permanent. The potential for organ damage is the reason you need to be in good health (other than your lymphoma), with your lungs, liver, and kidneys in good working order, to be a candidate for a transplant.

Total body irradiation (TBI) can irritate your lungs; although this irritation is usually temporary, it's a good idea to exercise to avoid developing a lung infection. Many transplant facilities have stationary bikes and other equipment available for patients undergoing transplants.

About 20 percent of transplant patients develop a liver condition called *veno-occlusive disease* (also known as sinusoidal obstruction syndrome). Veno-occlusive disease occurs when *fibrin*—a substance involved in blood-clotting reaction—becomes deposited in the blood vessels of your liver. This impedes the flow of blood out of your liver, causing liver swelling, pain, and impaired function. It is sometimes confused with graft-versus-host disease of the liver and is treated symptomatically until your liver has a chance to repair itself.

The kidneys are susceptible to damage by drugs in the conditioning regimen and by some antibiotics (like amphotericin) as well as some immunosuppressant drugs (like cyclosporine). For this reason, kidney function is very carefully monitored. If kidney problems occur, your drug dosages may need to be modified.

Long-term complications

Chronic graft-versus-host disease is the most common serious long-term complication of a stem cell transplant. It usually clears up within two or three years of the transplant, although it may last for as long as five years.

Myelodysplastic syndrome is another very serious potential complication. Myelodysplastic syndrome is a condition of ineffectual bone marrow. Your stem cells still grow and reproduce, but they don't develop into mature, functional blood cells. Serious in itself, it frequently develops into myelogenous leukemia. Although these conditions occasionally occur following other forms of chemotherapy, they are more common in people who have undergone autologous stem cell transplants. It is very unusual for people who have had allogeneic transplants to develop myelodysplastic syndrome.

The risk of developing myelodysplastic syndrome or myeloid leukemia may be greater if you have undergone TBI as part of the conditioning regimen or have taken the drug etoposide as part of a "priming" regimen to increase the levels of peripheral blood stem cells. At this point, the risk of developing myelodysplastic syndrome or leukemia is up to 5 percent of autologous transplantees by five years post-transplant and up to 10 percent of transplantees by ten years post-transplant. (The risk varies with the form of lymphoma you have and with the details of your conditioning regimen.)

Although myelodysplastic syndrome, myelogenous leukemia, and chronic graft-versus-host disease are the most serious long-term effects of a stem cell transplant, other potential long-term complications can influence your quality of life. Osteoporosis, a potentially life-threatening condition in which your bones become thin, fragile, and easily broken due to loss of calcium, is a frequent complication of bone marrow transplants. TBI may lead to development of cataracts. The lung and kidney damage discussed above may not be fully reversible. Many transplant patients lose their ability to have children. Children who undergo transplants may experience stunted growth. It's likely that you'll experience reduced energy and physical strength, as well as some abnormalities in immune function, for some time after the transplant.

Facing the real possibility of such serious complications can be discouraging. It's important to remember that, if your doctor recommends a transplant, it's because he or she thinks a transplant holds your best chance for a cure (or for long-term disease-free survival). If you are facing a transplant, it may be comforting to realize that a large study of people who had undergone transplants for various hematological conditions found that, of those surviving disease-free for two years after their transplant, about 90 percent went on to survive at least five more years. And that was people who underwent transplants over seven years ago! Since this is one area of oncology where advances continue to be made at a rapid pace, the outlook is even more positive for people undergoing transplants now.

I'm grateful to have survived eight years postdiagnosis without having to undergo a stem cell transplant. I sincerely hope that I never need one. But if I were to experience a relapse, with treatments for lymphoma in their current state, I'd unquestionably undergo an autologous transplant. It's not the greatest option in the world, but all things considered . . .

Nonmyeloablative, or reduced-intensity, transplants

An intriguing new approach to allogeneic transplants is the *nonmyeloablative*, or *reduced-intensity, transplant*, sometimes casually referred to as the *mini-transplant* or *transplant lite*. In contrast to the standard stem cell transplant, the conditioning regimen doesn't attempt to obliterate your own marrow. Instead, you are given a milder regimen and repeated infusions of stem cells. That way, the new stem cells can gradually take over the job of producing blood cells from your own marrow.

For indolent lymphomas, the conditioning regimen may include antineoplastic drugs that suppress normal lymphocytes (such as fludarabine), perhaps in combination with an immunosuppressant drug like cyclosporine. These drugs will inhibit your own lymphocytes from attacking and destroying the transplanted marrow. For aggressive lymphomas, additional antineoplastic drugs may be included—but not the superhigh-dose therapies that obliterate your marrow.

Reduced-intensity transplants not only may allow you to avoid some of the nastier side effects of high-dose chemotherapy but may also minimize the risk of graft-versus-host disease. Damage to normal tissue by high-dose chemotherapy can lead to release of cytokines. These cytokines may play an important role in activating the donor lymphocytes that attack your body. Since chemo-mediated damage will be minimized in the reduced-intensity procedures, production of such cytokines should be minimal as well.

Therefore, with the nonmyeloablative transplant, doctors hope to harness the graft-versus-lymphoma effect of allogeneic transplants without some of the more difficult side effects. This means that these transplants could be available to people who aren't strong enough to withstand the rigors of a standard allogeneic transplant. At this point, reduced-intensity transplants are a promising approach to lymphoma therapy and appear to be well tolerated. It remains to be seen whether they are curative as well.

SUGGESTIONS FOR FURTHER READING

Chao NJ, Emerson SG, Weinberg, KI. (2004). "Stem cell transplantation (cord blood transplants)." *Hematology* 2004:354–371.
Dykewicz CA. (1999). "Preventing opportunistic infections in bone marrow transplant recipients." *Transplant Infectious Disease* 1:40–49.
"Guidelines for preventing opportunistic infections among hematopoietic stem cell transplant recipients. Recommendations of CDC, the Infectious Disease Society of America, and the American Society of Blood and Marrow Transplantation." (2000). *Biology of Blood and Marrow Transplantation*, suppl., 6:659–713.
Horning SJ. (1997). "High-dose therapy and transplantation for low-grade lymphoma." *Hematology/Oncology Clinics of North America* 11:919–935.
Morrison VA, Peterson BA. (1999). "High-dose therapy and transplantation in non-Hodgkin's lymphoma." *Seminars in Oncology* 26: 84–98.
Salzman DE, Briggs AD, Vaughan WP. (1997). "Bone marrow transplantation for non-Hodgkin's lymphoma: A review." *American Journal of Medical Sciences* 313:228–235.

Online, BMT InfoNet provides a very useful resource, with a newsletter, a transplant center search form, patient-oriented books pertinent to stem cell transplants, and a program to put people facing a stem cell transplant in touch with others who have already gone through it. Note, however, that the version of the book on stem cell transplants available for free was published in 1992 (although later versions can be ordered): www.bmtnews.org/
Additional useful information is available at Blood and Marrow Transplantation Reviews mtr.cjp.com/

CHAPTER 7

Unconventional Therapies

Shortly after I was diagnosed with NHL, I started digging around on the Internet to try to find out my prognosis. The survival statistics I turned up were discouraging: they indicated that it was more likely than not that I'd be dead within the next few years. While my oncologist tried hard to sound encouraging, it was clear that she, too, thought the odds were stacked against me.

We've become so accustomed to the miracles that modern medicine regularly performs, it can be a shock to discover that, even with the best of care, sometimes the disease wins. It was hard to go from being a young, healthy person, planning to have a baby and embarking on the most exciting part of my career, to realizing that I probably wasn't going to survive the next few years. It's not surprising that, like many people faced with such a bleak scenario, I wanted to learn about alternatives. Once I got over the shock of the diagnosis, I was determined to do everything I could to tilt the odds in my favor. I decided to participate in the rituximab + CHOP clinical trial, and, in this same spirit, I decided to investigate the options that nontraditional complementary therapies had to offer.

Moreover, I was disgusted by the apparent lack of concern displayed by some of the medical professionals involved in my diagnosis. The first oncologist I saw laughed when he told me I had a tumor the size of a football and left me shivering in a hospital gown while he took a phone call setting up a poker game. His glib reassurances about the curability of Hodgkin lymphoma were no comfort once I was diagnosed with NHL.

Like many Americans, I had heard that practitioners of complementary medicine were caring and compassionate. Additionally, having read extensively about herbal medicine years earlier, I was convinced that a treasure trove of untapped knowledge about unconventional pharmacological therapies existed out there and could be useful. As a trained scientist, I hoped to be able to determine which of the unconventional approaches seemed the most promising. I have to admit that I ended up feeling disappointed with what I could find out about nontraditional approaches to cancer therapy. The main problem for me was the lack of solid scientific information about the efficacy of a given treatment. By *solid scientific information* I mean information obtained in *controlled clinical trials.*

In a controlled clinical trial, a group of patients is given the treatment under investigation, and what happens to them is compared with what happens to a similar group of people given the best standard therapy available. In a correctly designed clinical trial, patients with similar conditions are randomly assigned to the two groups prior to treatment. This serves to avoid biasing the results in favor of one treatment or the other. Also, trials should include a large number of patients to avoid the types of statistical flukes discussed in Chapter 11. It's also important to confirm the diagnosis of the people undergoing the trials pathologically and to have adequate follow-up and precise documentation of their response to treatment.

Unfortunately, much information on alternative cancer therapies hasn't been obtained this way (although this is now beginning to change). Many practitioners rely on anecdotal information based on their experiences with individuals outside a controlled setting. The problem with anecdotal evidence, such as "I knew a woman with lymphoma who started eating shiitake mushrooms and red grapes and has been in remission for twenty years," is that we're all individuals, with highly individualized circumstances.

Occasionally people undergo spontaneous remissions. That is, there is no apparent reason for the remission. If a given woman went into remission after adopting a given dietary regimen, it's possible that her dietary regimen cured her. It's also possible that she had a spontaneous remission, having nothing to do with her diet. And even if the regimen *did* cure her, it's possible that it was an idiosyncratic response that wouldn't work for anyone else. From an anecdotal report, there's no way of distinguishing between the various alternatives. It's only when we find that large numbers of people exposed to the same regimen respond in predictable ways that we can begin to accept that approach as valid. This doesn't mean that anecdotal evidence is *bad.* If I was convinced that a certain regimen was harmless, I might decide to try it based purely on anecdotal evidence (and, hey,

I *like* shiitake mushrooms and red grapes). However, it does mean that anecdotal evidence shouldn't be treated as a *valid alternative* to a conventional approach that has more evidence to back up its effectiveness.

Another problem is that some practitioners of unconventional therapies have failed to document their results in a way that allows them to be objectively evaluated. For instance, if you've never confirmed through a biopsy that a person has lymphoma, it's hard to know what to make of the observation that his or her lumps went away after a certain treatment. Maybe that treatment cured the person's lymphoma—or maybe the person didn't have lymphoma in the first place! And while it's great to learn that "Treatment X" made people feel better, it would be nice to know if they lived longer, too. And all too frequently, people who underwent conventional therapy as well as unconventional therapy are counted as "successes" for the unconventional regimen. There's no way to validly come to that conclusion under those circumstances.

In order to avoid feeling like a complete hypocrite here, I should add that, while conventional medicine generally relies on reliably obtained information and seems to be better at self-correcting in the long run than unconventional medicine, conventional cancer therapy, too, sometimes relies less on clinical trials than I'd like. Some doctors continue using therapies they "feel" have worked for their patients previously (essentially anecdotal evidence) rather than being guided by *evidence-based medicine* obtained in clinical trials. Evidence from trials called *comparison to historical controls* sometimes leads to adoption of new treatments that later turn out to be no better than the old ones. In these trials, the response of the treatment group to a new treatment is compared with what would be expected from people who have had the disease and have been studied in the past.

One experience with CHOP is a classic example of the type of pitfalls that await the unwary when they try to make treatment decisions in the absence of controlled clinical trials. In the 1980s, many oncologists abandoned CHOP for newer chemotherapy regimens because trials using historical controls indicated that the new regimens were superior. When controlled clinical trials were performed, however, it was found that CHOP not only was as effective as the newer regimens but also had fewer toxic side effects. Presumably the people in the earlier trials were in better shape than the average lymphomaniac, so their results were skewed toward better outcome. Or perhaps the centers where the early trials were performed were more experienced in treating lymphoma, so the participants received better overall care.

Although I cannot claim to be an expert on unconventional therapies, and since an exhaustive discussion of this area is beyond the scope of this book, I will offer my impressions of some unconventional approaches to cancer therapy. If you're interested in pursuing such options, I hope this discussion will provide a basic background to help you evaluate information in this area.

In this book, I consider unconventional or nontraditional therapies to be those that are out of the mainstream of conventional medical care. The therapies I discuss are *complementary therapies,* which are meant to be used *together* with conventional medicine. I do not discuss *alternative therapies*—therapies meant to be used *instead of* conventional medicine—for reasons I explain below. It may seem obvious, but it is worth stating that clinical trials are not included in the category of unconventional medicine. Although clinical trials utilize approaches that aren't yet accepted in mainstream practice (that's why they're called *trials*), they are designed to test the efficacy of a promising approach prior to including it in, or excluding it from, the mainstream. In this sense, they're part of the mainstream approach of conventional medicine.

My conclusions about unconventional therapies as applied to lymphoma follow.

First, I decided that it would be *very* unwise for someone with lymphoma to abandon conventional therapy and rely *exclusively* on unconventional therapies, which, under these circumstances, would be considered *alternative therapies.* It would be tragic if someone who could benefit from conventional medicine chose to take the unproved, alternative route and died prematurely as a result. This applies to people with less curable or even incurable (but still treatable) versions of the disease as well as to those of us with curable disease. We're getting close to the point where conventional therapies can prolong life until a real cure for these forms of lymphoma is found.

There is good reason to believe that some unconventional therapies can add to your quality of life when used as a *complement* to conventional therapy. Possibly some of the unconventional treatments may help prolong life as well.

Second, because the potential price of making an error is so very high, and because I realized, as a biologist, how very complex our bodies can be, I discussed any complementary therapy I was considering with my oncologist. She might not have answers to my questions, but she could at least steer me away from things that were *known* to be dangerous by the medical community. I also read as broadly in the medical literature as I could to try to make sure there was no possibility that anything I was considering might interfere with my conventional treatment (i.e., chemo, immunotherapy, or radiation).

My approach to unconventional therapies as a cancer patient was distinctly different from my approach to knowledge as a scientist. As a cancer patient, I was more concerned with saving my life than with determining the truth. I was less concerned with proving or disproving the validity of a given approach than I was with doing *anything* that might possibly help. As long as I was *convinced* it couldn't hurt me, I was willing to try anything that made sense (and even a few things that didn't) and wasn't painful, unethical, or financially unreasonable.

In all my research, I found no evidence of a cure for lymphoma among any of the alternative therapies I looked into. I think it's likely that there are herbal remedies that could be beneficial to us. I think they haven't been exploited yet because of a lack of sufficient credible information that would lead anyone to study them. I disagree very strongly with those proponents of unconventional medicine who believe that the "medical establishment" has suppressed information about potential cures out of motives of profit and greed. I am suspicious of the motives of charismatic practitioners of alternative cancer therapies who refuse to subject their methods to careful scientific scrutiny through clinical trials, claim they are victims of persecution by the establishment, or claim categorically to cure "cancer."

With this as a background, I'd like to discuss several complementary approaches to cancer therapy. Let me stress that you should *discuss any unconventional treatment you are considering with your physician.* The stakes are just too high to risk making a mistake because of a lack of accurate information.

For this discussion, I divide complementary approaches to cancer therapy into two general areas. The first, *lifestyle-oriented approaches,* includes exercise, diet, vitamin and mineral supplements, and psychosocial interventions. The second general area, *pharmacologically oriented approaches,* covers herbal medicine—including approaches that are currently popular in the United States and approaches that are practiced in other medical traditions. Somewhat arbitrarily, acupuncture is included in pharmacologically oriented approaches as a subset of traditional Chinese medicine.

Lifestyle-oriented approaches

In general, I feel more comfortable with lifestyle-oriented complementary approaches than with pharmacologically oriented ones. There are two reasons for this. The efficacy of several of these approaches, including those involving exercise and psychosocial intervention, in improving quality of life for people with cancer has been substantiated in clinical trials. Moreover, this group of therapies by its very nature seems less likely to pose unforeseen hazards than therapies that involve pharmacological agents like herbs.

Exercise

I was shocked to learn that Adriamycin, one of the antineoplastic drugs I'd be taking, could damage my heart. Moreover, I'd be getting radiation to my chest, which could also lead to heart damage. I'd always had low blood pressure, and it wasn't uncommon for the nurses checking it to tell me that I'd live to be a hundred.

Not only was the cancer a *direct* threat to the chances of that happening, but it began to look as though the *treatment* might be as well. It was obviously better to risk a heart attack somewhere down the line than to die of lymphoma within a few months, but it wasn't something I felt happy about. I decided to try to avoid this unwelcome prospect by getting my heart into the best shape possible. That meant exercise. Aerobic exercise. Enough to get my heart beating faster and my pulse rate up.

I also figured that if I began to put on weight once the chemo started to get my tumor under control, I'd rather that weight take the form of muscle than fat. That meant exercise, too. Overcoming my aversion to strenuous exercise, I asked my oncologist if it was OK for me to exercise while I was undergoing chemo, and she said it was a good idea and to go ahead.

My parents had given me a NordicTrack exercise machine for my birthday several years before so I could stay active once I stopped walking five miles a day. I had used it for six months or so and then gradually converted it into an exotic clothes hanger in a corner of the bedroom. As soon as my oncologist gave the go-ahead, Paul set it up, and I started a program of daily exercise.

When I started out, I could only Track for about a minute. Then, weak, exhausted, and out of breath, I'd lie down to recover. I set the machine so that there was *no* resistance to leg movement, and I didn't bother using my arms. I gradually worked up to thirty minutes a day, slowly adding leg resistance and arm movements. I diligently kept up my exercise regimen the entire time I was undergoing chemotherapy. Whenever I was tempted to skip a day, I'd think about my poor heart being attacked by the Adriamycin. That was always enough to get me going. By the time I completed chemotherapy, I felt better than I had in a long long time. I was stronger and had much more endurance. (Of course, much of this was due to resolution of the tumor.)

I didn't know it at the time, but undertaking a regular exercise regimen was probably one of the best things I could possibly have done for myself. While there have been relatively few controlled studies on the effects of exercise during chemotherapy and radiation, those few studies suggest that it *is* beneficial. Regular exercise may not only help prevent cardiac damage from drugs like Adriamycin but may also help reduce various unpleasant side effects of chemotherapy and radiation such as fatigue, pain, nausea, difficulty sleeping, and depression.

And, amazingly, a recent study showed that people undergoing high-dose chemotherapy in conjunction with autologous stem cell transplants who performed regular aerobic exercise had a shorter duration of neutropenia and a shorter duration of hospitalization than nonexercisers. Exercise seemed to help their new marrow take hold and start producing new white cells more rapidly. Since susceptibility to infection when your white cell counts are down is one of the most worrisome complications of bone marrow transplants, such an effect, if confirmed, could have very important implications.

Regardless of any effect on white cells, *anything* that makes you feel better while you're undergoing chemotherapy and radiation is worth considering. There are several studies suggesting that exercise can do that. As always, check with your oncologist to make sure there's no specific reason you should avoid exercise. And try to avoid getting blisters—which are a potential route for infection. If you get the go-ahead, exercise is a low-risk activity that may contribute substantially to your quality of life.

Diet

There's a lot of evidence suggesting that certain diets are linked to increased or decreased risks for developing certain forms of cancer. People who eat high-fiber diets may be less likely to get colon cancer than people who don't; people who eat lots of smoked meats or pickled vegetables tend to have higher rates of stomach and esophageal cancer than people who don't; smokers with a diet that's high in dark green and yellow vegetables are less likely to get lung cancer than smokers who hate vegetables. While links between *lymphoma* and diet are less clear-cut, what evidence there is suggests that the sort of diet generally accepted as reducing the risk of cancer is useful in preventing lymphoma as well.

Most generally accepted cancer preventive diets emphasize a few basic principles. These "basics" include getting much of your food from plant sources and limiting your intake of fat. Eating five or more servings of fruit and vegetables a day is desirable, as is eating whole-grain products (sorry, Atkins diet followers). It's important to include a *variety* of different foods from plant sources, rather than existing on a monotonous, highly repetitive diet. While it may be OK to consider ketchup one of your vegetables—in fact, tomato products are believed to help protect against prostate cancer—don't let it be your *only* vegetable. Eat high fiber foods—including whole grains, peas and beans, and most fruits and vegetables. (Both Thomas Hodgkin, of Hodgkin lymphoma, and Denis Burkitt, of Burkitt lymphoma, were early advocates of high-fiber diets.)

Vegetables in the cabbage family (such as broccoli, cauliflower, brussels sprouts), dark green leafy vegetables (such as spinach, kale, collards), and tomatoes contain substances that have been specifically linked to anticancer activity. Soy products (like tofu) and "oily fish" (like sardines, salmon, and tuna) may be beneficial as well.

High-fat food, particularly from (nonfish) animal sources—such as red meat—is considered undesirable, as is a diet high in salt-cured, smoked, and nitrite-preserved foods (bacon, corned beef, pastrami). While some dietary fat is necessary, fats from fish oils, olive oil, flaxseed oil, and nuts appear to be preferable to fats from animal sources or highly saturated plant fats—like hydrogenated margarine. (You can distinguish a saturated fat from an unsaturated fat by how likely it is to be solid at room temperature. Fats that are liquid tend to be less saturated than fats that are solid.) Drinking a lot of alcohol is discouraged.

A "cancer-prevention" diet is all very well and good for the population at large; the more important question for those of us who've already been diagnosed with lymphoma is whether such a diet is beneficial to us or simply amounts to locking the barn door after the high-fiber, β-carotene-rich tofu burgers have been stolen. This question turns out to be more complex than you might expect. There is no simple "yes or no" answer, but there are a number of points worth making.

People with lymphoma who are undergoing chemotherapy and radiation, particularly those who, like me, become profoundly cachectic and undergo severe weight loss and malnutrition before treatment, have special dietary needs. These needs are distinctly different from the needs of people on watch-and-wait or lymphoma survivors in remission. I'll discuss nutrition during therapy first and then diet guidelines in other circumstances.

Chemotherapy and radiation can be tough on your body. Not only the malignant cells you're targeting but also some normal healthy cells—including stem cells in your bone marrow and epithelial cells lining your intestines—are likely to be destroyed by the treatment. Maintaining a good diet can help you rebuild your body and repair any damage. It's important to get enough protein to be able to carry out this rebuilding. It's also important—particularly for people who are cachectic when starting treatment—to avoid losing more weight and becoming malnourished (not usually a problem for people undergoing regimens that involve prednisone!). Finally, you need to be careful about eating undercooked meat or raw "foods grown in earth" when you're neutropenic to avoid the risk of bacterial infection.

Some of the common side effects of chemo and radiation can make people avoid eating. These side effects range from nausea and changes in taste, which make food seem unappealing, to mouth sores and sore throats, which make food difficult to chew and swallow. Most oncologists believe that keeping up an adequate intake of calories—and particularly protein—is of paramount importance and outweighs any cancer-preventative value of the specific foods eaten. Thus, concerned about my emaciated state, my oncologist urged me to abandon my normal (reasonably healthy) diet and told me to gain more weight and eat everything Americans aren't supposed to eat.

The week spent vomiting on allopurinol before I went on chemotherapy left me with a very sore throat, and I found it difficult to get down any solid foods at all. For the first three weeks of chemo, I subsisted on small servings of oatmeal, cream of wheat, applesauce, lemon ice, and chicken broth. I drank one can of high-fiber Ensure or Sustacal a day. Desperate to get more calories into me, Paul smothered my oatmeal, cream of wheat, and applesauce in whipped cream.

Although many cancer survivors shudder in recalling their dietary experiences while undergoing chemotherapy, my food memories of this time are a pleasant haze of eating lots and lots of *doctor-sanctioned* whipped cream (which I generally avoid because of the fat content). *Note:* It's probably a good idea to avoid eating your favorite foods *right* before and after receiving chemotherapy so you don't associate them with the nausea you may feel at this time.

Someone I knew decided to go on a healthy, high-fiber diet while he was undergoing abdominal radiation. The ensuing diarrhea was so terrible, he considered terminating therapy! His oncologist advised him to hold off on the high-fiber diet until after the radiation therapy was complete. (But if you're on a potentially constipating chemotherapy regimen, like one including vincristine, it's important to eat enough high-fiber food. Pears, prunes, figs—or, if you can't eat solid food, high-fiber liquid supplements—will all work for this purpose.)

As I began to put on weight and get stronger, I returned to a more normal diet, eating a variety of vegetables and grains and keeping up my levels of dietary protein. Since, like many people who have become cachectic, my blood tests indicated that I was suffering from malnutrition, my doctor also recommended a daily multivitamin supplement.

Although people who are undergoing chemotherapy and radiation, and those whose lymphoma is actively progressing, need to be concerned about maintaining adequate supplies of protein and calories, this is less of an issue for those of us in remission or on watch-and-wait. For many of us, the question then becomes finding the optimal cancer-discouraging diet. Frustratingly, there's no clear way to go about this.

It seems reasonable to conclude that a diet that helps *prevent* cancer would be valuable to someone who already *has* cancer, but it ain't necessarily so. In fact, there's some evidence that certain vitamin supplements that may be cancer-protective might be the worst thing in the world for people who already have cancer (see "Vitamin and mineral supplements," below). While it's unlikely that diet alone can *cure* cancer once it has gained a foothold in our body, the balance of evidence favors diet playing some role in preventing cancer from developing. Since chemotherapy and radiation can themselves induce cancer, and since people with lymphoma have already proved that they're *susceptible* to cancer, it seems reasonable that those of us in remission might want to pay some attention to eating a healthy diet. Although the risk of chemo- and radiation-induced secondary cancers is low, there doesn't seem to be any good reason to *avoid* following the sort of diet that would tend to help you minimize your risks. You may wish to discuss the standard American Cancer Society–type cancer prevention diet with your oncologist and ask whether adopting such a diet plan (subject to modifications when you're actually undergoing chemotherapy and radiation) is a good idea.

Some practitioners of alternative medicine believe that more radical approaches to diet can be very beneficial—even curative—for people *with* cancer (including lymphoma). And that's another kettle of unpickled, oily fish entirely. This area is frustratingly difficult to research. There are tantalizing clues to suggest that some of these diets may be helpful, but there is no compelling evidence. While there are numerous anecdotal accounts of people who feel they've benefited from specialized dietary regimens and accounts of spontaneous remissions among people who radically changed their lifestyle (including their diet), this doesn't prove anything. We don't know everything *else* those people did; nor do we know how many people changed their diet and *didn't* have a spontaneous remission. Still, it's interesting.

In a few cases, researchers have attempted to organize such information into more formal studies. For example, studies of people with pancreatic cancer and prostate cancer have suggested that people who followed the macrobiotic diet survived longer than is typical for people with these conditions. Such results are intriguing—and made me wish that some carefully controlled research studies evaluating the macrobiotic diet had been performed—but these two studies were conducted and reported in such a manner that it was impossible to evaluate the efficacy of the macrobiotic diet. *Note:* The "general" macrobiotic diet is considered to be nutritionally adequate as long as you pay attention to getting enough vitamin D (primary sources: exposure to sunlight and fortified cow's milk) and vitamin B$_{12}$ (primary sources: animal products—such as fish—or yeast); it should not be confused with extreme variants that rely on grains alone.

Reading reports of attempts to validate unusual dietary regimens, I got the feeling that the reviewers who believed only in conventional medicine found them unconvincing, while the reviewers who already believed in unconventional medicine found them impressive. Not exactly the kind of rock-solid information you want to have when making a decision of this magnitude!

As long as you're careful to maintain adequate nutrition and check with your doctor first, and as long as you incorporate a variety of foods and don't flout the basic rules—for example, by eating raw "foods grown in earth" when you're immunosuppressed—most special diets are unlikely to hurt you and may help. If nothing else, following such a dietary regimen may allow you to feel like you're taking back control of your life from the lymphoma. That alone may be beneficial (see "Psychosocial interventions," below).

It's a good idea to talk over unconventional dietary regimens with a holistically oriented physician or someone with a Ph.D. in physiology or nutrition. Don't rely on friends or dietitians to understand all the nuances of diet that are important for people with lymphoma, particularly if you're undergoing therapy. If you experience rapid weight loss on a new diet, this may be a danger signal. Be sure to tell your physicians.

On the other hand, if the idea of subsisting on fruits and nuts and grains is anathema to you, and if you feel that life without sirloin steaks would be unbearable, don't let yourself be *forced* into such a regimen by well-meaning friends or relatives. Contrary to the view of alternative medicine practitioners as "kinder and gentler," some proponents of alternative medicine (fortunately a minority) preach the merits of "proper" diets with a strident fervor. I sometimes felt as though they were accusing me of having caused my own cancer by choosing to eat a rotten diet, failing to exercise enough, and having the wrong sort of personality.

Having always followed the sort of diet now considered healthy, and having walked miles a day for years (I couldn't do much about my personality), it was hard for me to avoid feeling betrayed. As I underwent chemotherapy, I noticed the media play given to various foods touted to prevent cancer. I also noticed how many of these "good" foods were part of my regular diet. Shiitake mushrooms! Red grapes! Green tea! Bean curd! Cruciferous vegetables! Tomatoes! Garlic! Sardines! Olive oil! It began to sound as though the newscasters had gotten hold of a copy of my grocery list.

"I did all the right things," I thought, "and I *still* got cancer."

I found myself becoming defensive when confronted with devotees of healthy lifestyles and started wondering whether some people became "true believers" in anticancer dietary regimens as a means of dealing with their own fears. If you can blame the cancer patient because of his or her lousy diet and careless ways, then you can believe that you, with your wholesome diet, are safe. I felt like screaming,

"I never ate a lot of hamburgers! Dealing with cancer is enough! I don't need this sort of guilt trip!"

And it's clear that diet can't be the whole cancer story. Some people with great diets get cancer; some people with lousy diets don't. While it's likely that diet plays a role in cancer prevention, it's not at all clear that this is true for lymphoma. And there's even less evidence that a cancer-prevention-type diet can really help those of us who already *have* lymphoma. Ultimately, the choice in this matter is yours.

Vitamin and mineral supplements

Vitamins and minerals are substances found in various foods that are required, in very small amounts, for our bodies to function optimally. Vitamins differ from minerals in that vitamins are organic—compounds made by living things that contain carbon—while minerals are inorganic (they don't contain carbon). Different vitamins and minerals have different roles. For instance, vitamin D helps the body absorb the mineral calcium and is required for strong bones, while vitamin A is required for good night vision (among other things). Many vitamins were identified because people with poorly balanced diets developed characteristic diseases that resulted from specific vitamin deficiencies.

Sailors at sea, for instance, who went for extended periods of time without eating any fresh fruits or vegetables developed the disease called *scurvy*, characterized by bleeding gums, poor wound healing, and severe bruising and hemorrhage. Many sailors died of scurvy before it was recognized that scurvy could be prevented by including citrus fruit, like lemons, limes, and oranges, in their diet; we now know that scurvy results from a deficiency in vitamin C and that citrus fruits are a good source of this vitamin. Vitamin C plays a critical role in the synthesis of a protein that is required for properly functioning blood vessels. If we don't eat enough vitamin C, our blood vessels become weak and easily damaged—leading to the symptoms of scurvy.

As I've already mentioned, a diet deficient in the mineral iron can lead to a form of anemia, since iron is required for the manufacture of *hemoglobin*, the red pigment in blood that carries oxygen to all your tissues. Similarly, diets missing other required vitamins and minerals can lead to other disease states because the body is unable to carry out whatever specific functions those vitamins serve. However, just because a little is good, it doesn't mean that a lot is better. *Excess* vitamins and minerals can be bad for you, too. Too much iron, for instance, increases your risk of heart attacks, and too much vitamin E can make you bleed more easily.

The epidemiological studies showing that people who ate diets high in vegetables, grains, and fibers were less likely to get cancer sparked a lot of interest in why this is so. Presumably, the results of these studies mean that substances found in these foods help protect us from cancer. Therefore, once certain foods were associated with a decreased incidence of cancer, researchers looked to see what substances were found in these foods at especially high levels. Some of the substances identified in "cancer-preventative" foods were vitamins and minerals; others had no known role in nutrition (other than possibly helping prevent cancer). If specific foods that appear to protect against cancer are high in certain substances, it makes sense to wonder whether these substances provide the protection.

In many cases, substances found in the foods that were associated with a decreased risk for developing cancer had properties that were consistent with a role in cancer prevention. For instance, many vegetables are high in colored compounds called *carotenoids*. Probably the most familiar of these carotenoids is β-carotene, a *precursor* to (a substance that is made into) vitamin A. β-carotene is found in dark green leafy vegetables, like spinach and kale, and deep yellow or orange vegetables and fruits, like carrots, pumpkins, and mangoes. As previously noted, smokers with diets high in these fruits and vegetables have lower rates of lung cancer than do smokers with diets low in such vegetables.

TREATING LYMPHOMA

How could β-carotene prevent smokers from developing lung cancer? A lot of attention has focused on β-carotene's ability to act as an *antioxidant*. Antioxidants are substances that can protect your cells against damage caused by a class of molecules called *free radicals*. Free radicals are highly reactive molecules that interact with—and damage—critical components of your cells including the DNA. Free radicals are normal by-products of cell metabolism, but they have also been implicated in the actions of many carcinogens. While *severely* damaged DNA will lead to suicide on the part of the involved cell, less severe damage can lead to the types of mutations that are involved in carcinogenesis.

Antioxidants like β-carotene, then, could help protect smokers from lung cancer by protecting their DNA from the damage caused by free radicals. And, excitingly, researchers have showed that antioxidants like β-carotene were beneficial in experimental models of carcinogenesis. The epidemiological findings that the risk of lung cancer was lower among people whose diets were high in β-carotene, together with a plausible mechanism of action, led to great excitement about the idea of using dietary supplements of β-carotene (and other antioxidants like vitamin C, vitamin E, and the mineral selenium) for cancer prevention. After all, if you live on bacon cheeseburgers, ice cream sundaes, and french fries, it's a lot easier to swallow a daily β-carotene vitamin pill than it is to switch to a high-grain, semivegetarian dietary regimen.

When this theory was actually *tested*, however, β-carotene didn't perform as advertised. In a large-scale trial of the effects of vitamin supplements on the risk of lung cancer in 29,000 Finnish male long-term smokers, there was an 18 percent *increase* in the incidence of lung cancer among the group given β-carotene. The smokers who took β-carotene supplements were more likely to get lung cancer than the smokers who didn't take supplements. Similarly, another large-scale study on the potential benefits of β-carotene on 18,000 smokers, former smokers, and asbestos workers was terminated early when it became apparent that the smokers who took β-carotene were getting lung cancer at higher rates than those who didn't. A third study, on 20,000 U.S. physicians, showed no effect one way or the other.

What could explain these results? Right off the bat, I can think of three possibilities. Either β-carotene doesn't help protect smokers from lung cancer but just happens to be present as a bystander in the cancer-protective foods, or β-carotene is protective only when it's eaten in combination with *other* substances found in β-carotene-rich foods, or β-carotene helps prevent free radicals from damaging DNA but, for long-term smokers, this is actually harmful rather than beneficial. That could happen if those smokers already had some cells with DNA damage (early localized cancer or precancerous cells) and, by minimizing *further* DNA damage, the β-carotene kept these moderately damaged cells from getting killed off. Whatever the explanation, if I were a long-term smoker, I don't think I'd take β-carotene supplements.

Just to confuse the issue a bit, a synthetic vitamin A derivative has been shown to protect against second cancers in high-risk people who previously have had head or neck cancers (this compound is fairly toxic and is therefore recommended only for people at high risk for getting cancer). A study of 30,000 people in China indicated that people taking *combinations* of antioxidants (including β-carotene) experienced a decrease in deaths from stomach cancer. Furthermore, the Finnish smokers who took vitamin E had a lower incidence of prostate cancer (not something the study set out to investigate). They also had a higher incidence of hemorrhagic stroke—so vitamin E isn't necessarily a panacea, either.

All of this research suggests that the effects of dietary supplements are complicated and that we really don't completely understand the interactions between cancer prevention and the different—presumably beneficial—compounds found in food. The bulk of the evidence suggests that it's a good idea to eat a diet that's rich in a variety of vitamins, minerals, antioxidants, and other presumed cancer-protective substances. Since people with cancer are frequently malnourished (sometimes as an effect of the cancer itself, sometimes as an effect of the treatment), it's probably a good idea to take a daily multivitamin supplement (ask your doctor first and use a reputable, well-known brand). But if you venture into the realm of self-treatment with large doses of dietary supplements, you're entering uncharted, potentially hazardous territory.

Many people realize that they need to be careful about taking large doses of the fat-soluble vitamins (A, D, E, and K), since these vitamins can accumulate in your body; indeed, the toxic effects of overdoses of vitamins A, D, and K are well known. However, for people with lymphoma, excessive intake of even the water-soluble vitamins, which are excreted daily in your urine, may pose some risk.

People who are severely deficient in folic acid (or folate), a water-soluble vitamin in the vitamin B complex, develop a form of anemia called *megaloblastic anemia.* In people with megaloblastic anemia, DNA synthesis (and therefore chromosomal replication and cell division) in developing red cells is inhibited. This leads to a reduction in the numbers of circulating red cells; those that are produced grow to be larger than normal, since cellular proteins continue to be synthesized even though the cell doesn't divide on schedule.

For a year or two prior to my diagnosis with NHL, I had been trying to become pregnant. Because I knew that folate deficiencies in pregnant women can lead to a birth defect in their children called spina bifida, I had started taking dietary supplements of folic acid. Vaguely remembering that there was some connection between folate deficiency and anemia, I increased my folic acid supplements as my anemia progressed. And, indeed, a series of blood tests taken when I was diagnosed showed a general state of malnutrition (consistent with my dramatic weight loss and problems absorbing iron) but very high levels of serum folate.

Shortly after my diagnosis, I read about the children whose leukemia got worse when they were given folic acid (see the discussion of methotrexate in Chapter 3). Horrified, I wondered if, in attempting to protect an unconceived child from spina bifida, I had somehow fostered the growth of a small, manageable tumor into the football-sized monstrosity with which I was diagnosed. This certainly seemed possible.

On the other hand, it's also possible that I protected the rest of my body from experiencing a folate deficiency as the tumor greedily used up my normal supplies of dietary folate. There's evidence suggesting that high intake of folic acid protects against some forms of cancer (breast cancer and colon cancer). And the high levels of folate in my body may have helped me rebuild populations of normal cells damaged during chemotherapy. In fact, animal studies suggest that rats with breast cancer are better able to cope with chemotherapy if they receive dietary supplementation with folic acid.

At this point, it's impossible to say whether those folic acid supplements helped me, hurt me, or had no effect at all. And if I became pregnant now, I'd certainly start taking folate supplements again. Still, the folic acid experience gave me a healthy respect for the possible unforeseen consequences of taking seemingly beneficial and presumably innocuous dietary supplements. Recent research has suggested that even vitamin C—long beloved by proponents of alternative medicine as a cancer preventative—may actually be taken up and *used* by some cancer cells. Therefore, before taking *any* dietary supplement as an adjunct to conventional therapy, I'd be sure to read as much about it as I could as well as discussing it with my oncologist.

Antioxidants during treatment

A question of particular concern to those of us undergoing chemotherapy or radiation is whether it's a good idea to take antioxidants—like vitamins A, C, and E and the mineral selenium—during cancer therapy. As I said a little earlier, antioxidants can protect us from the cellular damage caused by free radicals. Many chemotherapeutic agents (and ionizing radiation) promote free radical production inside cells. The DNA damage resulting from the action of these free radicals is probably involved in the worst long-term side effects of these therapies—secondary cancers. The cardiac damage caused by Adriamycin likely involves free radicals as well.

Some proponents of complementary medicine advocate taking antioxidants during treatment to minimize the chances of these potential side effects. This seems to make sense, and some evidence suggests that taking antioxidants during chemotherapy *can* protect you from heart damage (from Adriamycin), lung damage (from bleomycin), kidney damage (from cisplatin), neutropenia, and hair loss. Free radicals may, however, be involved in the *therapeutic* action of these drugs as well in their side effects. And you don't want to protect yourself from side effects at the expense of protecting your cancer from destruction.

I agonized over this decision the entire time I was undergoing treatment. I decided that I wasn't going to do anything that could possibly interfere with the efficacy of my chemotherapy. My doctor's statement that we had *one chance* to save my life had made a big impression, and I decided that I wasn't about to blow that chance. I thought about taking antioxidants during the middle week of the three-week CHOP cycle (after the chemo drugs had left my body, but not right before I got the next dose). I finally decided not to fool around with it: the risks of secondary cancers from CHOP are very low, and I figured I'd count on exercise to protect my heart from the Adriamycin. As for saving my hair at the risk of protecting my lymphoma—well, that was too absurd to even consider. I did continue to take a multivitamin supplement and to eat antioxidant-rich foods.

If I had an incurable lymphoma, though, and needed to take one of the alkylating agents for an extended period of time, I might revisit the idea of taking antioxidants during therapy. I'd talk it over very carefully with my oncologist before coming to any decision, however, and probably with a nutritionist as well.

The decision about whether to take antioxidants during radiation was much harder. After all, by the time I underwent radiation therapy, it wasn't clear that there was any viable tumor left. Why shouldn't I try to protect myself from potentially horrific side effects like lung cancer and breast cancer and thyroid cancer? Animal studies from the literature were sparse and had conflicting results. I could find very little information pertaining to humans.

"Why haven't researchers done these studies?" I thought. "What's wrong with the cancer establishment?" (It finally occurred to me that, once someone realized that taking antioxidants during therapy might be harmful, no one could ethically carry out these studies.)

I talked with my radiation oncologist.

"I don't know," she said; "*no one* really knows. But, if it were me, I wouldn't take them. I tend to be conservative."

I talked with the hospital dietitians.

"No, no, don't take antioxidants," they said; "they could protect the tumor." A little later in the same conversation they suggested that, if I developed mouth sores or a sore throat while undergoing radiation therapy, I should puncture a vitamin E capsule with a needle and let the contents drip on the mouth sores and down my throat.

"But vitamin E's an antioxidant!" I said in horror. "You just said *not to take antioxidants!*"

"Oh," they said, "that's right. Then don't take vitamin E. Try vegetable oil."

I sent out a question on the listserve. The one person who'd spoken with medical professionals said he'd been told to avoid antioxidants during radiation.

Here was an opportunity for me to actually do something positive for myself. I could take antioxidants and protect myself from getting a radiation-induced cancer. But what if I made the wrong choice? I was frozen with indecision. Should I take antioxidants to protect myself from secondary cancers? Or would I take antioxidants and end up protecting the tumor? I eventually decided not to take antioxidants during radiation. I decided to let the death rays do their work unmolested. I'd just have to hope that any secondary cancer would be curable by the time it surfaced.

Psychosocial interventions

Another complementary approach involves psychosocial interventions—that is to say, approaches to dealing with lymphoma that are aimed at influencing the person's state of mind. The idea behind psychosocial approaches is that the state of your mind can influence the state of your body (and vice versa). There's a fair amount of evidence to suggest that this basic idea is true: it's well known that people who've experienced severe losses—the death of a parent, spouse, or child—are at increased risk of dying themselves during the following year. People who are unhappily married tend to have more medical problems than those who are happily married.

It's not entirely clear why this should be. People who are grieving or chronically unhappy may be less likely to take care of themselves than usual, and the resulting changes in their behavior and lifestyle (eating poorly, driving carelessly, abusing alcohol or drugs, or sleeping less) may make them more likely to get sick or have an accident. This is an indirect way in which the state of your mind can influence the state of your body. However, at least part of the effect may involve a more direct influence of the mind on the body.

There's some evidence that psychological factors can play a role in influencing our body's ability to deal with cancer. Some research suggests that psychological factors like stress and depression can make it more difficult to fight cancer. Animal studies suggest that animals with cancer that were subjected to stress showed more rapid progression of their tumors than animals in relatively stress-free environments. A study of women with early-stage breast cancer found that the women who remained severely depressed and had sustained feelings of hopelessness were less likely to survive for five years than those who didn't. On a more hopeful note, there's some evidence to suggest that some psychologically or behaviorally oriented interventions can be beneficial for people with cancer.

Two controlled studies have indicated that people with cancer who participated in small groups focused on psychological support, stress management, and/or education about their condition lived longer than those who did not participate. (Everyone in both the control and experimental groups got standard medical therapy.) In the first study, women with metastatic breast cancer who participated in support groups approximately doubled their survival time compared with women receiving similar therapy who didn't participate in support groups. In the second study, more people with early-stage melanoma who participated in support and educational groups were alive after five or six years compared with the people who didn't participate in these groups.

Some of the benefits of attending support groups may have resulted simply from improved health habits or enhanced compliance with treatment. People in the support groups might have been more careful about taking at-home medications, keeping appointments with their doctors, and avoiding infections when they were undergoing chemotherapy. In fact, studies have shown that the *majority* of people with hematological cancers like lymphoma and leukemia slip up on taking medications at home unless they've undergone some sort of educational program.

A controlled study on the effects of educational programs on the survival of people with hematological cancers showed that such programs led to increased compliance with treatment. As you'd expect, survival was related to such compliance. These behavioral changes couldn't completely account for the observed increase in survival, however. This suggests that the psychological benefits of the educational program may have played some *direct* role in enhancing survival.

How could a psychological intervention like attending a support group influence ability to survive cancer? While the answer is not clear-cut, it could be that complex interactions between our brain, the endocrine glands that secrete hormones, and the cells of our immune system affect the course of disease. Researchers have been particularly interested in exploring how biological or psychological stress—and therefore anything that leads to stress reduction—can affect our body by influencing a part of the brain called the *hypothalamus.*

The idea of mind-body interactions becomes less mysterious when we remember that neurons—the cells that make up our brains—communicate with each other, as well as with the rest of the body, by means of chemical messages. Anyone who's ever taken an antidepressant or a tranquilizer, or even had a few drinks, knows that chemicals can affect our mind. These *psychoactive* chemicals interfere with the normal chemical signals that are passed between neurons. It's also possible that our state of mind may be reflected in the particular balance of chemical messages our neurons put out.

Our brain also controls our *body* by means of chemical messages. Some of these messages are *voluntary*—for instance, the messages that allow us to control the muscles that let us move around. Our decisions to send voluntary messages are conscious: right now I'm making conscious decisions to move the muscles in my hands, arms, and fingers that permit me to type this sentence. Other messages are *involuntary*—for instance, the messages that control our heart rate, blood pressure, digestive function, hormone levels, and so forth. These involuntary functions, which are generally *not* controlled by conscious decisions, are regulated by the *autonomic nervous system.*

The autonomic nervous system is largely controlled by the hypothalamus. The hypothalamus also regulates the function of various endocrine glands—glands, like the pituitary, thyroid, and adrenals, that secrete hormones—by means of chemical messengers secreted into the blood. The hypothalamus can bring about profound physiological changes in bodily function either through the autonomic nervous system or through regulation of the endocrine glands (or both together).

When we are confronted with an emergency, the hypothalamus sends "emergency" messages out through our *sympathetic nervous system*—the part of the autonomic nervous system that prepares our body to cope with danger. Our heart rate goes up to help pump blood to our muscles, the sugar concentration in our blood goes up to provide a source of ready energy, and our pupils dilate so that we can see better. Some of these responses result directly from the action of chemical messengers released from the nerves in our sympathetic nervous system on target tissues, while others depend on hormones released from our adrenal glands in response to sympathetic stimulation. Once the emergency has passed, our blood pressure and so forth return to normal.

Under conditions of prolonged stress, in which sympathetic stimulation becomes chronic, physical problems like high blood pressure, muscular tension, or irregular heart rate may develop. Moreover, the chronic effects of increased hypothalamic activity that are mediated through chemical messengers released into the blood can also lead to problems. These chronic hypothalamic signals lead to increased secretion of a class of hormones from the adrenal cortex—called *glucocorticoids*—that have profound effects on all the systems of our body.

Glucocorticoids influence carbohydrate, protein, and fat metabolism; they also reduce inflammation and suppress the immune response. Some biological stresses—like infection—can lead to massive release of cytokines by the cells of the immune system; a stress-induced increase in glucocorticoid secretion protects us from potentially catastrophic effects of this massive cytokine release.

Conceivably, the mind's effects on our health—including our ability to deal with cancer—could be mediated through this constellation of the hypothalamus, the autonomic nervous system, and the endocrine system. In this context, a great deal of attention has focused on glucocorticoid inhibition of the cells of the immune system. If our immune system *does* play a significant role in protecting us from cancer, then chronic elevation of our glucocorticoids (and a glucocorticoid-induced diminution of an immune response) could promote tumor growth.

In this scenario, the social support derived from attending a group therapy session could lower stress and therefore reduce production of glucocorticoid hormones. (It's likely that other psychological and physiological mechanisms are involved as well.) Similarly, practicing meditation can be a deliberate means of reducing stress and perhaps inducing a more beneficial state of bodily function.

Autonomic functions aren't ordinarily under our conscious control, but we can learn to regulate them. People trained in yoga have demonstrated amazing control over autonomic functions such as heart rate and temperature. More recently, Western medicine has made use of *biofeedback devices* to teach people to regulate autonomic functions like blood pressure. Such devices measure some specific aspect of autonomic function—like blood pressure—and "reward" you whenever you change it in the desired direction. Many people have learned to control their blood pressure with these biofeedback devices—even if they don't know exactly how they're doing it.

The success of techniques like biofeedback implies that we are able to exert some control over our "involuntary" functions. This isn't as surprising as you might imagine: while the hypothalamus itself isn't involved in conscious thought, it receives input from parts of the brain that are. The idea that our conscious thoughts could influence the state of our body has led some people to use mental imagery as a device to focus our mind on fighting our lymphoma. The idea behind imagery is that *thinking* about a particular activity can cause an appropriate physiological response. If thinking very hard about eating a delicious meal can make you feel hungry—and even salivate—maybe thinking about your immune system vanquishing your lymphoma could activate such a response from the immune system.

People who use imagery visualize their lymphoma being cleaned from their body. This visualization can be very concrete—the different cells in the immune system recognizing, fighting, and overcoming the lymphoma; more abstract—a wave of blue light sweeping through the body to cleanse it of malignant cells; or highly symbolic—a knight sweeping down to destroy a lymphoma dragon. It depends on what feels comfortable for you. Some people prefer to develop their own personal imagery; others prefer to use professionally prepared guided imagery tapes.

To summarize what I've learned about psychosocial influences on health, in general, and cancer, in particular: there's some evidence that cancer survivors who participate in support groups do better, on the whole, than cancer survivors who don't. This trend seems to hold true for the factors that influence the level of social support you experience in general—marital status, contact with family and friends, community ties. There's evidence that stress can decrease the immune response and influence tumor growth in animals. There's *some* evidence that stress and other psychological factors can influence the human immune response. Meditation, relaxation, and imagery can certainly help you feel more relaxed and less anxious and can help you control pain. There's also evidence that these techniques are beneficial in certain disease states.

Whether these techniques can help you conquer cancer is much less clear. Although it's likely that the immune system plays *some* role in protecting us from cancer, it's not clear how important a role this is. Many tumors have figured out ways to avoid even the most vigilant immune systems. And while stress can suppress the immune response, it's not clear that the *magnitude* of this effect is sufficient to make much difference in your ability to deal with cancer. On the other hand, the people in the support groups really *did* seem to do better—although other studies have failed to confirm an effect of support groups on survival.

I ended up filing psychosocial interventions in the "Can't hurt. Why not?" pile. My search for a support group led me to the NHL mailing list. For me, at that time, an electronic support group was probably even better than a face-to-face support group. I didn't need to venture out into the New England winter; I didn't need to worry about catching the flu when I was immunosuppressed. And I could write in at any hour of the day or night.

I don't know whether participating in the NHL mailing list helped me make it into remission. I do know that it was invaluable to find a community of people experiencing the same thing that I was: it kept me from feeling completely alone. This was particularly important for me, since I hadn't really developed a sense of home or community so soon after moving to start a new job. The people on the list were always available. I continue to correspond with some of the fellow lymphomaniacs I met on the NHL list and count them among my closest friends.

Additionally, I did everything I could to eliminate unnecessary stress from my life. I spent time talking with my family and old friends. I took up imagery and meditation: I spent about an hour a day doing a combination of guided imagery with a professional tape and my own personal imagery sequence.

It did occur to me that, given that glucocorticoids like prednisone act against not only normal lymphocytes but *malignant* ones as well, avoiding stress—and presumably stress-induced glucocorticoid production—might be just the wrong tack to take with lymphoma. Rather than stress out about this as I did about the antioxidants (creating *more* glucocorticoids, no doubt!), I decided, in this case, to simply go with what "felt right." I'd been under tremendous stress from my job in the two years before diagnosis. Since glucocorticoid suppression of immune responses is a purely speculative mechanism for the possible cancer-promoting effects of stress, and since one of the social support studies specifically involved people with lymphoma, I decided to trust my hypothalamus to respond to meditation, social support, and stress reduction by promoting the right chemical balance rather than the wrong one.

Going with what "felt right" led me to some unexpected places. After I finished chemo and radiation, Paul and I took a vacation at a hot springs health sanctuary. While we were there, I noticed a brochure for "Tibetan Singing Bowl

Healing." I assumed that this was some sort of meditation/relaxation technique and decided to try it.

After the session (which was indeed relaxing), the healer told me that she felt very strongly that I needed to meditate on my "karmic point," which she described as the area midway between the heart and the throat. Midway between the heart and throat is a pretty good description of the anterior mediastinum. This was where my lymphoma started and where the residual mass remained. I didn't know what (if anything) it all meant, but having ceased practicing my antilymphoma imagery once I was in remission, I took up Tibetan Singing Bowl meditation.

I have no idea whether any of the imagery/meditation/stress reduction techniques helped my cancer go into remission. And I certainly wouldn't use them *instead* of traditional medicine. I doubt that these mechanisms are powerful enough, on their own, to fight off an established cancer. Nor do I think they can cure an incurable one. On the other hand, I wouldn't be surprised to learn that they can help. A medically induced remission from aggressive lymphoma can last a lifetime or a scant few weeks. Who's to say that psychological influences couldn't help tilt the balance one way or the other? The factors that regulate remission duration of indolent lymphomas are poorly understood. Who's to say that shifts in the cellular environment similar to those produced by activation (or inhibition) of different autonomic responses might not prolong or even initiate such remissions?

Practicing meditation, relaxation, and imagery helped me feel happier and more at peace during this time than I would have otherwise. They helped lift me out of the depression I'd fallen into right after the diagnosis. And for me, these benefits alone were worth the time invested.

Pharmacological approaches
Herbal Medicine

In this section I discuss the types of herbal regimens that have become popular in the United States today, either because they've been advocated by an individual—such as the Essiac therapy developed by Rene Caisse or the Hoxsey treatment developed by Harry Hoxsey—or because they are part of a general trend toward using "natural" remedies to treat illness, particularly those believed to stimulate the immune system.

When I was in college, I wanted to be an ethnobotanist—someone who traveled to remote places in the world to speak with people of different cultures and learn how they used plants for healing. I read a lot of books about herbal medicine, learned to recognize the wildflowers that grew in my neck of the woods, and pictured myself floating down the Amazon learning about plants from the indigenous peoples. Treating illness with teas brewed from the plants that were traditionally used by people who lived close to nature somehow seemed more appealing than swallowing some pills from a bottle purchased in the pharmacy.

Somewhere along the line, I realized that I wouldn't make a good ethnobotanist. I'd lose my glasses in the thickest part of the jungle, float into piranhas while swimming in the Amazon, step on venomous snakes in remote regions of the world. I shifted gears, went to graduate school to learn neurobiology, and ended up doing my exploration within the four walls of the laboratory.

My interest in herbal medicine was reawakened when I got lymphoma and decided to look into alternative cancer therapies. Herbal medicine had become extraordinarily popular. The pharmacy aisles in the supermarket were lined with products featuring echinacea and ginkgo and Saint-John's-wort.

"Great," I thought, "there'll be lots of information on applying herbal medicine to cancer."

Unfortunately, while there *is* a lot of information about applying herbal medicine to cancer, so far there's little in the way of controlled clinical studies to document the benefits of herbal therapies (although this is now beginning to change). I was unable to come up with any herbal approaches to treating cancer that seemed unequivocally beneficial—or even unequivocally harmless. Therefore, in spite of my initial interest in herbal medicine, I discovered that I'd grown a long way from my pro-herbal roots. I eventually opted against using *any* herbal remedies against my lymphoma.

Unlike many detractors of herbal remedies, I don't dismiss herbs as worthless and ineffective. I think that herbs and related therapies can have *very* powerful effects on our body: long before I developed lymphoma, I discovered that I couldn't take ginseng because it disrupted my menstrual cycles. I drink cranberry juice when I have a urinary tract infection. Natural remedies can sometimes help with symptoms of cancer or side effects of treatment. Ginger tea (or candied ginger) may combat nausea, the beneficial bacteria in kefir and yogurt may help overcome yeast infections, and black cohosh may alleviate the symptoms of chemotherapy-induced menopause. It's critical, though, to discuss even such apparently innocuous remedies with your doctor: ginger can inhibit platelet function and therefore shouldn't be used by people who are anemic or have low platelet levels; people undergoing stem cell transplants are advised to avoid un-pasteurized dairy products and yogurt containing live cultures.

However, I'm not convinced that the herbs used in alternative therapy to treat cancer actually do what we want them to do. My concerns about people using herbs to treat their lymphoma center around two main issues: we have no real proof that they work, and we don't really know what they're doing. I'll consider both of these issues in turn.

Do they really work?

Many of the herbs used in alternative cancer therapies have shown effects that are consistent with anticancer activity. For instance, burdock root (which may be toxic at high doses) lowers the mutation rate in cells exposed to carcinogens. This effect suggests that burdock root could help prevent cancer from develop-ing in the first place or perhaps help inhibit progression from a low-grade can-cer to a more aggressive one. Other herbs have shown antitumor activity against animal cancers or on human cancer cells grown outside the body. In general, though, such antitumor effects have tended to be inconsistent—one study shows an effect and another doesn't—and not terribly impressive.

Regardless of the possible effect (or lack of effect) of herbs on cancer in ani-mals or on cells grown outside the body, the critical point is whether they work on cancer in living people. Unfortunately, there's very little evidence that they do. While advocates of some herbal regimens can produce anecdotes galore, at-tempts to systematically analyze the records of patients treated with these regi-mens by people who weren't involved in administering the treatments have been disappointing.

As an example of what I mean by this, I'll discuss Essiac, which is one of the best-known herbal cancer therapies. I don't mean to "pick on" Essiac here—I could use any one of a number of herbal regimens to make the same case—but it provides a good example, since the potential anticancer effects of the treatment were evaluated on a reasonably sized patient group by a presumably objective group of outside reviewers.

Essiac is a combination of herbs that was used by Rene Caisse, a nurse from rural Ontario, to treat cancer. Caisse, given the formula for Essiac by a patient who told her it was based on traditional American Indian herbal medicine, treated hundreds of cancer patients at various times between the 1920s and the 1970s. She reported that she had helped many cancer patients with Essiac. How-ever, an objective review by the Canadian Bureau of Human Prescription Drugs,

Health Protection Branch, Health and Welfare Canada, found little evidence that Essiac was beneficial.

For this review, physicians whose patients had been treated with Essiac submitted reports to the bureau. Of the eighty-six reports submitted, the bureau found evidence suggesting possible benefits of Essiac in fourteen. Of these fourteen patients, one showed a "subjective improvement" (presumably meaning that the patient felt better), and five required fewer analgesics. That suggests that six of the eighty-six patients treated with Essiac experienced some improvement in quality of life.

As far as possible effects on their *cancer*, four patients showed an "objective response" (presumably meaning tumor regression), and four others were in "stable condition" (presumably meaning their condition was getting neither better nor worse). In following up on these latter eight patients, the bureau found that disease was progressing in three and that two had died. The last three patients, who remained in stable condition, had received conventional therapy in addition to Essiac, and the bureau reviewers believed that the conventional therapy could account for these patients' stable conditions.

It's difficult to conclude from this review that Essiac has much real anticancer activity. On the other hand, six patients showed some improvement in their quality of life; five of these patients experienced relief from pain. Since there were no controlled trials, we can't be sure that this had anything to do with something in Essiac: even sugar pills can sometimes help relieve pain. Still, for someone battling cancer, a harmless regimen that may improve your quality of life is nothing to sneeze at. And if I were convinced that all herbal regimens were harmless, I'd put them in the same category as my Tibetan Singing Bowls. If the therapy resonates for you and makes you feel better, why not?

With herbal regimens, though, unless you have expert guidance, you could actually end up harming yourself. Many people have the idea that "natural" substances are always harmless simply because they're natural. That just isn't true. Poison ivy is perfectly natural, and so is strychnine, and so is the deathcap mushroom. I wouldn't want to eat any of them. Aspirin is safer for you than the natural substance from which it was derived. Some natural substances are good, and some are bad, and if you take too much of the bad ones, they can kill you.

Like any drug, even some of the "good" natural substances can be dangerous under the wrong circumstances. People have suffered serious—even fatal—side effects of natural remedies that they took without proper supervision. This brings me back to my second concern about herbal therapies: we don't necessarily know exactly what they're doing.

What are they actually doing?

One of my concerns in the "we don't really know what they're doing" area has to do with herbs that are supposed to stimulate the immune system. Stimulating the immune system became one of the most popular catchphrases of complementary and alternative medicine in the 1990s. Everywhere I turned, I'd hear that such-and-such a regimen was beneficial because it "stimulates your immune system." Herbs, vitamins, imagery, massage—I didn't need to look too far to find someone telling me that they were good for me because they'd stimulate my immune system.

The idea that stimulating the immune system might be beneficial for people with cancer grew out of what's been called the immune surveillance hypothesis of cancer. The idea behind this theory, first developed by the Australian Nobel Laureate MacFarlane Burnet in 1970, is that while our body continually produces cancer cells, these cancer cells generally provoke an immune response and are therefore rapidly eliminated by a normally functioning immune system. It's easy to extrapolate from this basic idea that, if cancer arises only in the presence of a defective immune response, stimulating the immune system should be a terrific thing for people with cancer.

There's some evidence to back up this idea. As you'd predict, people who are severely immunosuppressed have an increased risk of developing cancer. This is true whether they were born with an immunological deficiency (like the boy in the bubble) or acquired one later in life—for instance, by contracting AIDS or through being given immunosuppressant drugs to prevent tissue rejection after receiving an organ transplant. Moreover, animal experiments have demonstrated that the immune system can control some transplanted tumors. And biopsies of human tumors sometimes show infiltration by lymphocytes directed against tumor antigens. Presumably, these lymphocytes are in the process of mounting an immune response against the tumor.

But it has become clear that the immune surveillance hypothesis oversimplifies the complexities of both the immune system and the relationship between the immune system and cancer. For one thing, rather than the tremendous across-the-board increase in all forms of cancer you'd predict from the immune surveillance hypothesis, people who are severely immunocompromised tend to get certain specific forms of cancer. The most prominent of these are Kaposi's sarcoma and certain (but not all) forms of NHL. Rates of cervical cancer, anogenital cancer, certain skin cancers, and Hodgkin lymphoma also rise in some immunocompromised populations. These particular cancers have all been linked to specific viral infections. Human herpesvirus 8 has been linked to Kaposi's sarcoma and some forms of NHL found in immunocompromised people; Epstein-Barr virus has been linked to some forms of NHL and some cases of Hodgkin lymphoma; human papillomavirus has been linked to the others.

The fact that people who are immunocompromised tend to get cancers associated with viral infection suggests that, rather than an immunological defect in controlling *cancer*, these people may be experiencing an immunological defect in controlling cells infected by cancer-inducing *viruses*. If that's the case, immunosurveillance might be of little benefit in other forms of cancer. It's also possible that instead of cancer resulting from an ineffectual immune response per se, alterations in cytokine balance that occur as a result of a decrease in the numbers of certain classes of lymphocytes could promote the growth of such cancers. And it's a big jump in logic to go from the observation that people who are severely immunodeficient tend to get cancer to the conclusion that people who get cancer must be immunodeficient. Cancer cells have ways to evade even the healthiest immune system.

To understand how this can happen, we need to understand a little about how the immune system works. As discussed at length in Chapter 9, the immune system essentially consists of a bunch of cells that work together to protect us from harm. The cells of the immune system recognize substances that are "wrong" or "foreign"—that is, not usually found in the body. Since cancer cells tend to be genetically unstable, their DNA undergoes mutations at a much higher rate than normal. That means they're more likely than most cells to produce abnormal proteins that could elicit an immune response.

So far, so good. However, not all cancer cells actually express these abnormal proteins. Those that don't may not be recognized as foreign. Or the cancer cells may lose certain cell surface molecules that are necessary to allow a certain class of immune system cells—the cytotoxic, or "cell-killing," T cells—to interact with them. Or the tumor may synthesize cytokines that suppress the immune response. Under any of these circumstances, the tumor will be able to evade your immune system.

Why not go ahead and stimulate your immune system anyway? That way, if you have a tumor with abnormal proteins and the right cell surface molecules and so forth, you just might beat your lymphoma into submission. If you don't, no harm done. Indeed, "immune-system stimulation" is a key feature of many aspects of *conventional* cancer therapy (see Chapter 5). With these therapies, however, we know exactly what cellular response the treatment is intended to produce. With "immunostimulatory" herbs, this is rarely the case.

Before taking any herb purported to "stimulate the immune system," you need to remember that lymphocytes are the key players in the immune system and that malignant lymphocytes resemble normal lymphocytes in many ways. Therefore you need to learn, for any particular herb, what "stimulating the immune system" actually means.

For instance poke (also called poke root or pokeweed), a component of the Hoxsey herbal therapy, contains a substance called pokeweed mitogen. Pokeweed mitogen is well known to immunologists as a *B cell mitogen* or *polyclonal activator*. It nonspecifically stimulates B cells to divide. Other herbs (not an exhaustive list) that may stimulate lymphocyte proliferation include astragalus, echinacea, and ginseng. Since most herbs purported to stimulate the immune system haven't been exhaustively studied to *rule out* potential effects, I tend to consider any herb in this general category suspect.

Do astragalus, echinacea, and ginseng *really* stimulate lymphocyte proliferation if you drink extracts as a tea? I don't know. Does poke (or any of these herbs) stimulate *malignant* B cells to divide? I don't know. If they do, could I get enough of the active substance from drinking herbal teas to actually influence any of my lymphocytes—normal or malignant? I don't know. Would I be willing to do the experiment on myself or on anyone else with lymphoma without a lot more information? Absolutely not.

This is one of those areas where it seems best to err on the side of being conservative. In the absence of any real evidence that nonspecific stimulation of your immune system is actually *helpful* in fighting cancer, it hardly seems worth running the risk of stimulating your lymphoma cells to proliferate—however small that risk might be. Given that aggressive lymphomas tend to be independent of external growth signals, I'd suspect that the more indolent the lymphoma, the more likely it would be to respond to substances that stimulate normal lymphocytes. It's awfully hard to imagine *anything* stimulating a superaggressive lymphoma—like Burkitt's—to divide more rapidly than it does on its own.

However, I'm not exactly comfortable with the idea of people with aggressive lymphomas—either active or in remission—randomly trying to stimulate their immune system, either. There's evidence that the initial development of some forms of lymphoma involves abnormal proliferation of nonmalignant lymphocytes (see Chapter 11). And, because I've been in remission for several years, it seems likely that all my actual lymphoma cells (i.e., cells that are unquestionably malignant) have been destroyed, but I certainly wouldn't want to wantonly stimulate any abnormal *premalignant* cells that might still be quietly lurking in my body.

Dosage

What about herbs *known* to have anticancer activity? After all, vincristine and vinblastine come from the Madagascar periwinkle. Etoposide is derived from the mayapple. Paclitaxel, most commonly used to treat breast cancer, is derived from the bark of the Pacific yew. Why not take these herbs, and a few of the others, for which animal studies have indicated some anticancer effect?

In addition to the question of what *other* compounds might be present in these herbs, the idea of taking herbs containing known anticancer compounds brings up the question of dosage. Different batches of herbs may have grown under widely different conditions and may contain vastly different concentrations of the therapeutic compound(s). Standardizing drug dosage is one of the great advantages of extracting the active ingredients. While it might not seem like such a big deal, getting the correct dose of an anticancer drug is critically important. Taking either too high a dose or too low a dose can be problematic.

The potential pitfalls of taking too high a dosage of one of these toxic drugs are obvious. It could do serious damage or even kill you. What about taking a low dosage? In general, when oncologists treat cancer, they use the highest dose of antineoplastic drugs that you can tolerate. That's because lower doses of drugs, in addition to being less effective than higher doses, may actually foster the development of chemo-resistant cancer cells. Just as people who take inadequate doses of antibiotics can develop strains of superbacteria that are resistant to normal doses of antibiotics, taking ineffective doses of antineoplastic drugs could lead to chemotherapy-resistant cells.

Here's how it works. Cancer cells have an unusually high rate of spontaneous mutations. Some of these mutations might make the cells carrying them weaker and more susceptible to chemotherapy, while some might make the cells carrying them stronger and more resistant to treatment. If you take a high enough dose of antineoplastic drugs, you're hoping that *all* the tumor cells will be susceptible and will be destroyed. If you start out with a relatively low dose of some antineoplastic drug, all the weaker cells will be killed, but those with some resistance to your drug may be spared.

TREATING LYMPHOMA

This population of cells has what's known as a *survival advantage*, and they'll bequeath their drug resistance to their daughter cells. Since the population of cancer cells, on the whole, has been enriched with drug-resistant cells, you'll be more likely to develop cells with new mutations that increase their drug resistance further. Worst of all, some drug-resistant cells develop strategies that make them resistant to *many* drugs. For instance, they may develop very efficient mechanisms for pumping out all unwanted substances. That means they may become resistant to some of the drugs used in conventional chemotherapy.

The concern about suboptimal dosing applies mainly to people with indolent disease on watch-and-wait. While it is unlikely that *any* dosage of currently available chemotherapeutic agents will destroy all their malignant cells, the same basic idea—avoiding the development of drug-resistant cells—applies. You don't want to do anything on your own that could eventually increase your resistance to standard therapies that are known to be reasonably effective (i.e., able to put you into a remission). Developing drug-resistant cells as a result of taking low doses of herbal antineoplastic agents really isn't a concern if you take such therapies *while* you're undergoing chemotherapy. However, given that you're already taking high doses of toxic drugs, you'd want to think very seriously before doing anything that might increase the strain on your body and make it more difficult for you to tolerate the proven treatment. Moreover, some herbal remedies can interfere with the way your body handles the drugs used in chemotherapy so that you end up being exposed to higher or lower concentrations of these antineoplastic drugs than appropriate.

All these factors make me extremely wary about using herbal remedies to treat lymphoma. If you feel very strongly that herbs are a therapeutic route that you'd like to pursue, I'd go beyond my usual advice to talk it over with your physician. Most mainstream physicians don't know enough about herbal medicine to be able to evaluate the potential safety (or efficacy) of supplementing your conventional therapy with an herbal regimen. In this case, I would seek out an oncologist or hematologist who is both trained in conventional means of therapy *and* very knowledgeable about herbal remedies. Although it may be difficult to find such a person practicing near your home, it's worth seeking one out, if only for a consult, before embarking on this path.

Other medical traditions

I feel somewhat more comfortable about the idea of supplementing conventional Western medicine with the medicines of other traditions, such as traditional

Chinese medicine or ayurvedic medicine from India, than I do about using recently developed herbal therapies that do not stem from such a tradition. That's because it seems more likely that medical traditions that have evolved over thousands of years will have ended up with therapies that actually work (regardless of whether one agrees with the underlying rationale) as opposed to alternative approaches that haven't stood the test of time.

Moreover, there's a tremendous amount of research going on in China today (as well as in Japan, Korea, Canada, and the United States) related to traditional Chinese medicine. While I'm no expert on research going on in China, it's my impression from reading summaries of this research that some studies appear to be poorly designed but others seem likely to yield useful information.

It's beginning to appear as though there's a real role for traditional Chinese medicine—particularly acupuncture—in improving quality of life for people undergoing chemotherapy and radiation therapy. Acupuncture involves stimulating specific points on the body to achieve certain specific physiological effects. Most often, acupuncture involves inserting very fine needles into the stimulus points. Variations involve acupressure (applying pressure to the acupuncture points, either manually or through special elastic bands), moxibustion (burning the herb moxa, or mugwort, on or near acupuncture points), and applying electrical stimulation to the acupuncture points.

Clinical trials have indicated that stimulating the P6 acupuncture point (above the wrist) can alleviate the nausea associated with several chemotherapy regimens. The St36 and Sp6 points on your lower legs may work as well. Acupuncture is ineffective in treating nausea if it's given while you are under general anesthesia or if a local anesthetic is injected near the acupuncture point.

If you decide to undergo acupuncture and your therapist uses needles, make sure he or she uses disposable needles. It's probably best to avoid acupuncture if your white cells or platelets are depressed as a result of chemotherapy (to avoid infection and excessive bleeding, respectively). If you want to try self-acupressure, press rapidly and firmly on each point about thirty times, as though you were sending a telegraph message.

Some of the herbs used in traditional Chinese medicine may be helpful in alleviating side effects of chemotherapy and radiation. If you are interested in pursuing the herbal route, you should be aware that some Chinese herbal mixtures contain immunostimulatory herbs such as astragalus and ginseng and that some components of these mixtures may influence the handling of drugs used in chemotherapy (see discussion above). As with other complementary approaches,

I think anyone interested in using the therapies of other medical traditions *must* discuss this idea with his or her physician and *must* follow the guidance of someone with real expertise in the area. People have suffered severe side effects—including death—from improperly formulated mixtures of Chinese medicinal herbs. Again, it would be ideal if the person with expertise in the alternative tradition was an oncologist or hematologist as well.

SUGGESTIONS FOR FURTHER READING

Cassileth BR. (1998). *The Alternative Medicine Handbook: The Complete Reference Guide to Alternative and Complementary Therapies.* New York: W. W. Norton.

> *A comprehensive and objective description of various alternative and complementary therapies. Sections on traditional healing methods, dietary and herbal approaches, mind/body techniques, biological therapies (including unproven pharmacological methods), bodywork (e.g., acupuncture, massage), sensory enhancement (e.g., aromatherapy, music therapy), and therapy involving application of external energy sources (e.g., prayer, therapeutic touch, crystals).*

Dimeo F, Fetscher S, Lange W, Mertelsman R, Keul J. (1997). "Effects of aerobic exercise on the physical performance and incidence of treatment-related complications after high-dose chemotherapy." *Blood* 90:3390–3394.

Gerbitz A et al. (2004). "Probiotic effects on experimental graft-versus-host disease: Let them eat yogurt." *Blood* 103:4365–4367.

> *This study suggests that probiotic bacteria such as those found in yogurt may alleviate a mouse model of graft vs. host disease.*

Kabat-Zinn J. (1990). *Full Catastrophe Living.* New York: Dell.

> *An excellent book for those interested in pursuing meditation, stress reduction, and mind-body approaches, by the founder of the University of Worcester Stress Reduction Clinic.*

Ladas EJ, Jacobson JS, Kennedy DD, Teel K, Fleischauer A, Kelly KM. (2004). "Antioxidants and cancer therapy: A systematic review." *Journal of Clinical Oncology* 22: 517–528.

Lerner M. (1994). *Choices in Healing: Integrating the Best of Conventional and Complementary Approaches to Cancer.* Cambridge: MIT Press.

> *A compassionate and balanced introduction to the field that provides a thoughtful and objective analysis of both conventional and complementary therapeutic options for cancer survivors. My division of alternative therapies into pharmacologically oriented and lifestyle-oriented approaches was based on the categories Michael Lerner defined. It is perhaps worth noting that his interest in unconventional approaches to cancer therapy arose when his father was diagnosed with non-Hodgkin lymphoma.*

Rabin BS, Cohen S, Ganguli R, Lysle DT, Cunnick JE. (1989). "Bidirectional interaction between the central nervous system and the immune system." *Critical Reviews in Immunology* 9:279–312.

> *A general overview of brain/immune system interactions.*

Sparreboom A, Cox MC, Acharya MR, Figg WD. (2004). "Herbal remedies in the United States: Potential adverse interactions with anticancer agents." *Journal of Clinical Oncology* 22:2489–2503.

> *This recent review describes interactions between various herbal remedies and the mechanisms by which your body handles drugs used in chemotherapy that could reduce chemotherapy effectiveness.*

Spiegel D. (2001). "Mind matters—group therapy and survival in breast cancer." *New England Journal of Medicine* 345:1767–1768.

> *Five published randomized trials (two including people with lymphoma) have reported that psychotherapeutic interventions, such as support groups, prolonged survival in people with cancer. Five other published trials have failed to find any survival benefits from such approaches. David Spiegel, who conducted the initial study demonstrating prolonged survival in women with metastatic breast cancer, discusses possible reasons for these discrepancies and includes references to the original studies.*

U.S. Congress, Office of Technology Assessment. (1990). *Unconventional Cancer Treatments*, OTA-H-405. Washington, D.C.: U.S. Government Printing Office.

> *This publication, which provides an objective analysis of complementary and alternative therapies, is no longer in print but is available online (see below).*

Vickers AJ. (1996). "Can acupuncture have specific effects on health? A systematic review of acupuncture antiemesis trials." *Journal of the Royal Society of Medicine* 89:303–311.

Resources are also available online:

The University of Texas Center for Alternative Medicine's review of various alternative therapies: www.mdanderson.org/departments/CIMER/

Memorial Sloan-Kettering Cancer Center's site about herbs, botanicals, and other products: www.mskcc.org/mskcc/html/11571.cfm

PDQ Cancer Information Summaries on complementary and alternative medicine: www.cancer.gov/cancertopics/pdq/cam/

Kidney cancer survivor Steve Dunn's site: cancerguide.org/alternative.html

Choices in Healing online: www.commonweal.org/pubs/choices-healing.html

The Office of Technology Assessment's Unconventional Cancer Treatment Report: www.wws.princeton.edu/cgi-bin/byteserv.prl/~ota/disk2/1990/9044/9044.PDF or: www.quackwatch.com/01QuackeryRelatedTopics/OTA/ota00.html

Dr. Steven Barrett's very skeptical look at alternative therapies is well worth looking at if you are considering such an approach: www.quackwatch.com/00AboutQuackwatch/altseek.html

Guided Imagery tapes are available from various sources. I particularly like the *Health Journeys* series by Belleruth Naperstek (www.healthjourneys.com/).

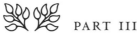 PART III

Understanding Lymphoma

P art III of this book is focused less on understanding what it is like to experience lymphoma and lymphoma treatment and more on understanding the underlying disease. Chapter 8, "Basic Cell Biology and Cancer," is an introduction to cell biology; I describe normal cells and explain how damage to an individual cell can disrupt the processes governing its behavior and lead to cancer. Toward the end of this chapter, I describe some of the specific cellular abnormalities that have been associated with lymphoma. In Chapter 9, "The Immune System," I discuss lymphocytes and the immune system in which they function. Understanding the development and behavior of normal lymphocytes helps us to understand the behavior of the malignant lymphocytes that make up lymphoma.

Armed with a basic knowledge of *normal* lymphocyte behavior, we can move on, in Chapter 10, "Lymphoma Classification and Staging," to an in-depth discussion of *abnormal* lymphocytes. In this chapter, I describe the different forms of lymphoma: how they are classified, how they differ from each other, and why lymphoma classification has traditionally been considered so confusing. Finally, in Chapter 11, I discuss the causes of lymphoma—the things we are exposed to that can damage a lymphocyte so that it turns cancerous.

The material in this part of the book is, necessarily, more technical than that in the first two parts. If you read the material carefully, however, and in the order in which it is presented, you will gain a true understanding of lymphoma. My goal is for readers to learn fundamental "lymphoma vocabulary" and concepts of the field, so they can make use of material about lymphoma found in the primary medical literature.

CHAPTER 8

Basic Cell Biology and Cancer

T his chapter describes basic cell biology and then looks closely at what goes wrong on the cellular level when someone develops cancer. Cancer arises when there is a disruption of the normal mechanisms that govern how frequently cells divide, how long cells survive, and where cells grow. Understanding the processes that determine the behavior of normal, healthy cells helps us understand how relatively small changes in the molecules that make up cells can lead to the abnormal behavior displayed by cancer cells. And the differences in the behavior and biochemical makeup of healthy cells and cancer cells make it possible for cancer treatments to work.

What is cancer?

Just as the different organs that make up a living organism must work together, the individual cells that make up the different tissues and organs of the body must fulfill *their* distinct functions and work together for the good of the whole. Although all the cells in an organism are derived from one original cell—the fertilized egg—they differentiate during development and become specialized to carry out their distinctive functions. The *differentiated properties* of a mature cell depend on both the inherent nature of the specific cell type and the cell's response to cues in its environment. Both of these factors influence the specific traits any individual cell displays.

Functional specializations are reflected in the appearance of the different cell types. Like so many tiny Bauhaus creations, living cells obey the "form follows function" rule. For example, nerve cells, or neurons, which are specialized to receive information and then pass it on, often have small, branching projections that gather incoming signals from other cells and one long "arm" to convey that information to target cells. The cells that line the intestines, on the other hand, which transport nutrients from the inside of the gut to the bloodstream, have highly folded membranes on the side facing the gut to maximize the surface area exposed to these nutrients.

Cells must not only carry out their appropriate functions but must also grow in the appropriate environment. A kidney cell, for instance, would be useless growing in the middle of the liver, no matter how faithfully it attempted to carry out the functions appropriate to kidney cells.

Each cell type also has a characteristic life span. Some cells, like the neurons in the brain, last for the lifetime of the organism and do not continue to divide and propagate themselves once development is complete. Others, like the cells that line the gut, have brief life spans and must be replaced. Some mature, fully differentiated cell types retain the ability to replicate themselves, but many lose this ability. These cell types need to be replenished from a population of *stem cells.* Stem cells are partially committed to a certain fate—the hematopoietic stem cells in the bone marrow, for example, may become different types of blood cells, but they will never differentiate into the cells that line the intestines. However, they retain the ability to divide and are not yet fully differentiated; they do not look like mature cells or carry out their functions.

When something goes wrong with the mechanisms that control the total numbers of a given cell's offspring, cancer may ultimately result. Cancer may develop either after a cell starts to divide too frequently or after a type of cell that normally propagates rapidly but does not normally survive very long begins to survive for a long time. Either of these two mechanisms will lead to an abnormal accumulation of that cell's offspring. A cell may begin to divide too frequently either because (1) it loses the ability to respond to external cues that slow down cell division or (2) it abnormally expresses some molecule that promotes cell division. Such aberrations in cell division and cell death are caused by *mutations* (see below).

To become unquestionably cancerous, a cell needs to acquire a number of such mutations. While cancer cells often resemble the cell type from which they arise and may retain some of the behaviors characteristic of that cell type, they don't express all the properties of the original cell. Not only do they grow and divide inappropriately, but they are also unable to carry out their proper function. Cancer cells often look abnormal, and they may not respond appropriately to cues in the environment—both those that control the rate of division and those that tell them where to grow. Thus cancer cells may grow in inappropriate sites, invading and destroying healthy tissue throughout the body. In general, the more mutations that accumulate, the greater the loss of differentiated characteristics, the more aberrant the behavior and appearance of the cell, and the more aggressive the cancer.

Normal cell structure and function

Around 1665, a man named Robert Hooke placed a thin slice of cork under a recently invented magnifying instrument called the compound microscope. Peering through the eyepiece, he discovered that the cork was filled with tiny little pores, or pockets, that reminded him of monks' small monastery cells. We now know that all living things are made up of these basic units Hooke called *cells.*

Very simple organisms, like bacteria and amoebas, are made up of single cells. Complicated organisms, like people, are made up of billions and billions of cells and are said to be *multicellular.* The different tissues and organs of our bodies can perform specialized functions because the individual cells that make them up have their *own* specialized shapes and functions.

However, all cells have certain elements in common, and all normal cells function together for the good of the organism. All cells have a boundary that separates them from their environment—called the *extracellular fluid.* If you were to put a bunch of grapes in a tub of water, the grape skins would form the same sort of boundary, separating the inside of the grape from the water in the tub. In people and other animals, this boundary is called the *cell membrane.* The cell membrane consists of a layer of fatty substances called *lipids,* which are interspersed with another class of substances called *proteins.*

Lipids and proteins are large molecules that have structural as well as functional roles; cells also contain *carbohydrates* and *nucleic acids,* as well as various smaller molecules. The four classes of large molecules (lipids, proteins, carbohydrates, and nucleic acids) differ from each other in terms of the smaller building blocks that make them up and in their specific functions for the cell and for the organism.

Cells are filled with a jellylike substance called *cytoplasm.* Located within the cytoplasm are small structures called *organelles;* different organelles have different specific functions. For instance, the *mitochondrion* (plural: mitochondria) provides energy for the cell, while *ribosomes* manufacture protein. The organelles fulfill the same role for the cell that organs like the lungs or the liver do for the whole

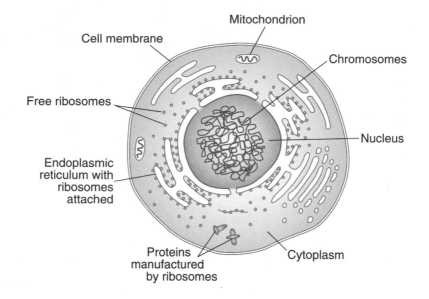

Figure 8.1. *A typical cell.* The cell membrane surrounds a jellylike substance called cytoplasm, which contains small structures called organelles; different organelles have different functions. Most cells in multicellular organisms have a large organelle called the nucleus, which contains the genome, organized into long strands of DNA. These long strands of DNA, together with associated proteins, are called chromosomes. Proteins are manufactured on ribosomes found either associated with the endoplasmic reticulum or free in the cytoplasm. A mitochondrion (plural, mitochondria) supplies energy to the cell, and the plasma membrane acts as a kind of "skin" separating the inside of the cell from the outside.

organism. All cells in multicellular organisms except red blood cells and platelets have a large organelle called the *nucleus* (fig. 8.1).

The nucleus contains the *genome*, essentially a blueprint that specifies how to construct and maintain a fully functional organism. The genome contains all the information that makes us human beings, as well as the specific details that make each of us slightly different from everyone else. Our genome not only specifies all the different kinds of molecules our cells need to make but also controls our development from a single cell—the fertilized egg—into a complete human being.

DNA, RNA, and protein

With the exception of the sperm cells and egg cells, which pass on our genetic information to our offspring, all our nucleated cells (the cells with nuclei) con-

UNDERSTANDING LYMPHOMA

tain our complete genome. The sperm and egg cells each contain *half* of the full complement of genetic information, so that we inherit half of our genome from each of our parents. The genetic information is encoded in long, double-stranded molecules called DNA (deoxyribonucleic acid). The two strands of the DNA molecule spiral around each other in a double *helix*, which looks like a long ladder that's been twisted around and around.

Each double-stranded molecule of DNA is a *polymer*—a large molecule made up of many similar or identical units; each DNA polymer consists of four basic units strung together into a long chain. The individual units—or *monomers*—that make up the DNA polymer are called *nucleotides*. They're called nucleotides because they are the building blocks that make up the *nucleic acids* (DNA and RNA), which are manufactured in the cell's nucleus. The nucleotides are considered DNA *precursors*, since they are necessary components of DNA that must be present before DNA can be synthesized. Each of the nucleotides contains a sugar-phosphate portion that's strung together with the sugar-phosphate portions of the other nucleotides to form the sides of the DNA ladder; each nucleotide also contains a ring-shaped base on the side to form the rungs. The sugar molecule in DNA nucleotides is called deoxyribose. The different nucleotides are named after their bases: adenine, thymine, cytosine, and guanine (abbreviated as A, T, C, and G).

The bases A and G have two rings in their side chain and are called *purines*, while C and T have a single ring in theirs and are called *pyrimidines*. A purine on one strand always matches up with a pyrimidine on the other so that the rungs of the DNA ladder are the same length. A always pairs with T, and C always pairs with G.

The genetic information carried by DNA—all the information required to transform a fertilized egg into a functioning human being—is encoded by the order of the nucleotides in the DNA molecules. Different sequences of nucleotides direct the cell to synthesize different proteins. Just as the nucleic acids are made up of chains of nucleotides, proteins are made up of chains of smaller building blocks, called *amino acids*. It is the amino acid sequence of a protein that determines its structure—and ultimately its function. Thus, whether a given protein acts as a structural element of the cell, an *enzyme* (which helps make some chemical reaction take place), or a *receptor* (which allows the cell to interact with molecules in its environment) depends on that protein's amino acid sequence.

Different sequences of three nucleotides code for different amino acids. For instance, the nucleotide sequence A, T, G codes for the amino acid *methionine*; the nucleotide sequence A, G, G codes for the amino acid *arginine;* and the nucleotide sequence G, C, A codes for the amino acid *alanine.* So, a strand of DNA with the nucleotide sequence ATG AGG GCA AGG AGG would code for a piece of protein with the amino acid sequence methionine-arginine-alanine-arginine-arginine.

Genes are sequences of DNA that direct the synthesis of individual proteins. (Some very large proteins, like antibodies, are made up of several smaller parts, each of which is coded for by a different gene.) Since nearly all your cells contain the entire genome, each cell has the *potential* to carry out the function of any other cell in that organism. The actual behavioral repertoire of any given cell is determined by which of its many genes are actively expressed.

In addition to the sequences of nucleotides that code for the order of amino acids that make up a given protein, each gene also contains sequences that regulate when a given protein will be made and in what quantities. The portion of a gene that specifies which amino acids are required to synthesize its protein is known as the *coding sequence;* the portion of a gene concerned with determining when a specific gene is turned on (and how rapidly it's made) is known as the *regulatory region.*

The regulatory regions are just as important as the coding sequences. They ensure that specific proteins are manufactured by the right cells at the right time. For instance, as you'll remember, only your B lymphocytes make antibodies. While all your nucleated cells *contain* the genes for antibody synthesis, only B cells *express* these particular genes. Resting B cells synthesize low levels of antibodies; they step up production in the presence of an invader. Therefore, not only do your B cells need to have some mechanism to tell them that they're the antibody-making cells, but they also need to have some mechanism to allow them to *increase* antibody synthesis when they've been signaled that a certain invader is present.

An entire gene—the regulatory region plus the coding sequence—is about 10,000 to 100,000 nucleotides long; individual genes are linked together into long double-stranded lengths of DNA called *chromosomes.* These chromosomes are covered with proteins. Many of these proteins bind to specific DNA sequences in the regulatory regions of genes and let the cell know whether it needs to make a specific gene's protein product at any given time.

The proteins that bind to regulatory regions and regulate gene activity are called *transcription factors.* Whether a given transcription factor acts on many genes or only a few depends on the specific sequences of DNA that it binds to and whether they're found in many or few genes. Transcription factors can either increase the expression of a given gene or repress it.

People have twenty-three pairs of chromosomes—or forty-six chromosomes total. Each of the twenty-three pairs of chromosomes is different from the others and contains a specific sequence of genes. One chromosome in each pair is inherited from your mother, the other from your father. With the exception of the two sex chromosomes, each of the two chromosomes in a pair contains the same set of genes. However, specific details of individual genes may differ a little.

For instance, the color of your eyes depends on the amount of melanin found in the iris (the colored part of your eye). If you had a gene on chromosome 19 that regulated an enzyme involved in melanin synthesis, that gene could influence your eye color. We can call this the *"eyecolor"* gene, and we can call the protein that it codes for the "Eyecolor" enzyme. (When biologists want to differentiate the name of a specific gene from that of its protein product, they commonly use italics for the gene and capitalize the protein.) So you would have a gene called *eyecolor* on the chromosome 19 you inherited from your mother and a gene called *eyecolor* on the chromosome 19 you inherited from your father. If you have brown eyes, your mother had blue eyes, and your father had brown eyes, it could mean that the Eyecolor enzyme you inherited from your father was more active than the one you inherited from your mother. On a molecular level, this would correspond to slight differences in the amino acid sequences of the two forms of the Eyecolor enzyme. On a *genetic* level, this would correspond to slight differences in the DNA sequences of the *eyecolor* genes. These slight differences in gene sequence are what make each of us an individual.

The other nucleic acid, RNA (ribonucleic acid), differs from DNA mainly in that the sugar component of its nucleotides is ribose, not deoxyribose. RNA is made up of nucleotides containing the bases adenine, cytosine, guanine, and uracil (U; uracil is substituted for thymine [T]) and generally exists as a single strand.

Since DNA is found in the nucleus and proteins are synthesized outside the nucleus, on the ribosomes, the cell needs to convey the information in the DNA to the ribosomes. That's what RNA does. When a cell needs to synthesize a certain protein, an enzyme called *RNA polymerase* binds to one of the DNA strands and copies the DNA strand into RNA, linking together nucleotides to form a strand of RNA that's complementary to the DNA strand. In other words, everywhere the DNA strand had an "A," the RNA strand would have a "U." Everywhere the DNA strand had a "T," the RNA strand would have an "A." Everywhere the

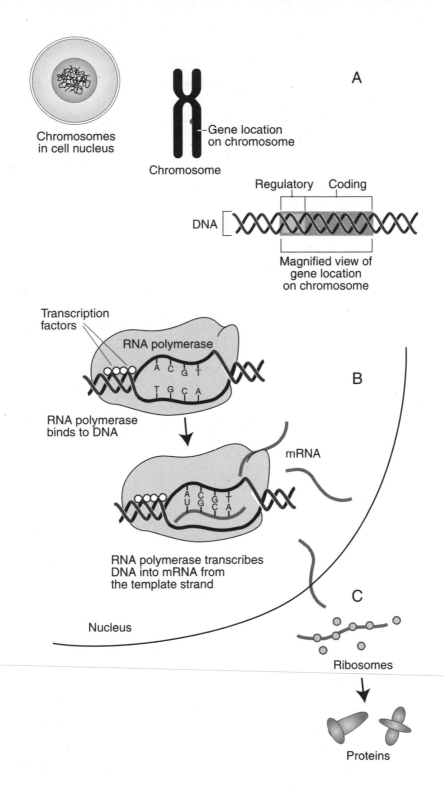

Chromosomes
in cell nucleus

Chromosome

Gene location
on chromosome

A

DNA

Regulatory   Coding

Magnified view of
gene location
on chromosome

Transcription
factors

RNA polymerase

A C G T

T G C A

RNA polymerase
binds to DNA

B

mRNA

A C   T
U G G A

RNA polymerase transcribes
DNA into mRNA from
the template strand

Nucleus

C

Ribosomes

Proteins

DNA strand had a "C," the RNA strand would have a "G." And everywhere the DNA strand had a "G," the RNA strand would have a "C" (fig. 8.2).

This process of copying the genetic information for a given gene from the DNA on a chromosome to a strand of RNA is called transcription. The information from the DNA *template strand* is copied—or transcribed—into the new molecule of RNA. RNA transcribed from the other strand of DNA, which is complementary to the template strand, wouldn't have the correct nucleotide sequence to code for the protein. Therefore, this strand isn't transcribed.

After the gene has been transcribed into RNA, the RNA, after undergoing some processing, leaves the nucleus for the ribosomes as messenger RNA (mRNA), where it directs the synthesis of the protein. This process is called *translation* because the DNA message contained in the gene is translated into the manufacture of a specific protein.

DNA replication and the cell cycle

In order to go from a single cell to a mature organism containing billions of cells, and in order to replace adult cells that become worn out, our cells need to divide many times. The sequence of events involved in duplicating a cell that spans the time between one cell division and the next is called the *cell cycle*. Abnormally rapid cycling is one of the hallmarks of some forms of cancer, including the aggressive forms of lymphoma. It's also critical to the success of several forms of chemotherapy. And it's mistakes in the processes involved in DNA duplication that ultimately lead to cancer.

Figure 8.2. *Transcription.* A. Each chromosome includes many genes linked together. An individual gene, which encodes an individual protein, contains both a coding sequence, which is the portion of the gene that specifies which amino acids are required to synthesize that gene's protein, and a regulatory region, which is the portion of the gene concerned with determining when it is turned on. B. Proteins called transcription factors bind to the regulatory regions and help determine when (and how rapidly) a particular gene is transcribed. When a cell needs to synthesize a certain protein, an enzyme called RNA polymerase binds to the DNA and copies one of the DNA strands (the template strand) into RNA, linking together nucleotides to form a strand of RNA that's complementary to that DNA strand. This process is called transcription. C. When the gene has been transcribed into RNA, the RNA leaves the nucleus and goes to the ribosomes, where it directs the synthesis of the protein.

The cell cycle can be divided into several distinct steps, or *phases*, depending on exactly what the cell is doing. The cell needs to accumulate enough building blocks to supply two daughter cells; then duplicate the DNA genome, so that each daughter cell receives a complete copy; and then physically divide in two. The period during which the cell is actually duplicating the genome is called *S-phase*—which stands for DNA synthesis phase. During S-phase, the two strands of the DNA helix unwind, and enzymes known as DNA polymerases copy each strand. It's similar to the process whereby DNA is transcribed into RNA: enzymes copy a strand of DNA by incorporating nucleotides one by one into a growing chain complementary to the strand of DNA being copied. However, unlike in the transcription of RNA, both DNA strands are copied during DNA duplication, and the entire genome is duplicated rather than just individual genes.

The other phase of the cell cycle that really stands out is called *M-phase* (for *m*itosis), when the cell splits in two. In addition to S-phase and M-phase are two periods when the cell gets ready for the upcoming challenge. These two phases are the *G-phases*—for *g*ap—because they form gaps in the cycle—one before DNA synthesis and the other before mitosis. During the first gap phase—G_1—which precedes S-phase, the cell gathers together the enzymes and nucleotide precursors that it will need to duplicate its DNA. It also makes whatever RNA and proteins it will need to supply the two daughter cells. During the second gap phase—G_2—the cell checks to make sure that DNA synthesis has proceeded correctly and that it has accumulated all the materials it will need for M-phase. During G_2, the cell actually has two complete sets of chromosomes!

Once the cell has completed G_2, it's ready for mitosis. The membrane around the nucleus dissolves, and the chromosomes are pulled to the opposite poles of the cell by a newly formed structure called the *mitotic spindle*. Once the two duplicate copies of the genome are at opposite poles of the cell, two new nuclei form—each with its very own copy of the complete genome. Following duplication of the nucleus, the cell splits in two—with a nucleus in each new daughter cell.

Following mitosis, the cell may return to G_1 and continue cycling, or it may exit the cell cycle and enter a "resting stage" called G_0. During G_0 the cell is fulfilling all its normal functions but isn't actively cycling. Some cell types—like mature nerve cells or muscle cells—remain in G_0 indefinitely. Others can be triggered by signals in their environment to return to active cycling. In many cell types, the mature, fully differentiated form of the cell can no longer divide. In these cell types, cell division is the hallmark of a young, undifferentiated cell that is still developing into its final form.

If you take a look at most normal, healthy tissues under a microscope, you'll see that very few of the cells are actually in mitosis at any given time. One of the features that characterizes aggressive lymphomas—like many forms of cancer—is that whenever you happen to look, you'll see many cells in mitosis. They are going through the cell cycle and dividing much more frequently than normal. In very aggressive lymphomas—like Burkitt lymphoma—nearly all the cells cycle continuously. In contrast, most indolent lymphomas have a relatively low rate of cell division.

This abnormally rapid progression through the cell cycle is one of the things that make cancer dangerous: cancer cells can overrun and crowd out normal cells and grab the necessary metabolic supplies away from more sedately dividing tissue. Since actively cycling cells are more susceptible to damage by radiation and many antineoplastic drugs, however, this too-rapid cycling of cancer cells is also an Achilles heel.

Some of the drugs used in chemotherapy are active against cells at specific phases of the cell cycle. For instance, cytarabine is closely related to the pyrimidine base cytosine and its sugar-containing derivative cytidine. If cytarabine is incorporated into newly synthesized DNA in place of cytidine, it disrupts the process of DNA replication. Cytarabine and other drugs that resemble the purine and pyrimidine bases can also bind to (and inhibit) the enzymes involved in DNA synthesis. Methotrexate, which inhibits the synthesis of nucleotide precursors of DNA, is also primarily active against cells undergoing DNA synthesis.

Vincristine and vinblastine, on the other hand, don't interfere with DNA synthesis at all. These two drugs are specifically active against cells in M-phase. They disrupt the mitotic spindle, the structure that develops during mitosis to pull the duplicated chromosomes apart so that one set ends up with each daughter cell. Trapped in midmitosis by destruction of the mitotic spindle, the cell dies.

Although they're not specific to any particular phase of the cell cycle, radiation therapy and some classes of antineoplastic drugs that damage DNA—like the alkylating agents—are also more active against rapidly cycling cells than they are against cells sitting quietly in G_0. DNA strands that are undergoing replication are more easily damaged, and this sort of DNA damage triggers intracellular pathways that lead to programmed cell death when the damaged cell enters

S-phase. Cells in G$_0$ have a lot of time to repair their DNA before the transition to S-phase occurs and are therefore more likely to survive than are rapidly cycling cells.

What is a mutation?

While the process of DNA replication is extremely accurate, mistakes do occur. Maybe ten to one hundred mistakes are made for every billion nucleotides copied. Since we have over a billion nucleotides in our genome, some mistakes in DNA replication are made *every time* a cell divides.

If you think of all the cell divisions that take place in our body, both during development and to replace worn-out cells, it's little wonder that small changes in the genome of individual cells continually occur. Changes in the genome, which can lead to changes in the proteins that the improperly copied genes code for, are called *mutations.*

Mutations that take place in our sperm and egg cells are passed on to our children. These mutations are ultimately responsible for genetic diversity—the reason we're all a bit different from one another. Mutations that take place in the rest of our cells won't be passed on to our children, but they can influence the function of the cell that bears the mutation. Since the mutation is now part of that cell's genome, it will be copied during all subsequent cell divisions, and all of that cell's daughter cells will carry the same mutation.

Mutations can take place in the coding sequence of a given gene, leading to production of an abnormal protein. They can also occur in the regulatory region. Mutations that occur in the regulatory regions can lead to lack of expression of a particular gene, or they can cause a gene to be expressed inappropriately so that it shows up in the wrong cell type or stays turned on at the wrong times.

There are many different types of copying errors. The simplest is substitution of one nucleotide for another. If a nucleotide substitution takes place in the coding sequence for a given gene, it can lead to substitution of one amino acid for another.

To go back to the example I used earlier, if a gene normally had the nucleotide sequence ATG and this was miscopied as AGG, the cell would make a protein in which arginine was substituted for methionine. Depending on the exact substitution that took place, this might or might not seriously affect the function of that protein (and the cell that makes it). Or you could end up with a nonsense nucleotide sequence that didn't code for any amino acid—in which case translation of the protein would be abruptly terminated.

　　　　　　　　　　　　　　　　UNDERSTANDING LYMPHOMA

A potentially more serious error occurs if one or more nucleotides are *skipped*. This is known as a *deletion*. Loss of a single nucleotide will disrupt reading of all the subsequent nucleotides in that gene. For instance, if our nucleotide sequence ATG AGG GCA AGG AGG, which codes for the amino acid sequence methionine-arginine-alanine-arginine-arginine, were to lose the second "A," it would read as ATG GGG CAA GGA GG, which would code for the very different amino acid sequence methionine-glycine-glutamine-glycine. If the normal amino acid sequence forms part of a protein that carries a "don't divide" message, such a major disruption of the protein's composition could permit the cell to divide more frequently than was appropriate.

Errors involving more than a single nucleotide can also occur. Large portions of a chromosome can be deleted, as well as single base pairs. Sometimes an entire chromosome is lost. Sections of a chromosome may be repeated many times. This is called *amplification,* and cells that have a portion of a chromosome that has undergone amplification have multiple copies of the genes present in the repeated area. In that case, the mutant cells may make too much of the protein those genes codes for. Sometimes the cell makes an additional copy of an entire chromosome, so there are three copies of that chromosome instead of the normal two. This is called *trisomy*. Sometimes part of one chromosome breaks off and becomes attached to another chromosome; this is a *translocation.*

Thus the different genetic mutations include substitution, deletion, amplification, trisomy, and translocation. Any given mutation may be beneficial, innocuous, or dangerous to the organism as a whole, depending on what genes are involved and what has happened to them. Frequently, different forms of lymphoma are associated with different specific mutations.

As I've just indicated, mutations can arise by chance simply because the DNA copying mechanism is imperfect. However, ultraviolet light, ionizing radiation, certain chemicals, and certain viruses can damage DNA and increase the probability that mutations will occur. Any chemical that damages DNA will increase the likelihood of a mutation; such chemicals act as *carcinogens*—substances that increase your chances of getting cancer. Other agents, known as *promoters,* don't damage DNA directly, but they do increase the chance that cancerous mutations will occur, simply by increasing the rate of cell division.

Mutations and lymphoma

Many mutations are harmless. Others are beneficial—we're human beings instead of single-celled organisms because of mutations that took place during evolution. Mutations can lead to cancer if they disrupt the normal processes of cell division and differentiation and lead to the abnormal accumulation of a group of dysfunctional cells.

This can happen if a given population of cells is forced to divide more rapidly than appropriate. In this case, a cell that is quiescent unless it is signaled to divide might somehow get its "divide" genes turned on in the absence of external stimulatory signals and lose the ability to respond to the inhibitory signals that tell it to cease dividing.

For instance, a given cell type may normally spend most of its time in G_0 but retain the ability to divide in response to a chemical message from a neighboring cell. Such messages are received when the messenger molecule binds to a *receptor* protein on the cell membrane. The receptor protein receives the external message, which triggers the receptor to pass along a "divide" signal to the inside of the cell. The "divide" message is conveyed to the cell nucleus (and ultimately to the DNA) through a complex intracellular signaling pathway (fig. 8.3).

Cancer can result if a cell starts inappropriately producing its *own* "divide" messenger molecules. For example, the malignant cells in adult T cell leukemia/lymphoma produce both abnormally high levels of a chemical called interleukin-2, which stimulates T cell division, *and* increased levels of the interleukin-2 *receptor*. They are forced to make abnormally high amounts of both interleukin-2 and its receptor by a virus that inserts its own genome into that of the T cells it infects. These cells are even more sensitive to interleukin-2 than normal T cells (because of increased production of receptors) and are continually stimulated to divide. Eventually they accumulate enough additional mutations to become malignant.

Cancer can also result from changes that take place farther along the cell division signaling pathways. Burkitt lymphoma involves abnormal production of a transcription factor called Myc. Like all transcription factors, Myc regulates genes with DNA sequences that it can bind to. Myc binds to the regulatory regions of various genes involved in cell division and turns them on. Ordinarily, production of Myc itself is very tightly controlled; it's turned on *only* when it's needed in response to the signals that tell the cell it's time to divide. However, in Burkitt lymphoma, the malignant B cells manufacture Myc protein incessantly. Expression of the *myc* gene is no longer regulated by signals from the environment.

This results from a chromosomal translocation. Parts of two chromosomes become interchanged, so that the coding sequence for the *myc* gene becomes at-

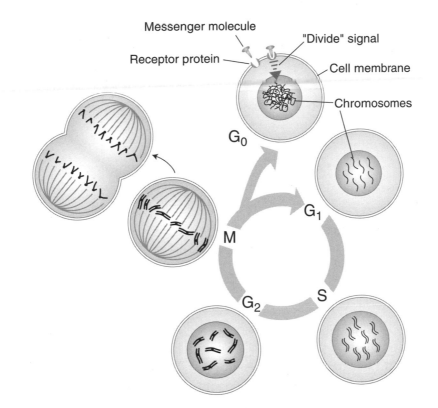

Figure 8.3. *Messenger stimulating cell division.* A cell that normally spends most of its time in G_0 can still retain the ability to divide in response to a signal from a neighboring cell. These signals are received when the messenger binds to a receptor protein on the cell membrane, triggering the receptor to pass a "divide" signal to the cell interior. The "divide" message is conveyed to the DNA through a complex intracellular signaling pathway. Some mutations can cause a cell to produce its own divide signal; others can bypass the external messenger entirely by activating a later step in the "divide" signaling pathway.

tached to the regulatory sequences for a gene involved in antibody production. Since the major role of B cells is to manufacture antibody, *those* regulatory regions are set up to carry on transcription constantly. And since the regulatory regions don't know that they're attached to the *myc* coding sequence instead of to the antibody coding sequence, they inappropriately stimulate *myc* transcription. The cell keeps churning out more and more Myc, which in turn binds to the genes it regulates, forcing the cell to continue to divide.

In general, a single mutation—no matter what it does—isn't enough to make a cell cancerous. A single mutation—like the translocation that turns on *myc*—

could cause a given cell and its progeny to multiply abnormally. However, that mutation alone wouldn't give those cells the ability to invade and destroy normal surrounding tissue, much less colonize regions of the body far away. The vast majority of cancer cells—if not all—contain *multiple* genetic abnormalities. While the enhanced rate of cell division alone increases the likelihood of further mutations, it appears that many cancer cells are far more genetically unstable than their normal counterparts.

This results from mutations in genes that act to safeguard the genome. Their jobs may be to prevent the cell from miscopying DNA, to repair any errors that slip through, or—if all else fails—to commit suicide. Some lymphomas involve mutations in genes that are involved in DNA repair. Others involve mutations in *tumor suppressor* genes. These genes keep damaged, potentially malignant cells from progressing through the cell cycle. One such gene, which appears to be involved in as many of 50 percent of human cancers, including several forms of lymphoma (Burkitt lymphoma and some follicular lymphomas that have transformed to diffuse large cell lymphoma) is *p53*.

p53 is activated in response to DNA damage. It acts as a transcription factor to keep the cell from progressing through the cell cycle (arresting it in G_I) until DNA repair processes are complete. If the damage is too extensive for repair, *p53* triggers apoptosis—programmed cell death—so that the damaged cell self-destructs. Both of these mechanisms prevent the damaged cell from propagating itself and limit the accumulation of mutations in a given cell. If, however, *p53 itself* is damaged—by so much as a single nucleotide substitution at just the wrong place—it no longer stops the damaged cell from propagating, and dangerous mutations can accumulate.

While mutations in growth-promoting genes like *myc* lead to inappropriately rapid cell division, cancer can also result when a cell that *normally* continues to divide is prevented from dying. Mutations in *bcl-2*, a gene that blocks apoptosis, are involved in most follicular lymphomas. Follicular lymphoma cells correspond to B lymphocytes at a specific stage in development when they are actively dividing. The majority of cells at this stage of development are slated for cell suicide pathways; only the cells that produce the best antibodies are supposed to survive and continue to differentiate. The malignant cells inappropriately express the *bcl-2* gene, which prevents them from undergoing apoptosis.

However, instead of differentiating into mature, nondividing, fully differentiated cells, the follicular lymphoma cells are stuck in a developmental stage at which it's appropriate for them to continue dividing. Therefore, as in other forms of cancer, a population of abnormal, dysfunctional cells starts to accumulate. Unlike the malignant cells in Burkitt lymphoma, the primary abnormality characterizing follicular lymphoma cells isn't that they're being forced to divide too frequently, it's that they're allowed to survive inappropriately.

These differences in the exact mutations that lead to the different forms of lymphoma are responsible for the very different behaviors of the affected cells. Ultimately, it's these genetic differences that determine not only the natural course of the different forms of lymphoma but also the likely response to different forms of therapy.

SUGGESTIONS FOR FURTHER READING

Alberts B, Johnson A, Lewis J, Raff M, Roberts K, Walter P. (2002). *The Molecular Biology of the Cell.* 4th ed. New York: Garland Publishing.
> *Probably the most comprehensive textbook on modern cell biology around, a book that is not only extremely informative but also astonishingly readable. While I am mostly recommending it for the wealth of material on basic cell biology, it's worth noting that the twenty-third chapter is on cancer and the last two chapters are on the immune system.*

Varmus H, Weinberg RA. (1993). *Genes and the Biology of Cancer.* New York: Scientific American Library.
> *A wonderful and extremely accessible introduction to cell biology as it applies to cancer written by two leading researchers in the field of genes and cancer.*

Weinberg RA. (1996). "How cancer arises." *Scientific American* 275 (3): 62–70.
> *A briefer discussion of the same basic themes.*

CHAPTER 9

The Immune System

Lymphoma involves a class of cells called *lymphocytes*. If you have lymphoma, it means that, at some point, somewhere in your body, a lymphocyte made an error in copying the genetic information that directs how that cell was supposed to look and behave. When the cell reproduced itself, it passed this error on to its daughter cells. After several such genetic errors accumulated, the cell's descendants became *malignant*, or cancerous, cells. They no longer played by the rules that allow all the cells of the body to work together in harmony. Instead they became dangerous and destructive.

As with many forms of cancer, the behavior of malignant lymphocytes echoes the behavior of the normal cells from which they arose. Malignant cells in the different kinds of lymphoma can resemble normal lymphocytes at different stages of development. Therefore, understanding how lymphocytes normally develop and function helps us understand the behavior of the abnormal lymphocytes found in lymphoma. This understanding has also helped researchers design therapies that target lymphoma cells.

Lymphocytes are an integral part of the *immune system*, which consists of a variety of different cell types and tissues that work in concert to defend us from disease. While understanding how normal lymphocytes behave helps us to understand lymphoma, understanding the function of the other cells that make up the immune system is less directly relevant. However, a basic understanding of immune system function is useful to people with lymphoma for several other reasons.

First, many of the therapies used to treat lymphoma affect other cells in the immune system. Understanding the basics of immune system function will help you understand the potential side effects of these treatments.

Moreover, some of the exciting new approaches to treating lymphoma, such as those using monoclonal antibodies or cancer-specific vaccines, depend on recruiting your own immune system into the fight. Basic immunology will help you understand how these therapies work and why they are more specific than older approaches to therapy. Finally, understanding the immune system is key to understanding the *immune surveillance hypothesis of cancer.* This hypothesis, which has received a lot of publicity in alternative health circles, suggests that malignant cells continually arise in your body but are kept in check by your immune system. Many people believe that stimulating the immune system should be beneficial if you have cancer, and these people may be interested in taking herbs and supplements that they hope will do this. Once you start thinking of the immune system as consisting of a group of different types of cells rather than as an abstract notion, however, you might question whether taking such substances, without understanding exactly *what* they're doing and *where* they're acting, is a good idea for someone with a cancer of the immune system itself, such as lymphoma.

This chapter focuses on understanding the immune system and how it works, paying particular attention to lymphocytes and those aspects of immune system development and function that are relevant to lymphoma and its treatment. Chapter 8 provides an introduction to cell biology and current ideas about cancer; the concepts introduced in that chapter may be helpful in understanding this chapter.

General overview of the immune system

Our immune system allows us to remain healthy in what might otherwise be considered a hostile, germ-ridden world. Without an immune system, our body would be easy prey for the multitudes of *pathogenic* (disease-causing) organisms that surround us. Our cuts would routinely become infected, and we'd have no better defense against mold spores than does the half-eaten peanut butter and jelly sandwich your four-year-old slipped behind the radiator a week ago. With an immune system, though, we do a remarkably good job of coexisting with most of the microorganisms we encounter.

In the broadest sense, the immune system includes such organs as the skin and the *mucous membranes* that line the airways and the *gastrointestinal tract* (stomach, intestines, and associated structures). These are the first lines of defense against potentially harmful invaders. However, the immune system is usually considered to consist of the cells involved in an active response to potentially harmful microorganisms rather than those that simply form a barrier to invasion. These actively responding cells include different types of white blood cells that circulate in the body's two interconnected vascular systems (the circulatory system, which carries blood, and the lymphatic system, which carries a colorless fluid called *lymph*) and reside in tissues.

White blood cells as a group are called *leukocytes*, from the Latin *leuko* for white and *cyte* for cell. Leukocytes can be divided into distinct cell types, including *granulocytes*, *monocytes*, and *lymphocytes*. These different kinds of leukocytes can be distinguished from each other under a microscope, and they have somewhat different functions.

The immune responses mediated by leukocytes can be broadly divided into two types: *innate* and *adaptive*. Some of the cells in the immune system participate in both innate and adaptive immune responses, while others are specialized to participate in adaptive responses only. Innate responses are nonspecific defenses that we are born with. They are the first defenses to come into play in response to a threat. They become activated nonspecifically—that is, in response to any perceived threat. In contrast, adaptive responses are acquired during the lifetime of an individual following exposure to specific pathogens.

During a battle against infectious organisms, the adaptive immune responses come into play later than the innate responses. The adaptive immune responses involve the lymphocytes, which receive signals from the cells participating in the earlier, innate response that there is a problem. Adaptive immune responses are the basis for the phenomenon of *immunological memory*, which is the biological mechanism underlying the effectiveness of *vaccination*, as well as the reason you can't get certain diseases more than once (fig. 9.1).

The *granulocytes*, which participate in innate responses, are composed of three different cell types, *neutrophils*, *eosinophils*, and *basophils*. As the general name implies, all three types contain little granular structures in their cytoplasm. The three types of granulocytes are named for the types of dye that stain these cytoplasmic granules.

Neutrophils, whose cytoplasmic granules stain salmon-pink, act as *phagocytes*. Phagocytes, or "eater cells," are cells that can *phagocytose:* they engulf, devour, and destroy bacteria and other pathogens. The neutrophils, sometimes called *polymorphs* or *polymorphonuclear leukocytes* because of the characteristic multilobed ap-

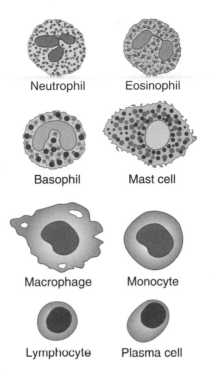

Figure 9.1. *White blood cells and related cell types.* The granulocytes include the neutrophils, the eosinophils, and the basophils. All the granulocytes participate in innate immune response; they can be distinguished from each other under a microscope by the types of dye that stain their granules. Mast cells, which are closely related to basophils, are found throughout the tissues of the body. Monocytes give rise to the macrophages; like neutrophils, they are eater cells that engulf and destroy bacterial invaders. Resting lymphocytes are small and have little cytoplasm. Plasma cells are a fully differentiated form of B lymphocyte.

pearance of their nuclei, are considered a first line of defense against bacteria. Many forms of chemotherapy suppress the production of neutrophils, leaving you more susceptible to bacteria. Therefore, people undergoing these forms of chemotherapy need to be very careful to avoid exposing themselves to bacterial infection. This is particularly true for people who've undergone high-dose chemotherapy in preparation for a bone marrow transplant, in which virtually all the neutrophils have been temporarily knocked out.

The eosinophils, whose large hamburger-shaped cytoplasmic granules are stained a sort of orangy pink by the acidic (negatively charged) dye eosin, are involved in defense against large parasites as well as some allergic reactions. Like a nihilist throwing a Molotov cocktail at an elephant, the eosinophils discharge the contents of their granules in the presence of certain parasites. This liberates an enzyme that attacks the parasite's cell wall. For reasons that are unclear but probably involve a response to substances released by the tumor cells, the levels of eosinophils circulating in the blood are sometimes elevated in people with Hodgkin lymphoma and some forms of NHL.

The function of the basophils, whose granules are stained a dark purplish blue by the basic (positively charged) dye methylene blue, is less well understood, though the basophils may be involved in allergic reactions. Some hematologists have joked that basophils—and *mast cells*, a similar cell type found throughout the body—exist mainly to make people with allergies miserable.

Like other types of white blood cells, the granulocytes can leave the circulatory system and migrate throughout the body. They are attracted to sites of infection by chemical messages released by other cells in the immune system and substances released from injured cells. An average granulocyte circulates in the bloodstream for several hours, then spends several days patrolling the body for infection, and then dies. This means that there is a constant demand for new granulocytes.

Monocytes, another type of leukocyte, circulate in the blood for about twenty-four hours before migrating into the tissue and developing into *macrophages*. Monocytes and macrophages, like neutrophils, are phagocytes (macrophage means "big eater"): they back up the neutrophils as a major defense against bacteria. In addition to their direct phagocytic role in controlling infection, macrophages help coordinate the response of the various cell types.

Like many other cells in the immune system (as well as elsewhere in the body), monocytes and macrophages release chemical messengers called *cytokines*, which influence immune function in various ways. Cytokines can produce very localized responses (such as stimulating nearby lymphocytes to divide or increasing the permeability of local blood vessels) as well as *systemic* responses (responses that influence the entire body, such as fever).

Macrophages, like granulocytes, participate in innate immune responses, such as the rapid inflammation that occurs in response to a local infection. They also act in coordination with the *lymphocytes* in adaptive immune responses. Monocytes manufacture a cytokine that stimulates some types of lymphocytes to divide; this chemically mediated interaction may have significance for some forms of lymphoma.

For historical reasons (it's *not* just to confuse the uninitiated), macrophages found in specific locations of the body are given special names: macrophages found in connective tissue are called *histiocytes;* macrophages found in the brain are called *microglia;* macrophages found in the liver are called *Kupfer cells;* and macrophages found in the bone are called *osteoclasts.* When macrophages are found in *lymph nodes* (small organs involved in generating adaptive immune responses), they are often called *tingible body macrophages.* (The tingible bodies are small pieces of dead lymphocytes that have been eaten by the macrophages.) In some of the older classification systems, certain forms of lymphoma are called histiocytic because the lymphoma cells were so large that the pathologists thought they were histiocytes. This type of lymphoma is now known as diffuse large cell lymphoma.

The two major classes of *lymphocytes* are *T lymphocytes* (*T cells*) and *B lymphocytes* (*B cells*). Both T and B lymphocytes participate in adaptive responses to disease— acquired responses that are specific to a given type of pathogen. B lymphocytes give rise to *plasma cells,* which secrete a class of proteins called *antibodies.* Antibodies are particularly important in controlling pathogens found outside cells rather than pathogens that have already succeeded in infiltrating a cell.

The other major class of lymphocytes, T cells, has a variety of functions, including killing cells that are infected with viruses and regulating the activity of the other cells in the immune system. Different kinds of T cells—*cytotoxic T cells, helper T cells, regulatory T cells,* and *inflammatory T cells*—carry out the different T cell functions. Cytotoxic T cells kill cells that have been infected with virus, while helper T cells, regulatory T cells, and inflammatory T cells act like conductors; they orchestrate the responses of the other cells in the immune system. Like the cytotoxic T cells, a third class of lymphocytes, called *natural killer cells* or *large, granular lymphocytes,* kills virally infected cells (and possibly cancer cells). Natural killer cells (NK cells) play roles in both innate and adaptive immune responses.

Although lymphoma was recognized as a disease of the lymphoid tissue in the nineteenth century, an understanding of the role of normal lymphocytes, currently considered central to the functioning of the immune system, has only recently emerged. Elie Metchnikoff, a flamboyant Russian-born researcher who developed calomel ointment for use against syphilis and advocated yogurt to extend life, described the phagocytic activity of macrophages in the 1880s. Emil von Behring, who worked on a cure for diphtheria, and Shibasaburo Kitasato, who investigated tetanus, recognized the existence of antibodies by 1890. However, as recently as 1960, the lymphocyte (then viewed as a single cell type) had no known function. Most of the remainder of this chapter explores the development and function of lymphocytes. Before discussing these cells, however, I describe the structure and organization of the lymphatic system and its relationship to the circulatory system in which blood is carried.

The human lymphatic system

The primary function of lymphocytes is to actively protect the body from infectious disease. They are like a patrolling police force that is constantly searching for criminals. All lymphocytes arise from precursor cells in the *bone marrow*—the spongy tissue found in the centers of our bones. During development, one class of lymphocytes—the B cells—continue to mature in the bone marrow. The second class of lymphocytes—the T cells—migrate to the *thymus* (an organ located above the heart in the upper middle part of the chest) to mature. It's easy to remember which is which: "B" for bone marrow and "T" for thymus. The bone marrow and thymus, the two organs where lymphocytes develop and mature in humans, are called the *central* (or *primary*) *lymphoid organs.*

Mature lymphocytes leave the central lymphoid organs (again, the bone marrow and the thymus) and pass through the bloodstream to several different tissues known as the *secondary* (or *peripheral*) *lymphoid organs.* The peripheral lymphoid organs include the *spleen,* the *lymph nodes,* and areas of lymphoid tissue associated with the *mucous membranes* that line bodily cavities. (Mucous membranes, or mucosa, line many areas of your body, including your lungs, mouth, throat, and intestines; they're called mucous membranes because they contain cells that secrete mucus.) *Mucosal-associated lymphoid tissue* (MALT), the lymphoid tissue associated with mucous membranes, is found in locations such as the *tonsils,* the *adenoids,* the *appendix,* and areas of the intestinal wall called *Peyer's patches.* The secondary lymphoid organs are the site of later stages of lymphocyte development, where immune responses to specific pathogens are generated. The spleen has the additional job of removing old red cells and damaged platelets from the bloodstream.

As the blood circulates through the body, it's under pressure. This pressure forces water and small dissolved substances through the spaces between the cells that make up the walls of the *capillaries*—the smallest class of blood vessels—and out into the *interstitial fluid* (the fluid surrounding all your cells). This flow of water- and bloodborne molecules out of the capillaries and into the interstitial fluid would create a condition of fluid imbalance if some mechanism didn't exist to return fluid back to the circulatory system. This mechanism is accomplished by the *lymphatic system.*

The interstitial fluid drains into the system of vessels that make up the lymphatic system. Interstitial fluid collects into small lymphatic vessels, at which point it's called *lymph*. The lymphatic vessels join together into progressively larger vessels and finally return the lymph into the circulatory system via the subclavian veins near the heart. On the way back to the circulatory system, the lymph passes through the lymph nodes.

The lymph nodes are small organs about the size and shape of a kidney bean that are found in the lymphatic system, typically at sites where lymphatic vessels join together. The lymph nodes and other secondary lymphatic tissues act like biological filters. If an infection is present, bacteria in the interstitial fluid are swept into the lymphatic system, carried back through the lymphatic system, and trapped in the lymph nodes. This contributes to the "swollen glands" you sometimes see with an infection—these are lymph nodes filled with trapped bacteria and bacterial debris (as well as rapidly dividing lymphocytes).

Similarly, pathogens entering the respiratory tract when you breathe encounter lymphoid tissue in the tonsils and adenoids. Bacteria brought into the digestive tract when you eat are trapped in the MALT in the gut, and bacteria that get into the bloodstream through cuts are trapped in the spleen. Lymphocytes continually recirculate through the blood, lymph, and peripheral lymphoid tissues. This constant recirculation, together with the strategic location of the peripheral lymphoid tissue, optimizes the chance that the lymphocytes will encounter a pathogen that they can recognize—and become activated to fight it.

Hematopoiesis: the development of the cells that circulate in the blood and lymph

All blood cells are descended from a cell type found in the bone marrow known as an *uncommitted* or *pluripotent stem cell*. In this context, the word *stem* implies an immature, undifferentiated cell that has not yet attained its final, fully functional form. You can think of it as analogous to the stem of a plant that can branch off into several directions. *Uncommitted* and *pluripotent* imply that, at this stage, the cell still has many different potential fates. It can continue to divide and create more stem cells, or it can differentiate into a mature blood cell. It is still capable of responding to various cues in its environment that will allow it to follow one of several pathways that ultimately lead to all the different differentiated blood cell types (fig. 9.2). The stem cell is like a gifted child who has a wide variety of careers accessible to him or her before various experiences and educational choices narrow the options.

The environmental cues that influence the stem cell include cytokines as well as molecules embedded in the external membranes of neighboring cells and in the *extracellular matrix* of the bone marrow. Cytokines, as you'll recall, are chemical messengers released from various cells in the body. Cytokines diffuse through the extracellular fluids to signal other cells. The extracellular matrix is a network of large molecules that forms a sort of framework—or scaffolding—outside the cells.

Cytokines and other environmental signals can speed up or slow down the proliferation of their *target cells*—the cells that are the recipients of these molecular messages. Cytokines can also signal the target cell to produce more or less

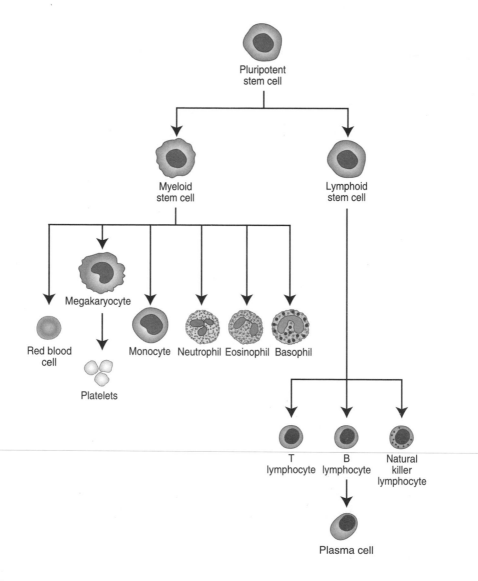

of a specific protein, which might induce it to develop along one or another of several possible pathways. The target cell is able to receive such cues through *receptors*, large proteins on the cell surface. Cytokines and other signaling molecules fit into their receptors like a key fitting into a lock.

Specific cytokines are produced by—and influence—all the cells of the immune system. Some are of particular interest to people with lymphoma. People whose bone marrow function is suppressed by chemotherapy, so that levels of circulating blood cells are reduced, may be given cytokines to speed up the production of one or more cell types. *Granulocyte colony-stimulating factor* is given to speed up neutrophil production, and *erythropoietin* may be given to increase the production of red cells. Cytokines are also used to increase the numbers of circulating stem cells in people who are preparing for a stem cell transplant. Some interesting new approaches to lymphoma therapy utilize substances from two cytokine families, the interferons and the interleukins (see Chapter 5).

Some cytokines have a very restricted range of target cells—acting on only one cell type (or subtype)—while others act on a variety of cell types. In each case, the specificity of action (or lack of specificity of action) is determined by the presence (or absence) of receptors on target cells. Different cell types—or even the same cell type at different stages in the differentiation process—have different receptors. A given signaling molecule interacts with a specific target

---

Figure 9.2. *Hematopoiesis.* All blood cells descend from a single progenitor cell, the pluripotent stem cell. The pluripotent stem cell differentiates in one direction or another depending on environmental cues from both the particular cells in its neighborhood and the growth factors to which it is exposed. Early in differentiation the stem cell becomes committed to developing into either a lymphocyte or another type of blood cell. Lymphoid stem cells give rise to the three types of lymphocytes (B cells, T cells, and natural killer cells), while myeloid stem cells give rise to red blood cells, platelets, monocytes, and granulocytes (neutrophils, eosinophils, and basophils). Both T and B lymphocytes participate in adaptive responses to disease—acquired responses that are specific to a given type of pathogen. B lymphocytes give rise to *plasma cells,* which secrete a class of proteins called antibodies. Antibodies are particularly important in controlling pathogens found outside cells rather than pathogens that have already succeeded in infiltrating a cell, while T cells can recognize and kill cells that harbor an unwelcome invader. Natural killer cells, unlike B cells and T cells, are involved in innate (rather than adaptive) immune responses. Dendritic cells (not shown) are also derived from the pluripotent stem cell (usually from the myeloid lineage).

receptor. Different types of receptors are shaped differently, which allows unique signaling molecules, or *ligands*, to bind to and interact with them. Each cell carries a large repertoire of receptors on its surface, allowing it to respond to a variety of different signals. The cell integrates all the different incoming signals it receives, and this determines its final response.

In response to some combination of environmental cues or signals, the pluripotent stem cell begins to proceed along one of several possible pathways. The next step along the developmental road is the *committed* stem cell, or *progenitor* cell. While still an immature form, the progenitor cell has become committed to either a *lymphoid* or a *myeloid* path. Its options have become more limited. Lymphoid progenitor cells will differentiate into one of several types of lymphocytes. Myeloid progenitor cells can differentiate into granulocytes (neutrophils, basophils, and eosinophils), macrophages, mast cells, erythrocytes (red blood cells), or platelets, proceeding along a specific pathway to a final cell type in response to various environmental cues.

Lymphocytes

A critical element of the immune response is the ability to recognize foreign or abnormal substances as wrong and target them for destruction. Substances that can elicit an immune response are called *antigens*. Antigens include proteins found on bacteria and viruses, toxic substances released from bacteria and viruses, and innocuous foreign substances like ragweed pollen. Many of the substances that make up the cells in your body would elicit an immune response if they were injected into another organism, but your own body perceives these "self" substances as harmless. These substances are sometimes called *self-antigens*, in recognition of their antigenic potential.

The lymphocytes are the true xenophobes of the immune system. If lymphocytes lived on Orwell's *Animal Farm*, they would post signs reading: "Self-antigens, good. Foreign antigens, bad." Individual lymphocytes recognize distinct antigens (i.e., a lymphocyte that recognizes and is active against a protein found on the smallpox virus would not recognize polio or flu viruses and so forth). As noted earlier, there are two main classes of lymphocytes: B lymphocytes (or B cells) and T lymphocytes (or T cells).

B cells

In the United States and Europe, most cases of lymphoma arise from B cells, the class of lymphocytes that synthesize the proteins called *immunoglobulins*, or *anti-*

bodies. These proteins bind specifically to particular antigens. (The word *antigen* comes from the term *antibody generating.*) They either exist in a membrane-bound form that remains associated with the cells that synthesize them, or they are secreted into the blood. Although the terms *antibody* and *immunoglobulin* are often used interchangeably, an antibody is defined by its ability to specifically bind antigen, whereas immunoglobulin refers to the general class of proteins. Here, I use *antibody* to refer to these antigen-binding proteins only after they have been secreted into the blood, and I use *immunoglobulin* to refer to either the secreted or the membrane-bound form.

Individual antibodies actually recognize relatively small portions of antigens. These antibody recognition sites are called *antigenic determinants,* or *epitopes.* Any given antigen has a number of distinct antigenic determinants and can be recognized by a number of distinct antibodies. A given antibody, however, will bind only to its specific antigenic determinant.

Since antibodies circulate in the blood and extracellular fluid and can act in isolation from the cells that manufacture them, B lymphocytes are referred to as the *humoral* limb of the adaptive immune system. (The word *humor* comes from the Greek for "fluid." Many years ago, disease was believed to originate from imbalances of four fluids termed *humors,* and blood and lymph are sometimes still called *humors.*)

Humoral immune responses are the immunological defenses that can be transferred via *plasma*—the liquid part of blood that is left after all the cells have been removed—to another person, such as when antiserum containing horse antibodies is given to people who have been bitten by venomous snakes. (The T cells represent the second limb of the adaptive immune system. T cell–mediated defenses involve direct cellular activity, so they cannot be transferred from one person to another by means of plasma.) Antibodies are an important part of the immune response, since they can both neutralize pathogens on their own and "tag" them for destruction by cells in the immune system.

B cells, like all the other blood cells, arise in the bone marrow. Their development can be divided into two phases. During the first phase, *B lymphopoiesis,* an uncommitted stem cell differentiates into a mature B lymphocyte that is capable of responding to antigens. This phase consists of the processes involved in basic development of the lymphocyte. When the cell has completed lymphopoiesis and has become a mature B lymphocyte, immunoglobulin molecules are found on the cell surface, where they can act as receptors that recognize and bind to their specific antigen.

The second phase of development, termed *immunopoiesis,* has to do with changes that take place after a mature B lymphocyte encounters antigen. The binding of an antigen to an immunoglobulin molecule on the surface of the mature B cell triggers further differentiation into either a plasma cell, which is the cell type that secretes antibodies, or a memory B cell. Thus, in immunopoiesis, a quiet, inactive, "unawakened" B cell develops into a tribe of identical daughter cells that can actively participate in the immunological defense against disease.

Differentiation and function of B cells

During fetal development, lymphopoiesis takes places in the liver and bone marrow. After birth, all B lymphopoiesis takes place in the bone marrow. During B lymphopoiesis, the stem cell passes through several developmental stages. These developmental stages include the pro–B cell, the pre–B cell, the immature B cell, and the mature B cell (or B lymphocyte). As the cell matures and passes through these stages, it undergoes a number of changes, including changes in its physical appearance and in the types of proteins it manufactures (including the specific receptors expressed on the cell surface), and development of an immunoglobulin unique to each particular developing lymphocyte.

Different cell surface receptors allow the B cell to interact with different molecules on neighboring cells, and to respond to different cytokines, at different phases of its development. These receptors also allow cells to recognize a particular environment in the body and thereby influence the specific sites to which lymphocytes "home" at different stages in their development. Homing, in this context, refers to the ability of lymphocytes, like homing pigeons or very small salmon, to return to certain tissues after exploring the rest of the body. Not only are surface receptors important to normal lymphocyte development, but they are also used in several approaches to lymphoma therapy (see Chapter 5).

Immunoglobulin molecules are shaped like the letter *Y.* They contain a *constant region* (the "stem" of the *Y*) and a *variable region* (the "arms" of the *Y*). The constant region controls the interaction of the immunoglobulin with the rest of the immune system. There are five different classes of immunoglobulins (IgM, IgD, IgG, IgE, and IgA); the constant regions of all immunoglobulins within a class are essentially the same (and the general structure of the constant region is similar even among the different classes).

The variable region is the part of the immunoglobulin molecule that recognizes and binds to its specific antigen. Different B cells manufacture immunoglobulins containing different variable regions. The acquisition of a unique immunoglobulin, with its own unique variable region, for each developing B lymphocyte allows each different lymphocyte to recognize and respond to the unique antigen that "fits" its particular immunoglobulin species.

During B cell development, different genes (DNA sequences) that code for portions of the variable region of the immunoglobulin protein (fig. 9.3) are rearranged and recombined to provide each B cell with a unique immunoglobulin. Think of shooting one hundred hours of film and then splicing together a few of these hours to make a movie. Pushing this analogy a little further, assume that all the movies ever made are generated from this same one hundred hours of film. Each movie is different because it is put together out of different specific film segments. Any given segment can be used in multiple movies, and there are strict rules requiring each movie to use the same total number of film segments.

Moreover, each movie must include segments taken from each of several general regions on the original roll of film. So each new movie requires a segment taken from the "possible beginnings" region of film, a segment from the "possible middles of the story" region, and a segment from the "possible endings" region. This process of genetic shuffling and splicing allows for the generation of an enormous diversity of specific antibodies from a relatively limited amount of DNA.

This shuffling is critical to the proper functioning of the immune system. Gene rearrangement and recombination permits the synthesis of an almost infinite number of antibodies, which can recognize and bind to the almost infinite number of possible antigens, without requiring an infinite supply of DNA. Such a supply of DNA would be unwieldy, to say the least, since huge, enormous nuclei would be required, and this would necessitate huge, enormous cells, which would . . . well, you get the picture.

As far as we know, only lymphocytes undergo this process of gene rearrangement, a process that is necessary because each new lymphocyte must be able to recognize a distinct antigen. Unfortunately, this process of lymphocytic gene shuffling is probably also involved in the development of lymphoma. The vast majority of lymphomas involve alterations in gene expression (see Chapter 8), which means either that a gene has *mutated* so that the protein product it codes for is abnormal or that the *regulation* of some gene has been disrupted so that more or less of its protein product is made than appropriate (or shows up in the wrong place or at the wrong time).

In many lymphomas, these abnormalities in gene expression result from disruptions of chromosomes, particularly *translocations* (part of one chromosome

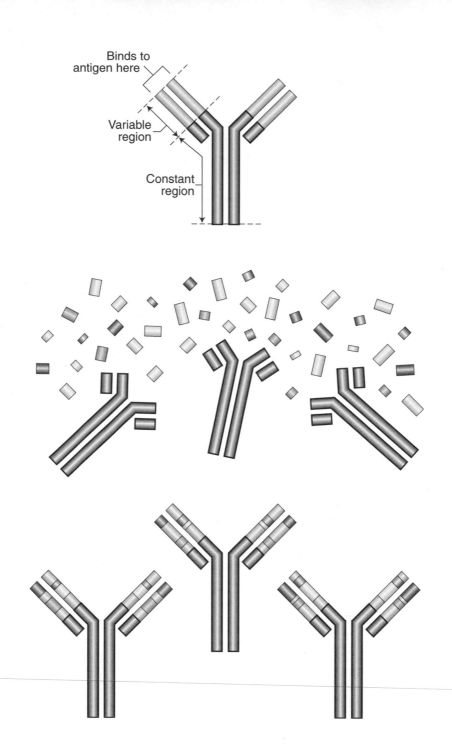

breaks off and becomes attached to another chromosome). Frequently, these translocations involve portions of chromosomes that contain those gene segments that code for portions of antibody variable regions. It's as though something went awry in the normal process of gene rearrangement, so that a set of genes winds up where it shouldn't be. To return to the film analogy, it's as though Han Solo and R2D2 suddenly showed up in the middle of *Gone with the Wind* and took over the rest of the story, while Scarlett and Rhett suddenly found themselves at the Death Star. Other chromosomal abnormalities that may be found in association with lymphomas are *deletions*, in which part of a chromosome is missing, and *duplications*, in which there is an extra copy of a specific chromosome (fig. 9.4).

The process of gene rearrangement and recombination, in which each developing B cell is equipped with its own unique immunoglobulin species, is irreversible. Although the immunoglobulin variable region can be modified so that it has an even greater affinity for an antigen that it recognizes, it cannot be restructured to recognize a different antigen. For instance, if a B cell has an immunoglobulin that recognizes a protein that is part of the smallpox virus but doesn't bind to it very well, this immunoglobulin can be modified so that it binds more tightly to the smallpox virus protein, but it can never be changed to a form that would recognize a different protein on a polio virus.

After the B cell has acquired a unique immunoglobulin, the new immunoglobulin species is displayed on the cell surface. In this way, the immunoglobulin molecules can act as receptors that recognize and bind to antigens in the environment. During this stage of development, while the B cell is still in the bone mar-

---

Figure 9.3. *Structure of antibodies and how they are made.* As shown in the top part of this figure, immunoglobulin molecules are shaped like the letter Y. The constant region (the "stem" of the Y) controls the interaction of the immunoglobulin with the rest of the immune system, whereas the variable region (the "arms" of the Y) is the part of the immunoglobulin molecule that recognizes and binds to its specific antigen. During B cell development, different genes that code for portions of the variable region of the immunoglobulin protein are rearranged and recombined to provide each B cell with its own unique immunoglobulin, as shown in the middle part of the figure. This process of rearrangement and recombination allows each developing B cell to synthesize its own unique form of immunoglobulin. As shown in the bottom part of the figure, these different forms of immunoglobulin have different variable regions and thus recognize and bind to different antigens.

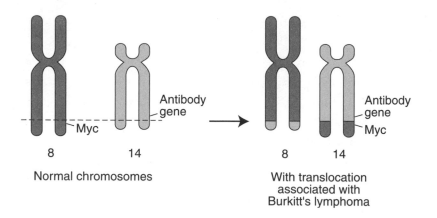

Figure 9.4. *Chromosomal abnormalities that can lead to lymphoma.* Many lymphomas result from disruptions of chromosomes, particularly translocations, in which part of a chromosome breaks off and becomes attached to another chromosome. In certain B cell lymphomas, these translocations involve portions of chromosomes that code for immunoglobulins (which are highly expressed in B cells). In most cases of Burkitt lymphoma, for instance, regulatory regions from antibody genes on chromosome 14 become attached to the portion of chromosome 8 that contains the gene for Myc, a transcription factor that is involved in the regulation of cellular proliferation. Other chromosomal abnormalities that can lead to lymphoma include deletions, in which part of a chromosome is missing, and duplications, in which there is an extra copy of a specific chromosome.

row, any B cell that encounters an antigen it recognizes—such as proteins on neighboring cells—is triggered to die by means of a process called *apoptosis*, or programmed cell death. Apoptosis eliminates cells that would grow up to produce antibodies against self-antigens. Eliminating these cells keeps the immune system from attacking normal constituents of the body. (Occasionally, circulating lymphocytes that recognize self-antigens are found. This leads to a condition known as *autoimmune disease*. As discussed in Chapters 10 and 11, people with certain autoimmune diseases are more likely to develop lymphoma than the general population.) At this point in B cell development, the cell carries a class of immunoglobulins called immunoglobulin M (IgM) and is considered an immature B cell.

Mature B cells carry an additional class of immunoglobulins, called immunoglobulin D (IgD), which has the same antigen specificity as their IgM and are ready to leave the sheltering environment of the bone marrow and go out into the body in search of foreign antigens. Malignancies that correspond to cells in the very early stages in B cell development, the stages that take place in the bone marrow, generally appear as leukemias, while most B cell lymphomas, except B cell lymphoblastic lymphoma, resemble B lymphocytes at later stages of development, after they have left the bone marrow.

The next stage of development, B immunopoiesis, occurs in response to contact with antigen, after the mature B cell has left the bone marrow. B immunopoiesis takes place in the secondary lymphoid organs: the lymph nodes, the spleen, and the mucosal-associated lymphoid tissue.

A mature B cell leaving the bone marrow is called a *naive* cell. It is inexperienced in that it hasn't yet encountered an antigen that its immunoglobulin recognizes. The innocent young B cell passes through the bloodstream into the lymph nodes and other peripheral lymphoid tissues. If it doesn't encounter a trapped antigen that it recognizes, it passes out of the lymph node into the lymphatic system, eventually being returned to the circulatory system (see fig. 2.1). A naive B cell continues to recirculate through the blood and lymphatic system in search of the antigen that will give meaning to its existence. Once it does encounter antigen that its immunoglobulin receptor recognizes, it becomes *activated*.

Activation means that interaction of the membrane-bound immunoglobulin receptor with its specific antigen triggers a series of intracellular reactions that lead to increased proliferation and further differentiation of the cell. The cell has been signaled that a foreign invader ("A foreign invader! A foreign invader! A foreign invader!") is present. To successfully combat this invader, the body will need more lymphocytes that recognize the same foreign antigen, and the B cell will need to develop into an active form in which it can participate in the defense of the organism.

Antigen binding is necessary for B cell activation. For a few classes of antigens, binding alone is sufficient to induce B cell activation. These antigens, called *thymus-independent antigens*, contain very repetitive structures, whereby the same structural motif is repeated over and over. At low concentrations, thymus-independent antigens react with a specific immunoglobulin receptor (just like other antigens). At very high concentrations, however, some of these thymus-independent antigens are able to activate B cells nonspecifically and can stimulate B cells to divide, regardless of whether their immunoglobulin receptors fit correctly. This type of thymus-independent antigen is called a *B cell mitogen* or a *polyclonal mitogen*, since it can stimulate B cells to undergo *mitosis*, or divide.

Most of the time, however, B cells need to receive a simultaneous signal from an activated *helper T cell* while they are binding antigen in order to become activated. Because of this requirement for a concurrent signal from a helper T cell,

B cell activation takes place in T cell–rich regions of the secondary lymphoid tissues (fig. 9.5). When the B cell binds an antigen, two series of events are triggered. First, when the immunoglobulin receptor becomes occupied, this signals the B cell that antigen is present and sets into play a series of intracellular events that will ultimately lead to activation.

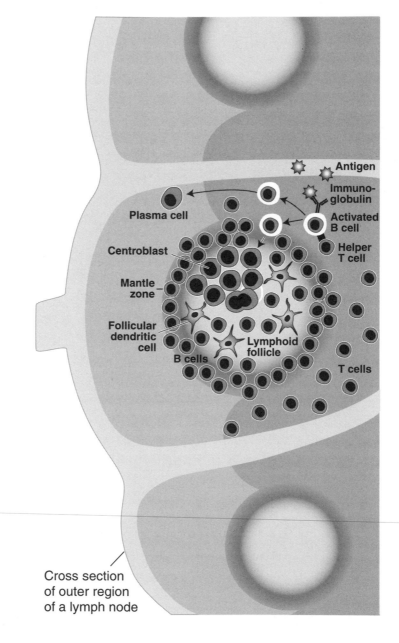

Cross section
of outer region
of a lymph node

Second, the B cell internalizes the receptor-bound antigen. It engulfs the whole immunoglobulin-antigen complex, swallows it, and chews up the antigen. Bits of chewed-up antigen are then carried back to the cell surface, where, like a child sticking out his or her tongue during lunch to elicit some response from a playmate, the bits of antigen are displayed together with some of the B cell's own cell surface proteins. In this semidigested form, the antigen can be recognized by helper T cells that are specific for that same antigen. These helper T cells respond by sending activating signals to the B cell.

A mature B cell that has both bound antigen *and* received an activation signal from a helper T cell starts to divide. Following activation, some B cells differentiate into plasma cells, which are capable of releasing antibody into the circulatory system, and can participate in the response to the infection. Other activated B cells migrate into a specialized region of the lymph node (or the other peripheral lymphoid tissue where activation is taking place) known as a *lymphoid follicle* (sometimes called a lymphoid *nodule*).

The follicle consists of a cluster of several different types of cells. These include resting B cells; *follicular dendritic cells*, which are a class of specialized cells with long branching processes (the word *dendrite* comes from the Greek for "branching" and can be recognized in such plant names as "rhododendron"); certain types of T cells; and the tingible body macrophages (remember these from the section on macrophages?). If you look at a slice of a lymph node under

---

Figure 9.5. *B cell activation and lymph node organization.* B cells generally need to receive a simultaneous signal from a helper T cell while they are binding antigen in order to become activated. Thus, B cell activation takes place in T cell–rich regions of the secondary lymphatic tissues that are adjacent to primary follicles (specialized regions of the lymph node that contain several different cell types, including resting B cells and follicular dendritic cells). Following activation, some B cells differentiate into plasma cells, while others migrate into lymphoid follicles and start dividing. Many kinds of lymphoma are believed to represent malignancies that correspond to B cells at particular stages of development, particularly those found in the secondary follicle. The centroblasts in the germinal center probably correspond to the cell that gives rise to the diffuse large cell lymphomas, the centrocytes correspond to the "small, cleaved cell" seen in follicular lymphomas, and cells normally found in the mantle zone correspond to the malignant cell in mantle cell lymphoma. Even the Reed-Sternberg cell is now believed to be derived from a germinal center cell.

a microscope, you can clearly discern the clumped cells in the follicle from the other parts of the lymph node, just as you can distinguish the raisins in a slice of raisin bread from the bread and the cinnamon.

Once they've entered a follicle, the activated B cells begin dividing into numerous daughter cells. Each of these daughter cells makes antibody to the same antigen as the parent B cell. (The actual process is more complex and involves antigenic determinants. For the sake of simplicity, however, I simply refer to antigens, with the understanding that specific lymphocytes actually recognize only portions of any antigen.) The proliferating cells become larger than a resting B lymphocyte, more of their total volume is taken up by cytoplasm, and the DNA in the nucleus is no longer tightly coiled as it is in resting cells but becomes spread out.

During this stage, the B cells are called *centroblasts,* and the portion of the follicle where the centroblasts are undergoing this rapid proliferation is known as the *germinal center.* (*Germinal* implies origin, as in seeds germinating to give rise to plants.) The centroblasts in the germinal center divide in two about every six hours. Other B cells in the follicle are pushed out of the germinal center into a more peripheral area called the *mantle zone.* The mantle zone is still considered part of the follicle but is distinct from the germinal center. A follicle that consists solely of "resting" cells is called a *primary lymphoid follicle;* one that contains a germinal center with actively dividing centroblasts is called a *secondary lymphoid follicle.*

While all the daughter cells produced during this period of rapid proliferation contain immunoglobulin specific for the same antigen as the activated B lymphocyte that migrated into the follicle, the genes coding for the immunoglobulin variable region undergo a period of mutation at this time. These mutations result in slight changes in the exact structure of the immunoglobulin, producing slight variations in the affinity of that immunoglobulin for its antigen. Therefore, different cells formed at this time carry immunoglobulin that binds to a given antigen more or less tightly.

The follicular dendritic cells have cell surface receptors that allow them to trap antigen. They carry antigen on their surfaces for a very long time—days, weeks, or even months. During the period of proliferation in the germinal center, the follicular dendritic cells present antigen to the centroblasts. There are a limited number of dendritic cell antigen-presenting sites, and the maturing centroblasts compete to bind to them. This competition is won by the centroblasts whose immunoglobulin is able to bind most tightly to its antigen.

Those centroblasts whose immunoglobulin has mutated to have a high affinity for its antigen (i.e., it binds very tightly to the antigen) move on to a different region of the germinal center. The cells then undergo structural and functional changes, becoming smaller and expressing different cell surface receptors and intracellular proteins. At this stage in development they are called *centrocytes.* The centroblasts that make low-affinity, weakly binding immunoglobulin (who lose out on the antigen-binding competition) undergo apoptosis, the process of programmed cell death. In this case, apoptosis eliminates the cells that are less qualified to mount an effective immune response.

Depending on the specific environmental signals that they encounter, the high-affinity centrocytes leave the germinal center to follow one of two different pathways. They can become *plasmablasts,* differentiating into mature antibody-secreting *plasma cells,* or they can differentiate into *memory B cells.* Plasma cells survive for about two weeks. A few remain in a specialized area of the lymph nodes called the *medullary cord,* but most migrate back to the bone marrow, where they pour out antibodies directed against any pathogens that bear "their antigen." Memory B cells, which survive for a much longer time, are available for rapid recruitment against a subsequent challenge with the same antigen. They become activated more rapidly than naive B lymphocytes, and, since they have already gone through the process of selection, they already carry higher-affinity immunoglobulin (fig. 9.6).

Although the other peripheral lymphoid structures like the spleen and mucosal-associated lymphoid tissues look different from the lymph nodes, their basic organization into different compartments that preferentially attract distinct cell types is similar, and the same basic processes of B cell activation take place. One distinction in the architecture of the spleen and mucosal-associated lymphoid tissues that should be noted, however, is the existence of an area surrounding the mantle zone, which is called the *marginal zone.* The marginal zone contains a distinct type of B cell, the marginal zone cell. Marginal zone–type cells are also found in the mantle zones of lymph nodes, but in lymph nodes the marginal zone doesn't constitute a distinct region surrounding the follicle.

T cells

The other major class of lymphocytes is the T lymphocytes, or T cells. Like B cells, T lymphocytes participate in adaptive immune responses. Unlike B cells, T cells are not part of the humoral immune system—the immunity that they confer is directly mediated by the cells themselves and cannot be transferred

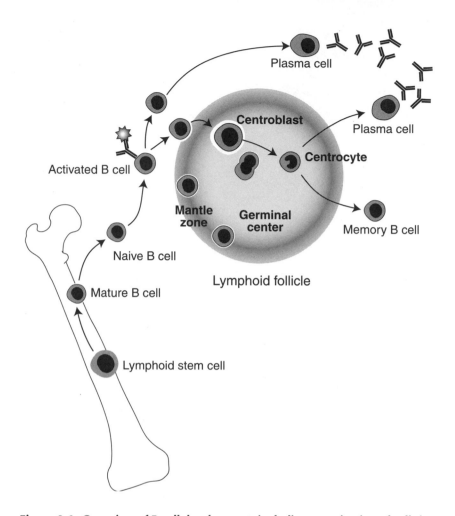

Figure 9.6. *Overview of B cell development, including organization of cells in a follicle.* Mature B cells leave the bone marrow as naive lymphocytes to circulate through the blood and lymphatic system. Activated B cells can differentiate into plasma cells or migrate into lymphoid follicles and start rapidly proliferating. These rapidly proliferating cells, which are larger than a resting B lymphocyte, are called centroblasts, and the portion of the follicle where the centroblasts are undergoing this rapid proliferation is known as the germinal center. Other B cells in the follicle are pushed out of the germinal center into a more peripheral area called the mantle zone. Centroblasts whose immunoglobulin has mutated to have a high affinity for its antigen move on to a different region of the germinal center to become centrocytes. The high-affinity centrocytes can leave the germinal center to become plasmablasts, differentiating into mature antibody-secreting plasma cells, or they can differentiate into memory B cells.

Types of Lymphoma Corresponding to Follicular and Postfollicular B Cells

Many forms of lymphoma correspond to B cells at the follicular and postfollicular stages of development. That is to say, the malignant cells look like, express the same proteins as, and act like caricatures of normal B cells at these stages of development. The follicular lymphomas grow in clumps that superficially resemble normal lymphoid follicles. If you look at a cross section of a piece of tissue from a follicular lymphoma under a microscope, you can see that the tissue is filled with cells clustered into these follicular clumps. This group of lymphomas is further classified by whether the malignant cells consist predominantly of small cells that resemble centrocytes or large cells that resemble centroblasts.

The large cells found in diffuse large B cell lymphoma also correspond to centroblasts. In this aggressive form of lymphoma, the cells are more abnormal than those found in the follicular lymphomas, and they no longer grow in a follicular pattern.

Many researchers think that the malignant cells in Hodgkin lymphoma correspond to a genetically damaged germinal center cell that made low-affinity, weakly binding immunoglobulin but somehow managed to escape apoptosis.

Marginal zone and mantle cell lymphomas are recognized as specific diseases. In some cases of mantle cell lymphoma, the malignant cells are found "ringing" apparently normal germinal centers in what would normally be the mantle zone.

The malignant cells found in lymphoplasmacytic lymphoma (immunocytoma), a form of lymphoma that is often associated with excess production of immunoglobulin, correspond to a very late stage in B cell development—just prior to the final differentiation into plasma cells. Because these cells are so close to differentiated plasma cells, they often secrete high levels of antibodies into the blood, which can lead to problems because of increased blood viscosity.

from one person to another by an injection of serum or plasma. Another basic distinction is that T cells cannot recognize isolated antigen found extracellularly—they recognize *only* antigen that is bound to a special class of cell surface molecules called the major histocompatibility complex (MHC). This allows T cells to act against cells that have been infected by intracellular pathogens like viruses.

MHC molecules are found on virtually all cells in the body. Most cells carry MHC class I molecules, but certain cells in the immune system carry a different class of MHC molecules (class II). Different people carry slightly different MHC molecules on the membranes of their cells; mature T cells recognize cells with *self*–MHC molecules. This means that they cannot act directly against bacteria or other extracellular pathogens (which don't carry self–MHC molecules) but that they can recognize and destroy cells that have been infected with virus.

All cells go through a process of chopping up and recycling intracellular proteins. Pieces of these chopped up proteins are displayed on the MHC molecules on the cell surface, where they can be examined by passing T cells. Most of these protein fragments come from normal cellular proteins; however, if a cell has been infected by a virus, fragments of the foreign viral proteins are displayed as well.

The presentation of proteins on the MHC molecule has been likened to a hot dog inside a bun. If an armed cytotoxic T cell finds a "foreign" hot dog inside a "native" bun, it destroys the cell that is carrying it. Between 1 and 10 percent of T cells recognize MHC molecules from other individuals as "foreign"; this is the mechanism underlying *acute graft-versus-host disease*, a potentially serious complication of certain types of bone marrow transplants. The group of proteins known as the *human leukocyte antigens* makes up the MHC. Before someone undergoes a transplant using marrow donated by another person, these proteins must be "matched" to avoid this complication (see Chapter 6).

Like B cells, T cells arise from stem cells in the bone marrow. Unlike B cells, they do not continue to mature in the bone marrow but migrate very early in their development to the *thymus*. The thymus, which is found under the breastbone in the upper middle part of the chest, is considered a primary, or central, lymphoid organ, like the bone marrow, since it is the site of T cell lymphopoiesis. Like mature B cells, each mature T cell carries many copies of a unique cell surface protein that allows it to recognize a foreign antigenic determinant. In the case of T cells, this membrane-bound protein is called the *T cell receptor.*

T cell lymphopoiesis is a little more complex than B cell lymphopoiesis because T cell receptors need to recognize both *self*–MHC molecules and *foreign* antigens. When early T cell precursors arrive at the thymus, they undergo a period of intense proliferation—they are now called *thymocytes.* Thymocytes pass through a series of developmental stages similar to B cell lymphopoiesis. During T cell lymphopoiesis, thymocytes rearrange the genes coding for the T cell receptor and express different cell surface markers and intracellular proteins.

These different stages occur in response to signals that the developing thymocytes encounter in the slightly different microenvironments within the thymus. They undergo *positive* T cell receptor selection for self-MHC recognition and *negative* selection so that T cells with receptors that recognize normal self-antigens are eliminated. So T cells that have receptors that *don't* recognize self-MHC receptors are eliminated, as well as those that have receptors that *do* bind to self-antigens.

The combined processes of positive and negative selection are so rigorous that only about 2 percent of developing thymocytes make it through the thymus as mature T lymphocytes. The rest are eliminated during development through apoptosis. The mature T lymphocyte leaves the thymus to circulate through the body in search of antigen. Mature T lymphocytes live longer than circulating B lymphocytes and make up the majority of circulating lymphocytes.

There are several different classes of mature T cells; each of these carries out its own set of functions. *Cytotoxic* T cells kill infected cells and some tumor cells. Other classes of T cells are important to B cell and macrophage activation. *Inflammatory* T cells recruit macrophages into the adaptive immune response, while *helper* T cells help activate B cells. (Sometimes the helper and inflammatory T cells are simply grouped together as helper T cells.) T cells also secrete numerous cytokines that affect the function of other T cells. *Regulatory* T cells secrete cytokines that inhibit the activity of other cells in the immune system.

Two marker proteins, CD4 and CD8, are frequently used to differentiate between the various classes of T cells. Very early during the process of maturation in the thymus, the developing T cells do not carry either of these markers and are referred to as CD4$^-$/CD8$^-$. At an intermediate stage of maturation the developing T cells carry both CD4 and CD8 and are referred to as CD4$^+$/CD8$^+$. In the mature T cell, however, only one of the two markers is expressed.

CD4 and CD8 are important in determining which class of MHC molecules a given T cell will recognize—MHC I or MHC II. Cells in which the CD8 marker is expressed recognize cells with MHC class I molecules and may function as cytotoxic T cells. Cells in which the CD4 cell surface marker is expressed recognize cells that carry MHC class II molecules; they therefore recognize those cells in the immune system that carry MHC II molecules and can function as helper T cells or inflammatory T cells.

Additionally, there are T cells with two slightly different types of T cell receptor proteins. These are known as αβ T cells (the "standard" form) and γδ T cells (the "variant" form).

Like B cells, mature antigen-specific T cells proliferate and differentiate into functional effector cells (see below) in response to antigen encountered in the peripheral lymphoid tissues (lymph nodes, spleen, and mucosal-associated lymphoid tissue). They also require a co-stimulatory signal from another cell to become activated. For T cells, antigen is presented and a class of cell called the professional antigen-presenting cell (honest, I'm not making these names up) delivers the co-stimulatory signal. Macrophages, B cells, and dendritic cells can all act as professional antigen-presenting cells. (Dendritic cells are also called *interdigitating reticular cells*; these are different from the follicular dendritic cells that interact with developing B lymphocytes in the germinal center.)

Since some self-antigens are specific to tissues outside the thymus, this requirement for a co-stimulatory signal is critically important to prevent destructive autoimmune responses. A mature T cell encountering a self-antigen on an ordinary cell that cannot deliver the co-stimulatory signal does not become activated. Instead, it becomes *anergic*—rendered unresponsive to that antigen.

If a tumor carries a specific antigen that isn't found on other cells in the body, this provides a mechanism whereby the immune system can potentially recognize it as "foreign" and therefore "bad" and mark it for destruction. However, the context in which T cells that recognize that antigen first come across it is critical. If the T cell first encounters the antigen in the presence of a co-stimulatory signal from a professional antigen-presenting cell, it will realize that cells carrying this antigen should be sought out and destroyed.

On the other hand, if the T cell first encounters the antigen on a tumor cell and *doesn't* receive the co-stimulatory signal, it will accept the antigen as "self," become anergic, and ignore the tumor. Not only that, but elements of the tumor environment may keep dendritic cells from maturing, so that dendritic cells found in tumors may fail to give the co-stimulatory signal and actually signal T cells to become anergic. Our recognition of the importance of the context in which T cells first encounter antigen has led to the development of a promising new approach to lymphoma therapy that involves removing some dendritic cells, exposing them to tumor antigens and other factors, and then returning them to the body (see Chapter 5).

Like naive B cells, mature naive T lymphocytes circulate through the blood, lymph, and the peripheral lymphoid organs. Most pass through the secondary lymphoid tissue without encountering antigen. Others encounter antigen on professional antigen-presenting cells and are induced to proliferate and undergo differentiation. Once a T cell has encountered an antigen it recognizes on the surface of a professional antigen-presenting cell and has received a co-stimulatory signal, it becomes activated. It begins to proliferate rapidly, giving rise to a *clonal* population of thousands of identical daughter cells over several days.

The activated T cell begins to synthesize and secrete a cytokine called inter-leukin-2 (IL-2) as well as the cell surface receptor that permits it to recognize and respond to IL-2. This secreted IL-2 is required for further proliferation and for the differentiation of T cells into *armed effector T cells* that are ready, willing, and able to participate in the immune response. The terms *effector* or *armed effector* imply that, like a cocked rifle, these T cells are now able to act against pathogens simply in response to the trigger of binding antigen and no longer need to undergo a period of proliferation and differentiation prior to taking action.

Once they have undergone differentiation into armed effector cells, T cells can recognize and act on any target cell that bears the specific antigen they rec-ognize—they no longer require the professional antigen-presenting cell or a co-stimulatory signal. Thus a cytotoxic T cell can recognize and destroy any cell that both expresses MHC class I molecules (most cells in the body) and displays an antigen recognized by the T cell receptor (say, part of a virus that has infected that cell).

Armed effector T cells not only circulate through the blood and lymph but also patrol through the tissues of the body in search of infection. T cell activa-tion also results in the production of memory T cells. Memory T cells home to the tissues in which they were first activated. Thus, a specific population of ma-ture T cells might preferentially patrol, say, the skin, while another T cell popu-lation might prefer to explore the mucosa of the gut.

Although the division into either CD4 or CD8 T cells has already taken place during lymphopoiesis in the thymus, the final functional differentiation of T cells—for example, into helper CD4 T cells or inflammatory CD4 T cells—occurs upon activation and may be influenced by local cytokines in their envi-ronment. T cells not only respond to many cytokines but also release them. T cell cytokines are critical in mediating specific local functions (activating a B cell or a macrophage or inhibiting viral activity) and can also act at a distance to help coordinate the activity and responses of the cells that make up the im-mune system.

Other lymphocytes and lymphocyte-like cells

While αβ T cells and "standard" B cells are the best understood and most stud-ied classes of lymphocytic cells, there are a few lymphocytic cell types that do not easily fit into these two categories. Some of these "exceptions" appear to be involved in certain forms of lymphoma. These include CD5 B cells, γδ T cells, and natural killer cells. All three of these cell types respond rapidly compared

T Cell Lymphomas

Just as B cell lymphomas correspond to cells at various normal stages of B cell maturation, T cell lymphomas correspond to T cells at different developmental stages. The majority of lymphoblastic lymphomas resemble early T cells at thymic or prethymic stages of development. These cells are characteristically either CD4$^+$/CD8$^+$ or CD4$^-$/CD8$^-$. Since the thymus is located under the breastbone, it's not surprising that lymphoblastic lymphomas tend to show up with large mediastinal masses. Among the T cell lymphomas that correspond to postthymic stages of T cell development, the CD4$^+$ class is more common than the CD8$^+$ class. Certain T cell lymphomas are found at specific locations in the body to which normal T cells home. For instance, mycosis fungoides is a T cell lymphoma that involves the skin. Intestinal T cell lymphomas have been described as well. Presumably, these malignant T cells bear some of the same specific receptors that allow normal T cells to home to specific regions.

with other lymphocytes, and, unlike "standard" T and B lymphocytes, they show little antigen specificity.

CD5 B cells represent a distinct lineage of B lymphocytes characterized by expression of CD5, a cell surface protein that is usually found on T cells and is not present on most B cells. Unlike "conventional" B cells, they do not appear to continuously arise from adult bone marrow but instead are believed to be descended from stem cells found in the fetal liver. They represent a small percentage of the total population of B cells found in adult blood and peripheral lymphoid tissue but are the major class of lymphocytes found in the peritoneal cavity. They show less antigen specificity than conventional B cells and may play a critical role in the humoral response to thymus-independent antigens.

Similarly, γδ T cells appear to represent a cell lineage distinct from that of the more common αβ T cells (although they also mature in the thymus). They constitute a small portion of total T cells and show a comparative lack of T cell receptor diversity. Although their specific function, if any, remains unclear, it has been proposed that they have evolved to defend the epithelial cells that cover the body's surfaces.

Finally, there are even some exceptions to the basic "B cells develop in bone marrow, T cells develop in thymus" rule. A small population of B cells, whose function remains poorly understood, inhabits part of the thymus, and recently classes of T cells that mature outside the thymus have been identified. Therefore, even people whose thymus has been obliterated can repopulate their body with T cells if this becomes necessary (e.g., after a stem cell transplant).

Natural killer cells (NK cells), a.k.a. *large, granular lymphocytes,* are large non-B, non-T lymphoid cells. They are classified as lymphocytes, although they have granules in their cytoplasm like granulocytes and don't display the surface antigens characteristic of either B cells or T cells. Unlike most lymphocytes, they act early and nonspecifically in response to infection. Natural killer cells kill cells that are "tagged" by antibody in a response known as *antibody-dependent cellular cytotoxicity.* Unlike cytotoxic T cells, natural killer cells can destroy virus-infected cells that do not display the MHC markers—in fact, they can be *inhibited* by the MHC molecules—and have been shown to kill tumor cells grown outside the body.

Summary

The immune system contains a variety of different cell types that work together to defend the body from disease. Immune responses can be divided into (1) nonspecific innate responses and (2) adaptive responses that are specific for a given infection. Lymphocytes, which include B cells and T cells, are primarily involved in adaptive responses and are responsible for immunological memory.

B cells undergo a series of developmental stages in the bone marrow prior to becoming mature B lymphocytes. They become activated to proliferate and differentiate into antibody-secreting plasma cells after encountering antigen in the peripheral lymphoid tissues. T cells, which mature in the thymus, are activated by antigen only when it is presented in the context of MHC molecules on the surface of professional antigen-presenting cells. Upon activation, T cells proliferate into a large population of clonal daughter cells and differentiate into one of several types of functional T cells.

The first cells that respond to a pathogen are the nonspecific phagocytic cells like neutrophils and macrophages. They attack the pathogen and chew it up. Sometimes this is enough to control the pathogen, but sometimes the adaptive immune responses are required as well. Macrophages and dendritic cells head for the lymph nodes and spleen, where they (1) send out cytokines to attract lymphocytes and (2) display antigenic pieces of pathogen to passing T cells.

A T cell that recognizes an antigen shown to it by a professional antigen-presenting cell is stimulated to proliferate and to differentiate into either a cytotoxic T cell or one of the regulatory T cells. A T cell that recognizes an antigen in the wrong context may be made anergic. Cytotoxic T cells head out into the body and start looking for cells carrying *their* antigen and the MHC I complex. They're now able to kill those cells. Helper T cells stimulate those B cells and cytotoxic T cells that recognize the same antigen to proliferate and differentiate. Inflammatory T cells recruit macrophages.

Naive B cells that both have found an antigen they recognize and have been signaled by a helper T cell migrate into the lymphoid follicles, start proliferating, and differentiate into either plasma cells or memory B cells. Plasma cells secrete antibodies that are specific for different antigens. Antibodies destroy pathogens through the action of a series of proteins found in the blood or by recruiting other cells, including phagocytic cells, like macrophages, or natural killer cells, the "nonspecific" class of lymphocytes.

The cells of the immune system communicate with each other, as well as with other bodily cells, both through direct cell-to-cell contact and by squirting cytokines into the blood and other extracellular fluids. All these messages are received by the target cell through receptors on the cell surface. When an appropriate signaling molecule occupies a cell surface receptor, some sort of response will be elicited from the target cell.

Although the different cell types that make up the immune system have distinct and specific functions, they all act together in the response against disease. Just as the individual muscle cells in the heart are coordinated to produce rhythmic contractions throughout the entire organ (rather than beating randomly in isolation from each other), so the individual cells in the immune system are coordinated to work in concert with each other to protect the body from disease.

While the malignant cells that constitute lymphomas have lost many of the controls that regulate the survival and proliferation of normal lymphocytes, the malignant cells still resemble normal lymphocytes in some ways, and they sometimes respond to the same signals. Different types of lymphoma correspond to different types of lymphocytes and may behave much like a given class of lymphocytes arrested at a particular stage of development.

SUGGESTIONS FOR FURTHER READING

Janeway CA, Travers P, Walport M, Shlomchik M. (2001). *Immunobiology: The Immune System in Health and Disease.* 5th ed. New York: Current Biology/Garland Publishing.
An advanced undergraduate-level textbook that covers everything you ever wanted to know about immunology.

For a somewhat briefer overview of immunology at more or less the same level, see the chapters on the immune system in:

Alberts B, Johnson A, Lewis J, Raff M, Roberts K, Walter P. (2002). *The Molecular Biology of the Cell.* 4th ed. New York: Garland Publishing.

For a very accessible, informal, undergraduate-level overview:

Sompayrac L. (2003). *How the Immune System Works.* 2nd ed. Malden, Mass.: Blackwell Publishing.

For in-depth coverage of several areas of particular interest to lymphomaniacs, see:

MacLennan ICM. (1994). "Germinal centers." *Annual Review of Immunology* 12:117–139.
Mapara MY, Sykes M. (2004). "Tolerance and cancer: Mechanisms of tumor evasion and strategies for breaking tolerance." *Journal of Clinical Oncology* 22:1136–1151.
Rudin CM, Thompson CB. (1998). "B-cell development and maturation." *Seminars in Oncology* 25:435–446.
Steinman RM. (1991). "The dendritic cell system and its role in immunogenicity." *Annual Review of Immunology* 9:271–296.
Particularly if you're thinking of going for a dendritic cell vaccine.

For a lively, entertaining, and enlightening history of immunological approaches to cancer therapy:

Hall SS. (1997). *A Commotion in the Blood.* Philadelphia: Henry Holt and Co.

CHAPTER 10

Lymphoma Classification and Staging

In this chapter I discuss the different types of lymphoma. I describe the different systems now in use to classify the lymphomas and describe the individual types of lymphoma in some detail. I also describe how the stage of disease—which defines how far lymphoma has spread through a person's body—is determined.

This is the most difficult chapter in the book: lymphoma classification has always been controversial and is considered confusing even by general oncologists. However, obtaining a detailed knowledge of the specific form of their disease is often helpful to people who want to understand, as much as possible, what's going on. Knowing which form of the disease you have, and something about the biology of the malignant cells and the clinical characteristics of that form of lymphoma, will also help you determine whether new therapies you hear about are likely to be helpful for you.

The material in Chapters 8 and 9 will be helpful as background to the material in this chapter.

The different types of lymphoma

There are over twenty different clinical entities—or specific diseases—known as lymphoma. These different kinds of lymphoma can be distinguished from one another by various characteristics including the appearance of the malignant cells under a microscope (known as their *histological* appearance or their *morphology*), the specific proteins that appear on the cell surface, the pattern in which the cells grow, the sites in the body that are likely to be affected, the population of people most likely to be affected, and the typical course of the disease. All the lymphomas are cancers that develop from lymphocytes; however, the different lymphomas resemble different types of lymphocytes at different developmental stages (see Chapter 9) and carry characteristic genetic mutations (see Chapter 8 and below). Perhaps the most fundamental of these distinctions is the cell type. Lymphomas can arise from B cells, T cells, or natural killer cells.

The different B cell, T cell, and NK (natural killer) cell lymphomas are distinguished from each other by how closely they resemble normal lymphocytes at different stages of development. For instance, the follicular lymphomas resemble germinal center B cells, while lymphoplasmacytic lymphomas resemble a B cell at a late stage of development—just before the transformation into a plasma cell. The different lymphomas are also distinguished by different mutations. For instance, both follicular large cell lymphoma and diffuse large B cell lymphoma correspond to *centroblasts* (see Chapter 9); the specific characteristics of these diseases depend on the specific genetic abnormalities found in the malignant cells.

Accurately classifying the different types of lymphoma is important for several reasons. First, different kinds of lymphoma follow different clinical courses— some grow very slowly and can safely be followed by "watching and waiting," while others grow rapidly and need to be treated right away (see below, under the WHO classification system). Second, different types of lymphoma respond to different treatment regimens: they are more or less responsive to radiation therapy or to specific chemotherapy regimens. Finally, effective use of the monoclonal antibody therapy—which is directed against specific proteins manufactured by the lymphoma cells—critically depends on appropriate classification of the disease.

Classification systems

Classifying all these different but closely related diseases has been a complex task. Over the years, physicians and researchers developed various classification systems, which have changed as researchers uncovered more information about both normal lymphocytic behavior and the specific forms of the disease.

The concept of lymphoma as a distinct disease (or group of related diseases) involving the lymphatic system emerged in the nineteenth century. Thomas Hodgkin, who wrote a paper in 1832 "on some morbid appearances of the absorbent glands and spleen," recognized what we would now call "lymphoma" as a disease characterized by enlargement of the lymph nodes and spleen. Initially, physicians focused on the clinical course of the disease (how it progressed in patients) and "macroscopic" appearance (for instance, enlarged lymph nodes) in defining the lymphoid disorders. During the twentieth century, classification schemes based on the microscopic appearance (histology) of the malignant cells became prominent.

The hope of such classification schemes is that the histological appearance of the cells will make it possible to distinguish distinct diseases that respond predictably to given therapeutic regimens. For any such classification system to function properly, the histological distinctions must be clearly recognizable (different pathologists viewing the same set of slides must come up with the same classification) and must correlate with the clinical course of the disease (different patients whose cells share specific histological traits show similar patterns of disease progression and respond similarly to a given treatment).

The Working Formulation and the concept of grade

Until recently, the Working Formulation was the classification scheme most widely used to classify NHL in the United States and Canada (the Kiel system was more popular in Europe). Devised in 1982 as a "translation" among several different classification schemes then in use, the Working Formulation became widely used as a classification system in its own right. It is based on the histological appearance of the malignant cells. Several properties that are clearly apparent in a specimen of the malignant cells under a microscope—cell size, cell growth pattern, and appearance of the cell nucleus—are used to classify NHL into ten kinds of lymphoma. The Working Formulation also recognizes several miscellaneous forms of lymphoma that do not fit readily into the general scheme. The ten basic clinical entities are organized into three groups. Each group defines a different clinical *grade* of the disease: *low grade, intermediate grade,* and *high grade* (table 10.1).

If we overlook the onslaught of unfamiliar terms (immunoblastic? nonconvoluted? histiocytic?), the basic plan of the Working Formulation is straightforward. The different types of NHL are placed in ten categories based on the histological appearance of the cells. Each of these categories belongs to one of three groups, which correspond to three different "grades" of lymphoma. The term *grade* as used in the Working Formulation simply implies the rapidity with which the untreated disease characteristically progresses.

Table 10.1. Working Formulation Classification of NHL

Low-grade
  A. Small lymphocytic
      Consistent with chronic lymphocytic leukemia
      Plasmacytoid
  B. Follicular, predominantly small cleaved cell
  C. Follicular, mixed small cleaved and large cell
Intermediate-grade
  D. Follicular, predominantly large cell
  E. Diffuse, small cleaved cell
  F. Diffuse, mixed small and large cell
  G. Diffuse, large cell, cleaved or noncleaved
High-grade
  H. Large cell, immunoblastic
  I. Lymphoblastic, convoluted or nonconvoluted cell
  J. Small noncleaved cell, Burkitt's or non-Burkitt's
Miscellaneous
  Composite, mycosis fungoides, histiocytic, extramedullary plasmacytoma,
  unclassifiable, other

Low-grade (sometimes called *indolent*) disease usually progresses very slowly. Most people diagnosed with low-grade lymphoma would be expected to live for years even if they were not treated. In contrast, high-grade (sometimes called *very aggressive*) disease typically progresses rapidly. Most people diagnosed with high-grade lymphoma would be expected to survive for weeks or months if left untreated. Intermediate-grade lymphoma (sometimes called *aggressive* disease) progresses at a rate between low grade and high grade, with survival of the untreated measured in months to a few years.

It is often appropriate to defer treating someone with low-grade lymphoma if the disease is not threatening to damage any vital organs or causing discomfort or disfigurement. This approach is called *watch-and-wait* or *watchful waiting*. These terms imply that it is safe to defer treatment (or wait) as long as you keep an eye out (or watch) for any developments that might require treatment. With the more aggressive forms of lymphoma, extended treatment delays are never appropriate. Since these forms of lymphoma progress rapidly, it is important to control the disease as rapidly as possible.

Classification into the ten basic categories is based on both the appearance of individual cells and the pattern of cellular growth. The terms *diffuse* and *follicular* refer to the *pattern* in which the cells grow. Lymph nodes and other lymphoid tissues contain clusters of cells called *follicles* (see Chapter 9). If you look at a slice of lymph node under a microscope, you can distinguish the follicles as discrete circular areas within the node.

During the process of normal B cell maturation, B lymphocytes go through a stage where they grow in follicles. When pathologists started classifying the different types of lymphoma, they noticed that sometimes the malignant cells retained this follicular growth pattern, becoming organized into rounded clusters of cells. In other types of lymphoma, the cells grew randomly. Lymphomas in which the cells show the follicular pattern are called *follicular lymphomas,* while lymphomas that don't show an organized pattern of cell growth are described as *diffuse.* All the high-grade lymphomas grow diffusely.

The terms *large* and *small* refer to the size of the malignant cell. Typically, normal (nonmalignant) lymphocytes going through a period of rapid proliferation are larger than lymphocytes that are not dividing. The rapidly dividing centroblasts in the germinal center are larger than either mature unstimulated B cells or the centrocytes that have survived the process of selection for high-affinity immunoglobulin. Similarly, immature lymphoblasts proliferating in the bone marrow are larger than naive circulating B cells.

This correlation of cell size with proliferation rate is loosely reflected in the histology of the lymphomas, with smaller cells generally being associated with the more indolent lymphomas. One exception to this "rule" is seen in Category J. The small noncleaved cells found in this group are the most rapidly dividing and aggressive of all the lymphomas. These cells differ from the other "small" cells because they have large nuclei, and, although smaller than the "large" cells in Categories G, H, and I, they are larger than the other types of cells called "small."

The other terms in the Working Formulation also refer to cell appearance. *Cleaved* and *noncleaved* refer to the cell nucleus. Cleaved cells display a pronounced indentation (or cleft) at the edge of the nucleus, as though it were starting to fold over on itself (informally referred to by pathologists as "buttock cell"). Noncleaved cells have a smooth nuclear contour.

Blast cells are immature cells undergoing a period of rapid proliferation. They are larger than resting lymphocytes, and the chromosomes in their nuclei are less tightly condensed, permitting more rapid access to the genetic information in their DNA required for the synthesis of the new proteins necessary for ongoing cell division. In both the Working Formulation and the WHO classification system (see below), *lymphoblasts* are blastic cells that correspond to an early stage of cell proliferation during lymphogenesis, while *immunoblasts* are cells that have been stimulated to proliferate following exposure to antigen. The cells in "lymphoblastic" lymphoma resemble cells in a very early stage in lymphoid differentiation. They are large cells that sometimes have a *convoluted* nucleus: the edges of the nucleus display irregular folds, or wrinkles, sometimes referred to as "crow's feet." "Immunoblastic" cells are typically large, with an oval nucleus containing a prominent nucleolus (a nuclear organelle).

The Working Formulation has two attributes that make it straightforward and easy to use. First, it uses readily recognizable aspects of the appearance of the malignant cells to group the various types of lymphoma into three easily identifiable clinical groups. Second, the specific disease entities within these three groups have similar prognoses and frequently respond to the same treatment regimens. The Working Formulation also has some drawbacks, however. The significance of some of the distinctions it makes has been questioned (for instance, classifying immunoblastic lymphoma as "high grade" compared with other diffuse large cell lymphomas classified as "intermediate grade"); it fails to recognize some of the more recently defined types of lymphoma; and there are those "miscellaneous" lymphomas that don't fit into any of the usual categories.

A fundamental issue is that the characteristics used to classify the different types of disease (cell size, cell growth pattern, whether the cell nucleus is cleaved or not) do not necessarily correspond to a specific cell type. For example, the Working Formulation category "diffuse large cell" lymphoma includes lymphomas that arise from B cells and also lymphomas that arise from T cells. Such distinctions might appear esoteric and of interest mainly to pathologists and lymphoma researchers. But as we learn more and more about lymphoma, the significance of these distinctions for therapy becomes clear.

Some of the categories recognized by the Working Formulation are heterogeneous: different clinical entities that resemble each other in terms of cell size and growth pattern are grouped into the same category. Not all of these diseases respond identically to the same treatment. This is a significant flaw: the ultimate aim of all such classification systems is to identify which forms of the disease respond best to specific therapies. If clinical trials demonstrate that a specific subtype of lymphoma responds to a specific treatment regimen, it is important to be able to accurately distinguish that type of lymphoma from superficially similar forms of the disease that do not respond as well to this treatment but that may respond to another therapy.

The REAL and WHO classification systems for lymphoid tumors

The specific repertoire of proteins displayed on a cell's surface constitutes its *immunophenotype*. Techniques that use antibodies that recognize different cell surface proteins have made it possible to identify the specific cell surface marker proteins found on the malignant lymphoma cells (see Chapter 2). The different types of lymphoma have characteristic immunophenotypes, and *immunohistochemical techniques* have permitted a more precise classification of distinct clinical entities and also a clearer understanding of the relationship between different types of lymphoma and the normal cell types to which they correspond. Since many aspects of a cell's behavior—for example, which environments in the body it homes to—are influenced by these same cell surface proteins, knowing the immunophenotype of a specific form of lymphoma may help researchers understand and predict its behavior.

Additionally, sophisticated techniques of genetic analysis have allowed researchers to identify some of the specific DNA mutations that contribute to certain forms of the disease and to correlate malfunctions in specific genes with development of certain kinds of lymphoma. These advances in understanding the biology of lymphoma have important implications for developing more effective and specific treatments. For example, using monoclonal antibodies to treat lymphoma depends on knowing that the malignant cells carry a cell surface protein that those particular antibodies recognize. Other new approaches to treatment involve using molecular genetic techniques to inhibit the activity of specific genes. To apply these new treatments appropriately, an accurate classification system, one that recognizes molecular distinctions between the different types of lymphoma, is essential.

Such issues led the International Lymphoma Study Group, composed of nineteen European and American pathologists, to devise a classification system that not only depends on histological criteria but includes information about immunophenotype, specific genetic lesions, clinical course of the disease, and the postulated normal counterpart of the malignant cell. Their proposed system, the Revised European-American Lymphoma (REAL) classification system, was published in 1994. It has since been modified and updated by the World Health Organization (WHO).

The WHO classification system, which includes myeloma (and related plasma cell disorders), neoplasms that may not represent true malignancies, and the lymphoid leukemias, as well as Hodgkin and non-Hodgkin lymphomas, divides the lymphomas into three basic categories: lymphomas of B cell origin, lymphomas of T cell (or of NK cell) origin, and Hodgkin lymphoma (table 10.2). Within the B cell and T cell (or NK cell) lymphomas, the WHO system distinguishes between two categories of disease: lymphomas in which the malignant cells resemble immature precursor lymphocytes, or *lymphoblasts*, corresponding to early antigen-independent stages of lymphocyte development, and those in which the malignant cells correspond to lymphocytes at later stages in development (see Chapter 9).

The REAL system has been criticized as being more relevant to the pathological classification of the disease than to clinical treatment and as being overly complex in light of the currently available treatments, splitting the lymphomas into numerous clinically irrelevant groups. And it's true that, right now, many of the different entities recognized by the REAL and WHO systems are treated clinically the same way. However, the categories in the REAL and WHO systems do define distinct clinical entities—diseases classified together under the REAL and WHO systems really do show similar clinical behavior, and the WHO-modified REAL system is now considered the "standard" lymphoma classification scheme. It is hoped that understanding which diseases respond best to currently available therapies will help oncologists pinpoint who can be successfully treated with current therapies and who would benefit most from new treatment regimens.

The WHO classification system does not explicitly split the diseases it defines into indolent and aggressive groups. This was deliberate: the pathologists who devised this classification system and the pathologists, hematologists, and oncologists who contributed to the WHO modifications believed that such a grouping is not clinically useful and were concerned that such groupings might mislead oncologists into overlooking important clinical features of the individual diseases. Not all indolent diseases respond to identical treatment regimens, and neither do all aggressive diseases.

Distinguishing between indolent and aggressive disease, however, is useful in a more general way in understanding the progression and likely response to therapy of the different forms of lymphoma. Because the response of slowly growing lymphomas to therapy is fundamentally different from that of the more rapidly advancing forms of the disease, several modifications of the REAL and WHO classification systems that highlight the split between indolent and aggressive disease have been published. In discussing the different types of lymphoma, I specifically group the different disease entities into slowly progressing

Table 10.2. The WHO Classification of Tumors of Lymphoid Tissue

B Cell Neoplasms
  Precursor B cell neoplasm
    Precursor B lymphoblastic leukemia/lymphoma
  Mature (peripheral) B cell neoplasms
    Chronic lymphocytic leukemia/small lymphocytic lymphoma
    B cell prolymphocytic leukemia
    Lymphoplasmacytic lymphoma
    Splenic marginal zone lymphoma
    Hairy cell leukemia
    Plasma cell neoplasms
      Plasma cell myeloma
      Solitary plasmacytoma of blood
      Extraosseous plasmacytoma
    Extranodal marginal zone B cell lymphoma of mucosal-associated lymphoid tissue
      (MALT lymphoma)
    Nodal marginal zone B cell lymphoma
    Follicular lymphoma
    Mantle cell lymphoma
    Diffuse large B cell lymphoma
      Mediastinal (thymic) large B cell lymphoma
      Intravascular large B cell lymphoma
      Primary effusion lymphoma
    Burkitt lymphoma/leukemia
  B cell proliferations of uncertain malignant potential
    Lymphomatoid granulomatosis
    Post-transplant lymphoproliferative disorder, polymorphic

and aggressive groups, based on modified versions of the REAL and WHO systems published by various authors.

Since many readers may be familiar with the Working Formulation classification of their disease but not the WHO-updated REAL classification, I include information so you can determine your classification if you have a pathology report that describes the immunohistochemical staining pattern of your lymphoma.

Your pathology report will indicate which of various marker proteins are present in your lymphoma cells. The specific pattern of markers is useful in determining which type of lymphoma you have. For instance, B cell lymphomas are almost always positive for CD19, while T cell lymphomas are not. Among B cell lymphomas, both mantle cell lymphoma and small lymphocytic lymphoma are generally positive for CD5, but small lymphocytic lymphoma is generally positive for CD23, while mantle cell lymphoma is not. In tables 10.3, 10.4, and 10.5

Table 10.2 *(continued)*

T Cell and NK Cell Neoplasms
  Precursor T cell neoplasms
    Precursor T lymphoblastic leukemia/lymphoma
    Blastic NK cell lymphoma
  Mature (peripheral) T cell and NK cell neoplasms
    T cell prolymphocytic leukemia
    T cell large granular lymphocytic leukemia
    Aggressive NK cell leukemia
    Adult T cell leukemia/lymphoma
    Extranodal NK/T cell lymphoma, nasal type
    Enteropathy-type T cell lymphoma
    Hepatosplenic T cell lymphoma
    Subcutaneous panniculitis-like T cell lymphoma
    Mycosis fungoides
    Sézary syndrome
    Primary cutaneous anaplastic large cell lymphoma
    Peripheral T cell lymphoma, unspecified
    Angioimmunoblastic T cell lymphoma
    Anaplastic large cell lymphoma
  T cell proliferation of uncertain malignant potential
    Lymphomatoid papulosis
Hodgkin lymphoma
  Nodular lymphocyte predominant Hodgkin lymphoma
  Classical Hodgkin lymphoma
    Nodular sclerosis classical Hodgkin lymphoma
    Lymphocyte-rich classical Hodgkin lymphoma
    Mixed cellularity classical Hodgkin lymphoma
    Lymphocyte-depleted classical Hodgkin lymphoma

and the following discussion, a particular marker is noted as $^+$ if it is found in more than 90 percent of people with that form of the disease, $^{+/-}$ if it is found more than 50 percent of the time, $^{-/+}$ if it is found more than 10 percent of the time but less than 50 percent, and $^-$ if it is found less than 10 percent of the time.

You will notice that most of the marker proteins used in characterizing the immunophenotype of the different forms of lymphoma are named "CD" followed by some number. "CD" stands for "clusters of differentiation," indicating that groups (or clusters) of different antibodies recognize given cell surface proteins, which are characteristic of specific cell types. CD19, CD20, and CD22 are typically found on B cells at various stages of development, as well as on most B cell lymphomas. They are often called the "pan–B cell markers." They are not found on stem cells in the bone marrow, fully differentiated plasma cells, or T cells.

CD2, CD3, CD5, and CD7 are typically found on normal T cells, as well as many T cell–derived lymphomas. They are often referred to as the "pan T cell markers." CD4 and CD8 characterize different classes of T cells (helper/inflammatory and cytotoxic, respectively). While the CD terminology doesn't imply any function, it's worth remembering that each protein does have a specific function that is significant for the cell type on which it is expressed. Some recognize and bind to other cells or the extracellular environment; others play a role in cell activation.

In the following pages, I discuss a number of different types of lymphoma individually, following the categories recognized by the WHO classification system. To discuss the different types of NHL, I first arrange them into (1) B cell and (2) T cell and NK cell lymphomas, subdividing these two categories into indolent and aggressive disease. I discuss Hodgkin lymphoma separately. I simplify the classifications where, for the purposes of this book, it does not appear useful to distinguish between specific diseases, and I do not discuss the leukemias (except where they overlap with the lymphomas), plasma cell disorders such as multiple myeloma, or the lymphoid neoplasms that are not clearly malignant.

Using tables 10.3, 10.4, and 10.5 to determine the WHO classification

If you have been told that you have low-grade, or indolent, NHL or any form of follicular lymphoma and do not have mycosis fungoides, your form of lymphoma should appear in table 10.3. You should be able to locate the most likely categories under the WHO system by locating the Working Formulation name of your form of lymphoma in table 10.3 and then comparing marker proteins in the table with those in your pathology report. If you've been told you have intermediate or aggressive NHL, look to see if your pathology report shows B cell markers ($CD19^+$, $CD20^+$, or $CD22^+$), in which case you should look for your type of lymphoma in table 10.3 or 10.4, or T cell markers ($CD3^+$, $CD4^+$, $CD7^+$, or $CD8^+$), in which case you should look for your form of lymphoma in table 10.5. If you have a T cell lymphoma, the specific characteristics of your disease (did it start in your intestines? in your nose?) may also help in determining the WHO name. Once you've determined the name, you should be able to locate your form of lymphoma in the appropriate section of "Description of various forms of lymphoma" (below). If you have Hodgkin lymphoma, you should be able to locate your form in the text, without needing to resort to tables, since there are only five types.

Description of various forms of lymphoma
B cell lymphomas

In the United States, about 85 percent of cases of NHL involve malignancies derived from B cells, and about 15 percent involve malignancies derived from T cells. Very rarely, lymphomas arise from NK cells. The vast majority of diseases classified as low grade in the Working Formulation derive from B cells. All follicular large cell (considered intermediate-grade) and small noncleaved cell (highly aggressive) lymphomas are B cell lymphomas, too.

Indolent lymphomas

As noted above, the indolent lymphomas are characteristically slow to progress. Some studies have found that median survival for people with indolent NHL is as long as eight to ten years after diagnosis. *Median* is a statistical term for the number that divides a group into two halves, so that one-half of the total population falls above the median and one-half falls below it. This means that half the people in these studies survived for *more* than eight to ten years (sometimes much longer), while half did not.

Indolent lymphomas can be cured if they are diagnosed when the disease is localized to a particular region of the body. Although advanced-stage low-grade lymphomas usually respond well to treatment, they are not generally curable with currently available therapies. In 1998, lymphomas classified as low grade according to the Working Formulation accounted for 22 percent of the lymphoma diagnosed in the United States. Most indolent lymphomas occur in people over the age of fifty.

Note on statistics: Different authorities cite different figures for the percentages of cases of lymphoma that fall into the different categories. There are many reasons for such variability, including differences in how different pathologists might classify a case, geographical differences in the incidence of certain subtypes of lymphoma, whether children were included in the population studies, and random chance [you would need an enormous sample size to obtain accurate breakdowns of the rarer forms of lymphoma].

When I consider changes in the incidence of lymphoma over time or cite incidence according to the Working Formulation, the figures I give are usually based on statistics gathered by the NCI's Surveillance Epidemiology (SEER) program, which collects information on the incidence of cancer at nine different

Table 10.3. Identifying Indolent B Cell Lymphomas

WHO Classification	Working Formulation Equivalent(s)	Characteristic Marker Proteins*	Probable Normal Counterpart
1. chronic lymphocytic leukemia (CLL)/small lymphocytic lymphoma (SLL)	small lymphocytic, consistent with CLL; small lymphocytic, plasmacytoid	surface IgM+ (weak); CD5+, CD19+, CD20+ (weak), CD22+ (weak), CD23+, CD43+, CD79a+, CD10−, SLL: CD11a+, CLL: CD11a−	circulating CD5+ B cell (naive); a subset may correspond to memory B cells
2. lymphoplasmacytic lymphoma (LPL)/ Waldenström's macroglobulinemia	small lymphocytic, plasmacytoid; diffuse, mixed small and large cell	surface IgM+, cellular IgM+, CD19+, CD20+ (variable), CD22+, CD79a+, CD5−, CD10−, CD23−	late-stage B cell (just before plasma cell)
3a. follicular lymphoma (FL),** grade 1	Follicular, small cleaved cell	surface Ig+ (strong), CD10+/−, CD19+, CD20+, CD22+, CD79a+, CD5−	germinal center B cell centrocyte
3b. follicular lymphoma (FL),** grade 2	Follicular, mixed small cleaved and large cell		germinal center B cell centrocyte/ centroblast
3c. follicular lymphoma (FL),** grade 3***	Follicular, large cell		germinal center B cell centrocyte/ centroblast
3d. diffuse follicle center lymphoma	Diffuse, small cleaved cell; diffuse, mixed small and large cell		germinal center B cell centrocyte

locations in the United States. A number of SEER cases are unclassified, so the total of indolent plus intermediate plus aggressive is less than 100 percent. Since the SEER statistics I used were classified according to the Working Formulation, I have occasionally extrapolated from the program's data to apply its statistics to clinical entities defined by the WHO classification system. For information on the incidence of diseases defined by the REAL and WHO systems, I have mainly relied on data accumulated for 1,403 cases of NHL gathered by the NHL Study Project (NHLSP) in eight countries between 1988 and 1990.

Chronic lymphocytic leukemia/small lymphocytic lymphoma

Diffuse small lymphocytic lymphoma (SLL; number 1 in table 10.3; most commonly small lymphocytic lymphoma consistent with chronic lymphocytic

Table 10.3 (continued)

WHO Classification	Working Formulation Equivalent(s)	Characteristic Marker Proteins*	Probable Normal Counterpart
4a. MALT lymphoma	*small lymphocytic,* small lymphocytic plasmacytoid; less commonly: diffuse, small cleaved or diffuse mixed small and large cell	surface Ig$^+$, cellular Ig$^{-/+}$, CD19$^+$, CD20$^+$, CD22$^+$, CD79a$^+$, CD5$^-$, CD10$^-$, CD23$^-$	marginal zone B cell (from MALT, lymph node, or spleen); possibly a memory B cell?
4b. nodal marginal zone B cell lymphoma (NMZL)			
4c. splenic marginal zone lymphoma (SMZL)			

Note: When different cases of a WHO entity could be classified under different Working Formulation categories, the most common Working Formulation classification is indicated by *italic* type.

*It should be noted that every case of lymphoma of a given type doesn't always bear all the markers characteristic of that type (see text). Cancer implies instability in gene—and hence protein—expression, and the specific immunophenotype found on the malignant cells from any individual may differ slightly from the pattern typical of his or her disease. I have not tried to make a list of all cell protein markers for the different types of lymphoma but have included those of potential therapeutic significance, as well as those useful in discriminating between different clinical entities. Where different authorities disagree on the likely correlation of a specific marker with a specific disease entity, I have followed the guidelines specified by the REAL classification system.

**Grade for FL, as used in the WHO system, is not equivalent to Working Formulation "grade." None of the FLs would be considered "very aggressive" disease. All the FLs have the same characteristic marker proteins.

***Follicular lymphoma, grade 3, generally progresses more rapidly than the other lymphomas included here. In the Working Formulation, follicular large cell lymphoma is classified as an intermediate-grade disease. I have included follicular large cell lymphoma here in order to discuss it along with the other follicular lymphomas.

leukemia in Working Formulation; B cell chronic lymphocytic leukemia/small lymphocytic lymphoma in REAL system) is one of the most slowly progressing of the different types of NHL.

Who gets it: The median age at diagnosis is sixty-five.

Incidence: The incidence of SLL (as defined by the Working Formulation) increased by about 50 percent between 1978 and 1993. In 1995, the incidence of SLL in the United States was about 1.3 cases diagnosed/100,000 people. As defined by the REAL system, it accounts for about 6 percent of all cases of NHL. If the closely related chronic lymphocytic leukemia (CLL; incidence of about 4/100,000 men and 2/100,000 women in the United States) is included together with SLL, this percentage is much higher.

Marker proteins: surface IgM$^+$ (weak), CD 5$^+$, CD19$^+$, CD20$^+$ (weak), CD22$^+$ (weak), CD23$^+$, CD43$^+$, CD79a$^+$, CD10$^-$; SLL: CDIIa$^+$; CLL: CDIIa$^-$

The majority of people with SLL are diagnosed with Stage IV disease, and most have some bone marrow involvement. Both of these factors are probably related to the homing characteristics of the malignant cells, which resemble naive, recirculating B lymphocytes. Progression of the disease results from a slow accumulation of malignant cells that may involve inappropriately long-term cell survival.

The malignant cell may be the counterpart of a naive $CD5^+$ B cell, a specific B cell type that arises early in development, is self-replicating, and may be involved in the response to thymus-independent antigens (see Chapter 9). No single genetic lesion has been consistently identified with SLL, suggesting that different molecular pathways may lead to this disease. In many patients, the malignant cells show a genetic abnormality called chromosomal duplication, however, which appears as *trisomy*, an increase from the normal two chromosomes/cell to three chromosomes/cell for a particular chromosome. In SLL, trisomy most commonly involves chromosome 12. Other people's cells show a genetic abnormality called a *deletion*, in which part of a chromosome is missing. The most common deletions in SLL involve chromosome 11 or 13.

SLL sometimes transforms into an aggressive, large cell lymphoma, a condition called *Richter syndrome.* Sometimes SLL appears to transform into Hodgkin lymphoma. This may represent coexistence of the two diseases, with regression of the SLL as the Hodgkin lymphoma "takes over."

SLL is very similar to chronic lymphocytic leukemia, which is the most common form of leukemia in adults. In fact, the WHO classification system considers them essentially the same disease. The two diseases are distinguished clinically by the extent to which the malignant cells are found circulating in the blood versus growing in the lymph nodes (the bone marrow is always involved in CLL and in 70 to 80 percent of cases of SLL). The appearance of individual cells (small, rounded lymphocytes with little cytoplasm and a rounded nucleus) and the pattern of growth in affected lymph nodes (generally diffuse, although there may be "pseudofollicles"—areas of larger, rapidly proliferating cells that superficially resemble follicles) is identical in SLL and CLL.

An immunohistochemical difference that appears to discriminate between SLL and CLL is expression of CD11a, a cell surface protein involved in cell-to-cell adhesion. This molecule is typically found in the membranes of the malignant cells in SLL but not in CLL. It is possible that the higher percentage of lymphocytes found circulating in the blood with CLL compared with SLL could be related to the absence of this molecule.

Cells in SLL proliferation centers sometimes stain for the growth factor interleukin-6 (IL-6), which can signal some lymphoma cells to proliferate. This suggests that growth of these particular lymphomas may involve a positive feedback system, with malignant cells both secreting and responding to this growth factor.

Lymphoplasmacytic lymphoma / Waldenström's macroglobulinemia

Lymphoplasmacytic lymphoma (LPL; number 2 in table 10.3; most commonly small lymphocytic, plasmacytoid, in the Working Formulation; lymphoplasmacytoid lymphoma/immunocytoma in REAL system) is a slowly progressing disease.

Who gets it: The median age at diagnosis is sixty-three; the majority of patients are in their sixties.

Incidence: In most areas of the world, the incidence is less than 1/100,000; this disease represents about 1 percent of cases of NHL.

Marker proteins: surface IgM$^+$, cellular IgM$^+$, CD19$^+$, CD20$^+$ (variable), CD22$^+$, CD79a$^+$, CD5$^-$, CD10$^-$, CD23$^-$

As in SLL, the malignant cells in LPL consist of small, diffusely growing cells, and most people are diagnosed with Stage IV disease. LPL can be distinguished from SLL by the histological appearance of the malignant cells and by the marker proteins they express. In LPL, the cells look like a cross between lymphocytes and plasma cells. The nucleus of a lymphoplasmacytic lymphoma cell resembles that of a lymphocyte, while the cytoplasm resembles that of a mature plasma cell.

CD20 expression is more variable than in most B cell lymphomas. This is consistent with the appearance of the cells, since mature plasma cells no longer express CD20, and suggests that the malignant cell in LPL corresponds to a late stage in normal lymphocyte development—the stage just before lymphocytes transform into plasma cells.

Consistent with this plasma cell-like appearance, LPL cells have immunoglobulin in their cytoplasm, and the disease is often associated with elevated blood levels of the specific antibody produced by the malignant cells, a condition called *Waldenström's macroglobulinemia.* If antibody levels become high enough, they lead to increased blood viscosity, or "thickening" of the blood, making it more difficult for the blood to flow through the circulatory system. This is aggravated by the tendency of the abnormal antibodies to circulate in clumps and can lead to various problems such as bleeding of the nose and gums, dizziness, headache, and sleepiness. Sometimes, these proteins come out of circulation at low temperatures, causing hives in chilled areas of the body.

LPL is usually widespread at diagnosis, and the bone marrow is usually involved. Enlargement of the liver and spleen are common symptoms, as is anemia. The anemia in LPL may arise because of the presence of malignant cells in the bone marrow or because of destruction of red cells by antibodies secreted by the malignant cells. People with LPL frequently experience weakness, fatigue, and weight loss. There is some evidence to suggest that LPL is associated with infection with the hepatitis C virus.

Follicular lymphomas

The follicular lymphomas are the most common form of indolent lymphoma and one of the two most common forms of NHL in adults. The WHO system recognizes several kinds of follicular lymphomas (FL, number 3 a, b, c, d in table 10.3). Confusingly, one of them involves cells that don't grow in the characteristic follicular pattern.

Who gets it: The median age at diagnosis is fifty-nine; most patients are diagnosed in their forties and fifties. FL seldom occurs in children.

Incidence: In the United States, the follicular lymphomas are a common subtype of NHL, accounting for about 16 percent of cases of NHL diagnosed in 1995 according to the NCI SEER statistics and about 22 percent of cases according to the NHLSP. Some studies suggest that the follicular lymphomas may account for an even larger proportion of the total cases of NHL.

The incidence of FL increased from about 2 new cases/100,000 people in 1978 to about 2.5 new cases/100,000 people in 1995, a much less dramatic increase than that of many other types of lymphoma. FL is a common form of lymphoma in other industrialized Western nations, but it is rare in China and Japan and in less developed countries.

Marker proteins: surface Ig^+ (strong), $CD10^{+/-}$, $CD19^+$, $CD20^+$, $CD22^+$, $CD5^-$

Most follicular lymphomas show a typical growth pattern: cells are clustered together so that they superficially resemble normal lymphoid follicles. The "follicles" of follicular lymphoma do not show the polarization of normal lymphoid follicles and lack a clear mantle zone (see Chapter 9). Involved lymph nodes may also contain areas of diffuse (disorganized, nonfollicular) cell growth. The types of follicular lymphoma that grow in a more or less follicular pattern are called *follicular lymphoma* (as distinguished from *diffuse follicle center lymphomas;* see later in this section) and are distinguished from each other either by the relative proportions of small cells with cleaved nuclei and large cells (with cleaved or noncleaved nuclei) or else by the number of large cells present in a typical high-powered microscope field (the latter is the favored method).

The predominantly small cell type (number 3a in table 10.3) consists mostly of small cleaved cells, which resemble centrocytes; zero to five large cells are present in a typical microscope field. This corresponds to the Working Formulation classification of follicular, small cleaved cell, and is the most common type of follicular lymphoma. The mixed cell type (number 3b in table 10.3) contains six to fifteen large cells in a typical microscope field and corresponds to the Working Formulation category of follicular, mixed small cleaved and large cell. The large cell type (number 3c in table 10.3) contains more than fifteen large cells in a typical field and corresponds to the Working Formulation category of follicular, predominantly large cell.

More than 70 percent of people diagnosed with follicular lymphomas survive more than five years, even though the majority of people are diagnosed with widespread disease. The small cleaved and mixed cell types of follicular lymphoma show reported median survival of up to ten years from diagnosis. The large cell type, which is the least common, progresses more rapidly and is considered an intermediate-grade disease in the Working Formulation.

It's controversial whether the more rapid progression of predominantly large cell follicular lymphoma is accompanied by the potential curability seen with other advanced-stage intermediate-grade lymphomas. Likely some of this controversy comes from differences in the classification of different specimens by different pathologists, as well as from variability in different parts of any tumor, with one part of a tumor having (say) an average of ten large cells in each microscopic field and another part of the same tumor having (say) an average of twenty large cells in each field. While pathologists have no trouble identifying a given specimen of lymphoma as follicular, even lymphoma experts may disagree about the specific subclassification. Follicular large cell lymphoma is also more likely to present as localized disease, at a stage when all lymphomas are potentially curable. Failure to distinguish between people with different stages of disease in reporting cure rates may have confused the issue still further.

Since large cell follicular lymphoma may be curable with current chemotherapy regimens and progresses more rapidly than the other follicular lymphomas, it is generally treated as an aggressive disease. Some physicians advocate handling mixed cell follicular lymphoma as an aggressive disease as well.

The WHO classification recognizes a variant form of FL (number 3d in table 10.3) in which the malignant cells grow in a diffuse pattern (this would correspond to a subset of diffuse, small cleaved cell lymphoma in the Working Formulation). These are classified as *diffuse follicle center lymphomas* because of the appearance of the small cleaved cells, the presence of follicular cell marker proteins, and the presence of a specific molecular lesion characteristic of the follicular lymphomas (see below). Another variant, cutaneous follicle center lymphoma, is localized to the skin (and can be treated with local therapies).

In all the FLs, the malignant cells look like normal centrocytes and centroblasts, and, like normal cells at these developmental stages, they have high levels of surface Ig. Since the malignant cells are clonal—they are all descended from a single aberrant cell—they all carry Ig of the same specificity. This forms the basis for therapies based on creating vaccines directed against this Ig (see Chapter 5).

As with many other types of cancer, FL is associated with a specific genetic abnormality. When the DNA of malignant FL cells is examined, most people's cells show a translocation of chromosome 14 and chromosome 18 (see Chapter 8). Parts of chromosome 14 and chromosome 18 are switched with each other so that two hybrid chromosomes, each containing part of chromosome 14 and part of chromosome 18 (called 14;18 hybrids), occur. This translocation juxtaposes a gene that codes for part of the immunoglobulin molecule with a gene that codes for a protein called Bcl-2.

Since activated lymphocytes are supposed to manufacture immunoglobulin, the immunoglobulin gene is "turned on." When the FL 14;18 translocation occurs, the *bcl-2* gene is regulated as though it were immunoglobulin. So the *bcl-2* gene, which is normally active only during certain stages of B cell development, is kept turned on as well. Bcl-2 protein blocks the process of *apoptosis*, or programmed cell death. The inappropriate expression of Bcl-2 in FL therefore leads to inappropriate survival of the malignant cells. Since some anticancer therapies work, at least in part, by initiating apoptotic pathways that lead to death of the malignant lymphocytes, cells that express Bcl-2 may be resistant to treatment.

The chromosome 14;18 translocation is found in most cases of FL; however, this mutation alone is not sufficient to produce the disease, since the same translocation can be detected in lymphoid tissue from people who do not have cancer. This indicates that development of FL, like other cancers, requires multiple genetic abnormalities. However, by creating a population of long-lived cells that continue to divide, the 14;18 translocation may increase the probability that other mutations could occur in the affected cells. Like most other low-grade lymphomas, follicular lymphomas may become more aggressive over time, as additional mutations accumulate, and can transform into an aggressive diffuse large cell lymphoma or I Iodgkin lymphoma.

FL cells retain the ability to respond to some signals. The cytokine interleukin-3, among other immune system signals, can stimulate them to proliferate. This responsiveness to normal signaling molecules may contribute to the spontaneous waxing and waning of FL that often occurs.

Marginal zone lymphomas

In mucosal-associated lymphoid tissue (MALT) and in the spleen, the marginal zone is a region surrounding the mantle zone of lymphoid follicles. While no distinct marginal zone is apparent in lymph nodes, marginal zone cells are mixed with mantle zone cells in the mantle zone. The WHO classification recognizes three categories of lymphoma arising from marginal zone lymphocytes that are distinguished by the general location in which they arise (number 4a, b, c in table 10.3).

MALT lymphomas (4a) are marginal zone lymphomas that arise in mucosal-associated lymphoid tissue outside lymph nodes and thus are considered *extranodal* disease. Marginal zone lymphomas arising in lymph nodes themselves (NMZL; 4b) are often called monocytoid B cell lymphomas because the morphology of the malignant cells can resemble that of a monocyte (another type of white blood cell; see Chapter 9). Splenic marginal zone lymphomas (SMZL; 4c) involve the spleen.

Who gets it: The median age at diagnosis for MALT lymphoma is sixty; for NMZL, fifty-eight. NMZL is slightly more common in women than in men.

Incidence: MALT lymphomas are the most common of the marginal zone lymphomas, accounting for about 5 percent of NHL; NMZL accounts for about 1 percent of NHL. Splenic marginal zone lymphomas are rare.

Marker proteins: surface Ig$^+$, cellular Ig$^{-/+}$, CD19$^+$, CD20$^+$, CD22$^+$, CD79a$^+$, CD5$^-$, CD10$^-$, CD23$^-$

MALT lymphoma and nodal NMZL are closely related: the malignant cells are similar in appearance and express the same cell surface marker proteins. In cases of MALT lymphoma in which lymph nodes become involved by the disease, the pathology of the affected nodes resembles those found in NMZL.

Although most of the malignant cells resemble normal marginal zone cells, malignant cells corresponding to various other stages of B cell differentiation—such as plasma cells—frequently occur.

Both MALT lymphoma and NMZL would most commonly be classified as SLL or LPL in the Working Formulation; less commonly, they would be classified as diffuse small cleaved cell or mixed small and large cell lymphoma. These diseases generally occur in adults and may be associated with triplication of chromosome 18.

MALT lymphoma is more common than nodal NMZL, accounting for about 5 percent of cases in the NHLSP. More than 50 percent of MALT lymphomas are diagnosed at Stage I or II, and close to 80 percent of patients survive eight years or more. MALT lymphomas may arise in a wide range of extranodal sites, reflecting the very widespread distribution of mucosal tissues (the tissues that line bodily cavities), as well as the tendency of certain lymphocytes to home to such mucosa. MALT lymphomas commonly occur in the gastrointestinal tract, lung, skin, thyroid, and salivary glands. The gastrointestinal tract—particularly the lining of the stomach—is the most common site.

Both MALT lymphoma and NMZL are more likely to be localized to a single site than are the other low-grade lymphomas; in these cases, the disease can be treated with localized therapy (surgery and/or radiation). Localized MALT lymphoma of the stomach is one of the few forms of NHL in which surgical removal of the involved tissue is a common form of treatment.

MALT lymphomas frequently arise in tissues that are chronically inflamed in response to either autoimmune disease or chronic infection. The coexistence of MALT lymphomas with autoimmune disease and chronic infection suggests that chronic stimulation of a population of lymphocytes may predispose to the development of this form of lymphoma. MALT lymphomas of the thyroid are often associated with an autoimmune disease called "Hashimoto thyroiditis," and MALT lymphomas of the salivary glands are often associated with an autoimmune disorder called "Sjögren syndrome."

Autoimmune diseases arise when a self-antigen is considered "foreign" and triggers an adaptive immune response, leading to damage of the attacked tissue. Since the instigating antigen cannot be cleared from the body, one would predict that autoimmune diseases would involve chronic stimulation of the population of reactive lymphocytes. This, in turn, would lead to increased proliferation of those lymphocytes that recognize the offending self-antigen.

The majority of gastric MALT lymphomas (MALT lymphomas found in the lining of the stomach) are associated with chronic infection of the stomach by the bacterium *Helicobacter pylori* (also associated with ulcer development). Eliminating the bacterial infection with antibiotics may cause the lymphoma to regress. Researchers believe that *Helicobacter pylori* infection stimulates a population of T cells and that cytokines released by these T cells promote the growth of the malignant B cells in the MALT lymphoma, which are initially dependent on T cell cytokines. This keeps the tumor localized to the area of chronic inflammation, where the T cells responding to the infection congregate. When the infection is cured, the population of stimulated T cells subsides. Deprived of their source of T cell cytokines, the malignant B cells stop proliferating, unless they have undergone further mutations so that they are now independent.

Like MALT lymphoma and NMZL, most splenic marginal zone lymphomas (SMZL) would be categorized as SLL in the Working Formulation. Patients with SMZL typically have an enlarged spleen, and although most people have bone marrow involvement, the disease can often be controlled simply by removing the spleen. In some splenic marginal zone lymphomas, the malignant cells have processes projecting from the cell surface. This is called "splenic lymphoma with villous lymphocytes."

Splenic lymphoma with villous lymphocytes is sometimes confused with a rare lymphoid malignancy called hairy cell leukemia, which also involves the spleen and in which the malignant cells also have "hairy" projections. However, the two entities tend to involve different regions within the spleen, and hairy cell leukemia can be further distinguished from splenic lymphoma with villous lymphocytes by the presence of the CD103 cell surface protein.

Aggressive lymphomas

The aggressive lymphomas progress much more rapidly than the indolent lymphomas. The median survival of people with untreated aggressive B cell lymphomas ranges from about six months to about two years. However, people with these lymphomas are more likely than people with the slowly progressing lymphomas to have localized disease, and even disease that is widely disseminated throughout the body is potentially curable.

The behavior of the malignant cells found in aggressive lymphomas is more aberrant than that of the malignant cells associated with slow growing lymphomas. The cells in aggressive lymphomas do not grow in an organized pattern in a part of the lymph node appropriate for the corresponding normal cell, such as the germinal center or the mantle zone; instead they grow diffusely and invade and destroy normal tissue.

Aggressive lymphomas are more common than indolent lymphomas in children and in people who are immunocompromised, are less subject to normal regulatory cues, and divide rapidly. They are more likely to invade areas of the body, such as the brain, where lymphocytes aren't normally found. The cell nuclei are large, and the cells may have a distinctly abnormal appearance.

Lymphomas classified as intermediate and high grade in the Working Formulation include both B cell and T cell lymphomas. The majority of Working Formulation diffuse large cell and immunoblastic lymphomas, as well as all the highly aggressive small noncleaved cell lymphomas, are of B cell origin.

Most diffuse, mixed small and large cell and lymphoblastic lymphomas are T cell lymphomas. About 40 percent of lymphomas diagnosed in 1995 would be considered intermediate grade. Of these, about 75 percent were diffuse large cell lymphomas. Lymphomas considered high grade in the Working Formulation accounted for about 9 percent of lymphomas diagnosed in 1995. Of these, less than 10 percent were lymphoblastic (predominantly T cell) lymphomas.

Precursor B lymphoblastic leukemia/lymphoblastic lymphoma

More than 80 percent of lymphoblastic lymphomas are derived from malignant T cell precursors. Since the cells of B cell lymphoblastic lymphoma are indistinguishable in histological appearance from the cells of T cell lymphoblastic lymphoma (they can be distinguished by the immunophenotype) and the two types of lymphoblastic lymphoma are treated the same way, precursor B lymphoblastic lymphoma is discussed with the T cell lymphomas.

Diffuse large B cell lymphoma

Diffuse large B cell lymphoma (DLBCL; number 2 in table 10.4), which includes most of the lymphomas classified as diffuse large cell lymphoma in the Working Formulation, as well as the majority of those classified as immunoblastic large cell lymphoma, is the most common subtype of NHL.

Who gets it: The median age at diagnosis is sixty-four. However, DLBCL has been found in children as young as ten and in people in their eighties.

Incidence: In 1995, diffuse large cell lymphomas (as defined by the Working Formulation) accounted for about 30 percent of cases of lymphoma diagnosed,

Table 10.4. Identifying Aggressive B Cell Lymphomas

WHO Classification	Working Formulation Equivalent(s)	Characteristic Marker Proteins*	Probable Normal Counterpart
1. precursor B lymphoblastic leukemia/ lymphoblastic lymphoma	lymphoblastic	CD10$^+$, CD19$^+$, CD79a$^+$, CD20$^{-/+}$, surface Ig$^-$	pre–B cell (lymphoblast)
2. diffuse large B cell lymphoma (DLBCL)	*diffuse, large cell;* large cell, immunoblastic; less commonly: diffuse, mixed small and large cell	CD19$^+$, CD20$^+$, CD22$^+$, CD79a$^+$, surface Ig$^{+/-}$, CD10$^{-/+}$	proliferating peripheral B cell, possibly of germinal center origin
Subtypes: mediastinal large B cell lymphoma (Med-DLBCL); primary effusion lymphoma (PEL); intravascular large B cell lymphoma		mediastinal: CD45$^+$, surface Ig$^-$, CD5$^-$, CD10$^-$	mediastinal: thymic medullary B cell
3. mantle cell (MCL)**	diffuse, small cleaved cell; less commonly: small lymphocytic; follicular, small cleaved cell; diffuse, mixed small and large cell; rarely: diffuse, large cleaved cell	surface IgM$^+$ (strong), CD5$^+$, CD19$^+$, CD20$^+$, CD22$^+$, CD10$^-$, CD23$^-$	mantle zone B cell
4. Burkitt lymphoma subtypes: endemic sporadic immunodeficiency-associated	small noncleaved cell, Burkitt's	surface IgM$^+$, CD10$^+$, CD19$^+$, CD20$^+$, CD22$^+$, CD5$^-$, CD23$^-$	unclear (several possibilities have been proposed)

Note: When different cases of a WHO entity could be classified under different Working Formulation categories, the most common Working Formulation classification is indicated by *italic* type.

*See notes to table 10.3.

**Mantle cell lymphoma is not recognized by the Working Formulation. Although its response to chemotherapy is similar to that of the indolent lymphomas, it is generally considered an aggressive disease.

according to SEER. Working Formulation immunoblastic lymphomas constituted another 9 to 10 percent of cases. The incidence of these two categories (considered as a single group) doubled from 1978 to 1995. In the NHLSP, DLBCL accounted for 31 percent of cases.

Marker proteins: CD19$^+$, CD20$^+$, CD22$^+$, CD79a$^+$, surface Ig$^{+/-}$, CD10$^{-/+}$

DLBCL progresses rapidly. Median survival, if the disease is left untreated, is less than two years from diagnosis, even though about a third of people are diagnosed with localized disease. Extranodal disease—cancer growing outside the lymph nodes—is common, although only about 10 to 20 percent of people with DLBCL have disease in their bone marrow. As the name implies, the malignant cells are large—with nuclei twice the size of a small lymphocyte—and grow in a diffuse, disorganized pattern.

DLBCL can be cured even when the disease has spread throughout the body, although cure rates are higher when the disease is localized. With present treatment regimens, about half of the people diagnosed with DLBCL are cured. While this is better than the cure rates for many forms of cancer, it raises an enormously important question: "What differentiates those who are cured from those who aren't?" At this point, it appears likely that DLBCL represents a heterogeneous group of diseases and that appropriate division into distinct treatment groups will need to await a clearer understanding of the differences.

Individual cases of DLBCL differ from each other in the morphological appearance of the cells, the immunophenotype, and the underlying genetic lesions, as well as in the clinical behavior and the response to therapy. Twenty to 30 percent of DLBCLs carry the 14;18 chromosomal translocation seen in follicular lymphomas. These particular DLBCLs may have started out as FLs that transformed prior to diagnosis.

Thirty to 40 percent of cases involve abnormalities in chromosome 3 that lead to dysregulation of a gene called *bcl-6*. Bcl-6 protein, which may be involved in cell differentiation, is normally found in germinal center B cells but not naive B cells or postgerminal center cells such as memory B cells or plasma cells. It has been proposed that sustained expression of *bcl-6* in lymphoma cells prevents them from undergoing further differentiation. Genetic lesions that lead to abnormalities in *bcl-6* expression correlate with a good response to therapy and a favorable prognosis.

Translocations involving chromosome 8 are found in 15 to 20 percent of DLBCLs. These lead to dysregulation of a gene called *myc* (discussed in the section on Burkitt lymphoma, below). A number of other chromosomal abnormalities have also been associated with DLBCL. For many of these, the affected gene(s) remain(s) unknown.

At this point, there is no clear correlation between the specific genetic lesion and the immunophenotype and histological appearance of the cells. The WHO classification recognizes six morphological variations of DLBCL, based on the microscopic appearance of the malignant cells, and three clinically distinct subtypes. All the morphological variants of DLBCL are treated similarly.

One clinical subtype of DLBCL recognized by the WHO classification is mediastinal (thymic) large B cell lymphoma (Med-DLBCL, called primary mediastinal large B cell lymphoma in the REAL system), which constituted 2 percent of cases in the NHLSP. Although the morphology and immunophenotype are similar to those of other DLBCLs, cells often lack surface Ig, and the disease is believed to arise from a population of B cells found in the thymic medulla.

The underlying genetic lesions leading to the disease appear to be distinct as well. Clinically, the disease can be distinguished from other DLBCLs by its predilection for "young females," occurring most commonly in women between the ages of thirty and forty, as well as by the location of the primary tumor in the anterior mediastinum (the area under the breastbone, between the lungs and in front of the heart and the associated great blood vessels). It is the form of lymphoma with which I was diagnosed.

Med-DLBCL is an aggressive disease that can grow into a very large tumor that tends to invade the surrounding tissue. It may metastasize to sites outside the lymphatic system, such as the liver, kidneys, and central nervous system. When Med-DLBCL was first recognized as a distinct disease in the 1980s, it was believed to have a poorer prognosis than other DLBCLs. However, more recent studies have suggested cure rates similar to those of the other DLBCLs.

DLBCL is one of the forms of NHL frequently found in people who are immunocompromised—including people infected with HIV. Frequently, DLBCLs in immunocompromised people are associated with Epstein-Barr virus infection, and these often appear as the immunoblastic form of the disease (one of the six morphological variants). An unusual subtype of DLBCL called primary effusion lymphoma (PEL) appears as a fluid filled with malignant lymphocytes inside body cavities. PEL, which is found primarily in people with HIV, is also associated with infection with a virus called human herpesvirus 8 (see "Viruses and the pathogenesis of lymphoma" in Chapter 11). Intravascular large B cell lymphoma is a rare subtype in which the lymphoma cells are found growing only inside small blood vessels.

Although it is not currently considered a distinct clinical entity, a morphological variation of DLBCL known as T-cell/histiocyte-rich B cell lymphoma (TCRBCL) is also worth mentioning. TCRBCL is characterized histologically by a mixture of large malignant B cells and either small, nonmalignant T cells or histiocytes, and accounts for some cases classified under the Working Formulation category of diffuse mixed small and large cell lymphomas. In TCRBCL, the T cells are normal and are attracted to sites of disease by cytokines manufactured and secreted by the malignant B cells. Specimens of TCRBCL may contain very large cells that resemble the Reed-Sternberg cells seen with Hodgkin lymphoma.

Because of these features, TCRBCL can resemble a T cell lymphoma or Hodgkin lymphoma when a specimen of the lymphoma is simply viewed under a microscope. However, it can be distinguished from a T cell lymphoma or classical Hodgkin lymphoma by determining the immunophenotype of the malignant cells. This is one instance in which obtaining an accurate immunophenotype is critical: TCRBCL treated as NHL has a cure rate similar to other DLBCLs, while patients with TCRBCL treated as Hodgkin lymphoma respond poorly to therapy.

Mantle cell lymphomas

Most mantle cell lymphomas (MCL; number 3 in table 10.4) fall into the Working Formulation category of diffuse, small cleaved cell lymphoma. This is a Working Formulation intermediate-grade category, and MCL has features characteristic of both indolent and aggressive lymphomas.

Who gets it: The median age at diagnosis is sixty-three; the disease is more common in men than women.

Incidence: Mantle cell lymphoma accounts for about 6 percent of NHL.

Marker proteins: surface Ig$^+$(strong), CD5$^+$, CD19$^+$, CD20$^+$, CD22$^+$, CD10$^-$, CD23$^-$

MCL progresses more rapidly than most low-grade lymphomas. The median survival is three to five years, although some people with MCL have survived over ten years. This implies slower progression than most of the truly aggressive lymphomas, however, and, unlike the aggressive lymphomas, advanced stage MCL does not appear to be curable with currently available therapies. It is therefore sometimes classified with the indolent lymphomas.

Perhaps consistent with its clinical behavior, the malignant cells characteristic of MCL are larger than those typical of SLL but smaller than those found in the large cell lymphomas. They are homogeneous in appearance and generally grow in a diffuse pattern, although they sometimes ring apparently normal germinal centers, consistent with a mantle cell derivation.

MCL is usually diagnosed at an advanced stage, frequently with involvement of the spleen, liver, and bone marrow and occasionally with involvement of the gastrointestinal tract. It is slightly more common in Europe than in the United States. MCL is associated with a chromosomal translocation involving chromosomes 11 and 14 that leads to inappropriate expression of a gene called *bcl-1*, which is involved in regulating the cell cycle.

Researchers have speculated that dysregulation of *bcl-1* in MCL leads to inappropriate passage through the cell cycle and hence abnormal propagation of a normally quiescent cell type. This is a very different mechanism for abnormal cell growth than that proposed for *bcl-2* in FL, although both will ultimately lead to inappropriate accumulation of a clonal population of malignant cells. The 11;14 translocation in MCL does not appear, by itself, to be sufficient to cause malignancy.

Burkitt lymphoma

Burkitt lymphoma (number 4 in table 10.4) is the most aggressive of the lymphomas.

Who gets it: Burkitt lymphoma is one of the forms of lymphoma found in children. In adults, the median age at diagnosis is about thirty. It is one of the types of lymphoma most commonly found in people with AIDS. It is much more common in males than females.

Incidence: While Burkitt lymphoma accounts for only about 3 percent of lymphomas in the United States and Europe (less than 1 percent of cases in the NHLSP, which primarily involved adults), it constitutes more than a third of NHL in children.

Marker proteins: surface IgM$^+$, CD10$^+$, CD19$^+$, CD20$^+$, CD22$^+$, CD23$^-$

Although this disease is described in the Working Formulation as "small noncleaved cell, Burkitt type," the cells are small only in comparison with large noncleaved cells and are larger than those that are called "small" in other "small cell" lymphomas. If you look at a specimen of Burkitt lymphoma under a microscope, you will see that virtually all the cells are passing through the cell cycle. There is also a high rate of spontaneous cell death, but it is not fast enough to contain the growth of the disease. The cells are similar to each other in appearance and grow diffusely.

"Endemic" Burkitt lymphoma is the most common childhood malignancy in equatorial Africa (Burkitt lymphoma also occurs at high rates in Papua, New Guinea, and parts of South America), accounting for more than 50 percent of childhood cancers, with incidence rates as high as 22 cases/100,000 boys in some regions. (Compare this with an incidence of 16 cases/100,000 people of *all* types of NHL in the United States as of 1995.)

Noticing that the pattern of incidence seemed to be influenced by variations in climate, Denis Burkitt, an Irish missionary doctor, speculated that an insect-borne virus caused the disease. Michael Anthony Epstein (called Tony), Yvonne Barr, and Bert Achong investigated this possibility and in 1964 isolated a new virus in the herpesvirus family from Burkitt lymphoma cell lines. This virus, which became known as Epstein-Barr virus, is familiar in industrialized countries as the cause of infectious mononucleosis, a disease of B lymphocytes that is common among college students.

Meanwhile, Alexander Haddow, a researcher in Uganda, noticed that the distribution of Burkitt lymphoma corresponded to regions in which malaria was common, suggesting a possible role for malaria in development of the disease. At present, endemic Burkitt lymphoma in Africa has been linked to infection with both Epstein-Barr virus and malaria. The combination of infection with *both* malaria *and* Epstein-Barr virus predisposes a subset of children to developing Burkitt lymphoma.

Since not everyone who is infected with both diseases also develops Burkitt lymphoma, other factors are likely involved as well. The nature of these other factors remains poorly understood, although it is possible that certain plants used in traditional African herbal medicine may contribute to the development of the disease.

Other pathways besides infection with Epstein-Barr virus and malaria can also lead to development of Burkitt lymphoma. "Sporadic" Burkitt lymphoma occurs in areas of the United States and Europe where malaria is uncommon. The extent to which Epstein-Barr virus infection plays a role in sporadic Burkitt lymphoma is unclear.

Both endemic and sporadic Burkitt lymphoma are associated with disruption of chromosome 8. This most commonly takes the form of a translocation involving chromosomes 8 and 14, although translocations of chromosomes 2 and 8 and of chromosomes 8 and 22 are also observed. In each case, the DNA sequences on chromosome 8 that code for a gene called *myc* are juxtaposed with DNA sequences on chromosomes 2, 14, or 22 that regulate immunoglobulin expression. Therefore, all three of these translocations lead to inappropriate expression of *myc*, which is involved in the regulation of cellular proliferation and differentiation (see Chapter 8).

Although dysregulation of *myc* function appears to be necessary for the development of Burkitt lymphoma, it isn't sufficient; other genetic lesions must also be present. Another genetic lesion commonly found in Burkitt lymphoma involves disruption of the *p53* gene. *p53* is believed to act as a *tumor suppressor gene*, and disruption of *p53* permits the survival of abnormal cells with damaged DNA that would otherwise be eliminated (see Chapter 8).

Although endemic and sporadic Burkitt lymphoma are indistinguishable histologically, there are some differences in the clinical patterns of the disease. The incidence of endemic Burkitt lymphoma peaks in children between the ages of five and ten, and the disease usually involves the jaw and the abdomen. Sporadic Burkitt lymphoma is more common in older children and adolescents, and while the abdomen is generally involved, the jaw is not. Both endemic and sporadic Burkitt lymphoma respond well to chemotherapy.

Similar to the rather peculiar definition of NHL as those lymphomas that aren't Hodgkin lymphoma, the WHO classification recognizes a morphological variation of Burkitt lymphoma as atypical Burkitt/Burkitt-like. This corresponds to a subset of cases in the Working Formulation category of small, non-cleaved cell lymphoma, non-Burkitt's.

The cell morphology in Burkitt-like lymphoma is intermediate between that of Burkitt lymphoma and that of DLBCL. The cells tend to be more variable in appearance than those found in Burkitt lymphoma. Like Burkitt lymphoma and some types of DLBCL, Burkitt-like lymphoma is a type of lymphoma commonly found in people with AIDS.

T cell and natural killer cell lymphomas

The classification of the T cell– and natural killer cell–derived lymphomas has been more controversial than that of the B cell–derived lymphomas. In part, this is because, in the United States and Europe, these lymphomas are much less common than B cell lymphomas, accounting for only about 15 to 20 percent of all lymphomas. Additionally, with some notable exceptions, such as T lymphoblastic lymphoma and mycosis fungoides, histological and immunophenotypic differences between the various T cell lymphomas are less distinct than those between the B cell lymphomas. Lymphomas that resemble natural killer cells have also been described but are far less common than even T cell lymphomas.

About 80 percent of lymphoblastic lymphomas as defined by the Working

Formulation are derived from T cells, as well as about 65 percent of diffuse, mixed small and large cell lymphomas and about 25 to 30 percent of large cell immunoblastic lymphomas. A much smaller percentage (less than 10 percent) of the Working Formulation categories diffuse large cell and diffuse small cleaved cell lymphomas are also derived from T cells. Mycosis fungoides, a form of T cell lymphoma involving the skin, is included among the "miscellaneous" varieties of lymphoma.

While it seems natural to classify the B cell lymphomas according to their normal developmental counterparts (e.g., naive B cell vs. activated centroblast vs. mantle zone cell), attempting such a classification scheme for the T cell lymphomas is more problematic. In the WHO classification, T cell lymphomas are broadly divided into precursor T cell–derived disease (lymphoblastic lymphomas/leukemias) and mature, post-thymic (peripheral) T cell lymphomas/leukemias.

The WHO classification further distinguishes between a number of peripheral T cell– and natural killer cell–derived lymphomas based on a combination of morphological, immunophenotypic, genetic, and clinical features—including the anatomic sites commonly involved. Since mature T cells tend to home to specific areas of the body (see Chapter 9), it is not surprising that several kinds of T cell lymphoma tend to involve very specific disease sites. Some of these diseases are discussed below.

Indolent T/NK cell lymphomas

Of the three categories of T cell lymphomas that generally grow slowly, two, T cell prolymphocytic leukemia and large granular lymphocyte leukemia, are primarily leukemias. A small number of cases of adult T cell leukemia/lymphoma (characterized as chronic or smoldering) are also indolent. These are discussed with the majority of adult T cell leukemia/lymphomas under "Aggressive T/NK cell lymphomas" (see below).

Mycosis fungoides

The third category of indolent T cell lymphoma is mycosis fungoides (number 1 in table 10.5), which is recognized as a miscellaneous subcategory in the Working Formulation.

Who gets it: The median age of diagnosis for mycosis fungoides is between fifty-five and sixty, and the disease is more common in men than women.

Incidence: Although mycosis fungoides is the most common type of lymphoma

Table 10.5. T Cell and NK Cell Lymphomas

WHO Classification	Working Formulation Equivalent(s)	Characteristic Marker Proteins*	Probable Normal Counterpart
1. mycosis fungoides	mycosis fungoides	$CD2^+$, $CD3^+$, $CD4^+$, $CD5^+$, $CD8^-$	post-thymic CD4 T cell that homes to skin
2. precursor T lymphoblastic leukemia/ lymphoblastic lymphoma	lymphoblastic	$CD2^{+/-}$, $CD3^{+/-}$, $CD5^{+/-}$, $CD7^+$, $CD4^+/CD8^+$ or $CD4^-/CD8^-$	precursor T cell, either prethymic or corresponding to a thymic stage of development
3. adult T cell leukemia/ lymphoma (ATLL)	*diffuse, mixed small and large cell; large cell, immunoblastic;* diffuse, small cleaved cell; diffuse large cell	$CD2^+$, $CD3^+$, $CD4^+$, $CD5^+$, $CD7^-$, $CD8^-$ (very rarely $CD8^+$)	post-thymic CD4 T cell
4. anaplastic large cell lymphoma (ALCL)	large cell, immunoblastic	$CD30^+$, epithelial membrane antigen	activated cytotoxic blast cell
5. angioimmunoblastic T cell lymphoma (AIL)	*diffuse, mixed small and large cell; large cell, immunoblastic*	$CD2^+$, $CD3^+$, $CD5^+$, $CD7^+$, $CD4^+>CD8^+$	post-thymic T cell
6. extranodal NK/T cell lymphoma, nasal type	*Diffuse, mixed small and large cell; large cell, immunoblastic;* diffuse, small cleaved cell; diffuse, large cell; small lymphocytic	$CD2^+$, $CD56^+$	natural killer cell, post-thymic T cell
7. enteropathy-type T cell lymphoma	Diffuse, mixed small and large cell; *large cell, immunoblastic;* diffuse, small cleaved cell; diffuse large cell	$CD3^+$, $CD7^+$, $CD103^+$, $CD4^-$, $CD8^{+/-}$	post-thymic T cell that homes to the lining of the gut

Note: When different cases of a WHO entity could be classified under different working formulation categories, the most common working formulation classification is indicated by *italic* type.
*See notes to table 10.3.

that involves the skin, there are only about 3 cases/1,000,000 people per year in the United States.

Marker proteins: $CD2^+$, $CD3^+$, $CD4^+$, $CD5^+$, $CD8^-$

Mycosis fungoides (which, peculiarly, means "fungal, fungal disease") is a form of lymphoma that arises in the skin. It can take different forms: ranging from scaly patches resembling psoriasis, to unmistakable tumors, to generalized reddening of the skin. The person who named mycosis fungoides thought the tumors looked like mushrooms.

Most frequently, mycosis fungoides starts out as scaly patches or plaques (patches refer to discolored areas of skin; plaques are patches that are elevated) often associated with very intense itching. At advanced stages, other organs, such as the lungs or the liver, may become involved. If there are abnormal cells circulating in the blood, mycosis fungoides is known as Sézary syndrome. Typically, people with Sézary syndrome have generalized skin redness and flakiness and don't develop skin tumors.

"Pure" mycosis fungoides is extremely indolent: people who are diagnosed with Stage I disease do not usually die of lymphoma. If people are diagnosed with Sézary syndrome or massive skin or visceral involvement, progression is more rapid.

Aggressive T/NK cell lymphomas
Precursor T lymphoblastic leukemia/lymphoblastic lymphoma

Lymphoblastic lymphoma (number 2 in table 10.5) is one of the most aggressive forms of lymphoma.

Who gets it: It is one of the types of lymphoma most commonly found in children and adolescents, accounting for 30 to 50 percent of pediatric NHL. It is more common in males than females; the median age at diagnosis is twenty-eight.

Incidence: According to NCI statistics, lymphoblastic lymphomas accounted for less than 1 percent of lymphomas diagnosed in 1995; according to the NHLSP it accounted for 2 percent of cases. Other studies have found a slightly higher incidence—lymphoblastic lymphoma constituted about 4 percent of cases in the study that led to the development of the Working Formulation. The incidence of lymphoblastic lymphoma has remained steady over the past twenty years.

Marker proteins: $CD2^{+/-}$, $CD3^{+/-}$, $CD5^{+/-}$, $CD7^+$, $CD4^+/CD8^+$ or $CD4^-/CD8^-$

Lymphoblasts are immature proliferating lymphocytes, which are larger, with relatively larger nuclei, than quiescent lymphocytes. The term *lymphoblastic lymphoma* is reserved for lymphomas in which the malignant cells correspond to *precursor* lymphoblasts—dividing cells at an early stage of development, when they haven't yet been exposed to antigen.

Most lymphoblastic lymphomas (about 85 percent) correspond to precursor T cells (developing T cells found either in the thymus or in the bone marrow).

Since most T cells mature in the thymus (see Chapter 9), it is not surprising that many cases of T cell lymphoblastic lymphoma are characterized by the presence of a large tumor in the anterior mediastinum. Consistent with the immunophenotypic patterns of developing T cells, T cell lymphoblastic lymphomas are usually CD4$^-$/CD8$^-$ or CD4$^+$/CD8$^+$. This is different from peripheral T cell lymphomas, which tend to be either CD4$^+$ *or* CD8$^+$ (consistent with the immunophenotypic patterns of mature T cells).

Some lymphoblastic lymphomas are derived from precursor B cells. However, precursor B cell–derived malignancies tend to develop as leukemias, with prominent involvement of the bone marrow. Lymphoblastic malignancies derived from pre-B, pre-T, very early lymphoid stem cells in the bone marrow most commonly appear as leukemias as well. Lymphoblastic lymphomas of NK cell origin have also been described. Unlike the REAL classification system or the Working Formulation, the WHO classification recognizes a rare type of lymphoma called blastic NK cell lymphoma, which typically involves the skin. Although the cells look like lymphoblasts, their developmental stage is not clear; nor is it certain that they are actually derived from NK cells.

The malignant cells in T cell and B cell lymphoblastic lymphoma are indistinguishable from each other, and from the malignant cells in acute lymphoblastic leukemia, by appearance alone. The cells grow diffusely and are larger than the cells in small lymphocytic lymphoma but smaller than the cells in diffuse large cell lymphoma. The distinction between acute lymphoblastic leukemia and lymphoblastic lymphoma is the degree of bone marrow involvement. Little or no bone marrow involvement is defined as a lymphoma, and more than 25 to 30 percent bone marrow involvement is defined as a leukemia.

All the lymphoblastic leukemias/lymphomas are highly aggressive and tend to spread to the central nervous system (CNS; the brain and spinal cord). Cancer in the CNS can be difficult to treat, so treatment of lymphoblastic lymphoma begins rapidly after diagnosis and usually involves taking measures to protect against spread to the CNS. All the lymphoblastic lymphomas can potentially be cured by chemotherapy; at present, cure rates for children are higher than those for adults.

Adult T cell leukemia/lymphoma

Adult T cell leukemia/lymphoma (ATLL; number 3 in table 10.5) is one of the few forms of lymphoma that is clearly associated with a specific cause: childhood infection with a virus called HTLV-I (for human T cell lymphotrophic virus I).

Incidence: ATLL is most common in southwestern Japan and in the Caribbean, locations where HTLV-I is also more common. In these regions, ATLL represents about half of the lymphomas in adults. It is far less common in the rest of the world.

Marker Proteins: CD2$^+$, CD3$^+$, CD4$^+$, CD5$^+$, CD7$^-$, CD8$^-$ (very rarely CD8$^+$)

While HTLV-I is clearly associated with ATLL, only about 4 percent of people infected with the virus develop the disease. Moreover, it takes years between viral infection and developing lymphoma. Therefore, other factors besides infection with HTLV-I are likely involved in the progression to lymphoma. ATLL is, by definition, a disease of adults. However, the peak age of onset in Japan (around age sixty) differs from that in the Caribbean (mid-forties); this observation may ultimately lead to clues as to what other factor(s) are involved in developing the disease.

The exact mechanism by which HTLV-I infection leads to ATLL is unclear, although research has suggested a role for interleukin-2, a cytokine that is involved in the proliferation of normal activated T cells (see Chapter 9). The production of other cell regulatory proteins is also disrupted, and likely some of these also play some role in the development of malignancy. Mutations involving the tumor suppressor gene *p53* are not uncommon in advanced stages of the disease.

Most people diagnosed with ATLL are very ill, with elevated (leukemic) white blood cell counts, enlargement of the liver and spleen, bone lesions, and metabolic abnormalities, such as elevated levels of blood calcium. Many patients have skin rashes and infections. However, the clinical presentation varies between chronic, slowly progressing, forms of the disease and aggressive, acute forms of the disease. Acute ATLL appears most often as a leukemia, less often as a lymphoma with a few abnormal cells circulating in the blood. The pattern of lymph node involvement is diffuse. As the multitude of possible Working Formulation classifications indicates, the histological appearance of individual malignant cells is variable, although in the leukemic form of the disease, cells with many-lobed nuclei circulating in the blood are common; these are poetically referred to as "flower cells" or "clover-leaf cells."

Anaplastic large cell lymphoma

Who gets it: Anaplastic large cell lymphoma (ALCL; number 4 in table 10.5) occurs most commonly in children and young adults, although it has been diagnosed in people in their nineties. The age at diagnosis with ALCL clusters around two peaks: the larger peak occurs in adolescence; a second peak appears after age sixty. Over two-thirds of cases occur in men.

Incidence: It is the second most common form of T cell lymphoma (2 percent of cases in the NHLSP).

Marker Proteins: CD30+, epithelial membrane antigen

ALCL is characterized by a specific cell surface protein, CD30, which is also called Ki-1. CD30, which is found on activated lymphocytes (lymphocytes that have been stimulated to proliferate by exposure to antigen), also appears on the malignant Reed-Sternberg cells of Hodgkin lymphoma (see below) and in some nonmalignant diseases involving abnormal proliferation of lymphocytes, such as infectious mononucleosis.

ALCL cells typically carry several other antigens characteristic of lymphocyte activation, as well as several (although usually not all) of the pan–T cell markers. They may also display membrane antigens that are not typically found on lymphocytes, such as epithelial membrane antigen (EMA), which is usually found on the epithelial cells that line the bodily cavities. Some CD30+ ALCL cells carry cytogenic markers consistent with derivation from B cells (these cases are considered to fall in the "DLBCL" category); some lack either B cell– or T cell–specific proteins. Some cases of ALCL involve a translocation of chromosomes 2 and 5.

The malignant cells in ALCL are very large, typically several times the size of the cells found in diffuse large B cell lymphoma, and look unusual. These large cells have abundant cytoplasm and oddly shaped, sometimes multiple, nuclei. They grow in clumps, invading the sinuses of lymph nodes.

The appearance of the cells is unusual enough that the disease may be misclassified as a malignancy of histiocytes (macrophages found in connective tissue), as some types of Hodgkin lymphoma, or as a carcinoma, which is a cancer arising from epithelial cells. This misleading histological appearance can be compounded by the presence of abnormal marker proteins such as EMA, so it is very important to run a full spectrum of immunohistochemical markers when making the diagnosis.

Although ALCL is aggressive and people are often diagnosed with widely disseminated disease, it frequently responds very well to chemotherapy. It has the best overall and disease-free survival rates of all the aggressive lymphomas; over 70 percent of patients surviving for more than five years. A more indolent variant of ALCL that predominantly involves the skin has also been described.

Other post-thymic T cell lymphomas

To quote the pathologists who formulated the REAL classification system: "We find, as have others, that peripheral T-cell lymphomas can be difficult to understand and subclassify. Problems include their rarity in Western material, their apparent heterogeneity, and the difficulty of identifying the neoplastic cell population." The REAL and WHO systems stress the importance of clinical behavior, rather than cell appearance, in classifying these diseases.

While the WHO system defines several distinct clinical entities, the majority of other peripheral, post-thymic T cell lymphomas are simply classified as *peripheral T cell lymphomas, unspecified*. This group of diseases typically contains malignant cells that grow diffusely and is the most commonly diagnosed post-thymic T cell entity defined by the WHO system, accounting for about 6 percent of cases in the NHLSP. The malignant cells are variable in size and shape, so many of these diseases fall into the Working Formulation category of diffuse mixed small and large cell lymphoma; some are immunoblastic in appearance and may be placed in that category.

These diseases are often widespread at diagnosis—about 65 percent are diagnosed at Stage IV—and clinically aggressive. Cells generally display some, but not all, of the characteristic T cell membrane proteins, including CD2, CD3, CD5, and CD7. $CD4^+$ cells are more commonly found than $CD8^+$ cells in this group of lymphomas.

One of the more widely diagnosed of the other post-thymic T cell diseases is *angioimmunoblastic* lymphoma (AIL; number 5 in table 10.5). The median age of diagnosis with AIL is about sixty; the disease is more common in men than women. Patients generally have advanced-stage disease: there is usually widespread enlargement of the lymph nodes, often enlargement of the liver and spleen, and various symptoms of systemic illness such as fever, weight loss, night sweats, skin rash, and increased susceptibility to infection.

Lymph nodes show an obliteration of their normal structural features, although lymph node sinuses are preserved or even enlarged. Even the normal boundary of the lymph node is lost, with the diseased areas extending from the affected node into the surrounding tissues. There is a characteristic proliferation of small, branching blood vessels surrounded by clumps of follicular dendritic cells. There are clusters of lymphoid cells of various different morphologies, including a characteristic cell with clear cytoplasm. In a reverse of the scenario seen in the variation of DLBCL known as T-cell/histiocyte-rich B cell lymphoma, the malignant T cells in AIL secrete cytokines that attract and stimulate B cells, leading to abnormal proliferation of normal B cells in areas of disease.

Extranodal NK/T cell lymphoma, nasal type (number 6 in table 10.5, called angio-centric lymphoma in REAL classification) most commonly starts with a tumor of upper airways, involving the nose and palate. The median age of diagnosis is fifty; the disease is more common in men than women and is more common in Asia than elsewhere in the world. Epstein-Barr virus is likely involved in the pathogenesis of the disease. The morphological appearance of the malignant cells is heterogeneous, and inflammatory cells may be mixed in with the malig-nant cells, which are either natural killer cells or T cells.

The disease frequently involves an apparent attack of the lymphoma on blood vessels. The malignant cells surround and invade the walls of blood vessels, choking them off so that they can no longer carry blood to and from neighbor-ing tissues. This leads to death of both the normal and cancerous cells supplied by those blood vessels.

Enteropathy-type T cell lymphoma (number 7 in table 10.5, intestinal T cell lym-phoma in the REAL system) involves the small intestine. Patients are typically in their forties through sixties and are often malnourished because they develop problems in absorbing nutrients across the intestinal wall. There are usually mul-tiple ulcers of the lining of the small intestine, which may eat through the intes-tinal wall. A tumorous mass may be present as well.

Abdominal pain or the symptoms of an abdominal emergency following either perforation of the intestinal wall or blockage of the intestines by a tumor usually precede the diagnosis. The disease is usually aggressive, although it gen-erally remains confined to the abdomen (local lymph nodes may or may not be involved).

Although it is a lymphoma of mucosal-associated lymphoid tissue, enteropa-thy-type T cell lymphoma is distinct from the low-grade B cell MALT lym-phomas and should not be confused with them. As with most of the post-thymic T cell lymphomas, there is a mixture of malignant cells of various sizes and shapes; however, the CD8+ immunophenotype is more common in enteropathy-type T cell lymphoma than in the other peripheral T cell lymphomas.

Enteropathy-type T cell lymphoma is frequently associated with a long-standing history of celiac disease, a disease of the small intestine that is associ-ated with an abnormal sensitivity of the cells lining the intestine to gliadin (part of gluten, the major protein found in wheat). In people with *celiac* disease, also called *celiac sprue* or *gluten enteropathy*, eating products that contain gluten damages these cells, and a chronic inflammatory state arises. This leads to problems absorbing nutrients, which can result in severe malnutrition, chronic diarrhea, loss of calcium from the bones, and anemia. It is not uncommon for people who are sensitive to gluten to develop a burning, itching skin rash as well. The symptoms of celiac disease generally clear up rapidly when products containing gluten (wheat and rye flour) are eliminated from the diet.

People with a history of celiac disease, particularly those who developed the syndrome as adults rather than as children, are at increased risk (fifty to one hundred times) of developing enteropathy-type T cell lymphoma. It is not clear whether the constant irritation and inflammation of the intestinal lining caused by the response to gluten make someone more likely to develop enteropathy-type T cell lymphoma, analogous to the role of infection with *Helicobacter pylori* in gastric MALT lymphoma, or whether adult-onset celiac disease might actually represent a premalignant state, in which local lymphocytes have already taken the first genetic steps down a road that may ultimately lead to malignancy.

Hodgkin lymphoma

There are several characteristics that distinguish Hodgkin lymphoma enough from NHL to justify classifying it separately. The first of these distinguishing features concerns the composition of the tumor. A tumor biopsy from someone with NHL generally consists mostly of malignant cells. A biopsy from someone with Hodgkin lymphoma shows mostly nonmalignant cells. The malignant cells typically constitute less than 1 percent of the tumor. The cells making up the bulk of the tumor in Hodgkin lymphoma consist of a mix of various immune system cells. T cells, B cells, macrophages, plasma cells, neutrophils, eosinophils, follicular dendritic cells—they're all along for the ride. These nonmalignant cells are recruited to the tumor by cytokines: chemical messengers released by the malignant cells.

Hodgkin lymphoma also differs from NHL in several clinically important ways. First, by and large, Hodgkin lymphoma is much more curable with the therapies currently at hand. Second, Hodgkin lymphoma generally spreads in a predictable pattern, moving from one involved region to the adjacent lymph nodes. In contrast, NHL often jumps to far-flung lymph node regions, skipping the areas in between. This means that you're more likely to "catch" any hidden disease with localized therapies (like radiation) in Hodgkin lymphoma, since it's unlikely that malignant cells would be hiding outside the radiation field.

The symptoms tend to be different as well. People with Hodgkin lymphoma are more likely to experience systemic symptoms, like generalized itching, weight loss, fevers, and night sweats. Similarly, while people with both Hodgkin and non-Hodgkin lymphoma may develop diminished immune responses, generally, people with Hodgkin lymphoma lose T cell activity while people with NHL commonly have diminished B cell activity. The diminution of T cell response in Hodgkin lymphoma has certain characteristic effects. For instance, people may fail to show an immune response when given the tine test (to detect tuberculosis) even if they have encountered TB. The loss of T cell activity also leads to increased susceptibility to certain fungal and viral illnesses.

Another distinction between Hodgkin lymphoma and NHL is who gets it. With a few exceptions involving the rarer forms of NHL—like Burkitt lymphoma, which is often diagnosed in children; lymphoblastic lymphoma, which occurs in adolescent boys; and mediastinal large B cell lymphoma, found in women in their thirties—NHL tends to strike older adults rather than young adults or children. The incidence increases as people get older. With Hodgkin lymphoma, on the other hand, at least in industrialized countries like the United States, there's a peak of incidence in young adults in their twenties followed by decline, before another increase in people over fifty. Someone in his or her twenties is at least as likely to get Hodgkin lymphoma as someone in his or her seventies and more likely than someone in his or her forties. With the exception of nodular sclerosis Hodgkin lymphoma, which affects men and women equally, Hodgkin lymphoma tends to be more common in males.

Perhaps the most significant difference, however, is that the chemotherapy regimens that are most effective against Hodgkin lymphoma are distinct from those that are most effective against NHL.

In spite of these differences, I find the division of lymphoma into Hodgkin lymphoma and NHL somewhat arbitrary. Some forms of NHL seem to have as much in common with Hodgkin lymphoma as with other forms of NHL. For instance, mediastinal large B cell lymphoma seems more similar to nodular sclerosis Hodgkin lymphoma than it is to mycosis fungoides or SLL. However, the difference in therapeutic approach makes the Hodgkin's/NHL distinction clinically useful.

There are five different types of Hodgkin lymphoma. There is a fundamental difference between the form of Hodgkin lymphoma called *nodular lymphocyte predominant Hodgkin lymphoma* and the other four categories—which are considered *classical Hodgkin lymphoma.*

Nodular lymphocyte predominant Hodgkin lymphoma

Nodular lymphocyte predominant Hodgkin lymphoma is a rare form of the disease, accounting for about 5 percent of cases of Hodgkin lymphoma. It occurs primarily in boys and young men—the peak incidence occurs between ages twenty-five and forty-five.

The malignant cell is called an L&H cell, which is informally called a "popcorn cell" because the pale, multilobed cell nucleus resembles a kernel of popcorn (popped). L&H cells differ from the malignant cells found in "classical" Hodgkin lymphoma not only in appearance but also in immunophenotype: the pattern of cell surface proteins they express. L&H cells correspond to malignant germinal center B cells (see Chapter 9).

Most of the cells making up the tumor are normal, mature lymphocytes. They are generally organized into *nodules*—something like large irregular follicles—although there may be diffusely growing areas. A ring of T cells often surrounds the malignant L&H cells. The rest of the nodule consists of follicular dendritic cells and B cells, with maybe a few T cells and macrophages. T cells and macrophages are frequently found in regions of tumor outside the nodules.

This form of Hodgkin lymphoma is often diagnosed at an early stage: about 70 to 76 percent of cases are diagnosed at Stage I or Stage II. It is most frequently found in lymph nodes in the neck or the armpits. "B" symptoms are rare. Nodular lymphocyte predominant Hodgkin lymphoma typically progresses very slowly; however, relapses after treatment are not uncommon.

Many oncologists consider lymphocyte predominant Hodgkin lymphoma a form of NHL; some believe that it is closely related to TCRBCL, with TCRBCL representing a more aggressive form of the same disease.

Classical Hodgkin lymphoma

The other four entities defined by the WHO system, nodular sclerosis, mixed cellularity, lymphocyte-depleted, and lymphocyte-rich, are all considered "classical Hodgkin lymphoma." The malignant cells are known as Hodgkin or Reed-Sternberg cells. Reed-Sternberg cells are giant cells (at least several times the size of a small lymphocyte). They typically have two nuclei or else a single nucleus divided into two lobes. These nuclei display large organelles (called nucleoli), giving the cells an "owl-eyed" appearance. Appearance of typical Reed-Sternberg cells, surrounded by other cells of the immune system (including lymphocytes, particularly T cells, eosinophils, macrophages, and plasma cells), is *pathognomonic* for classical Hodgkin lymphoma—that is to say, required to make a diagnosis.

There are some nondiagnostic variants that include giant cells with only a single nucleus (Hodgkin cells), giant cells with multiple nuclei (or a single nucleus with multiple lobes), and lacunar cells, with a single, multilobed nucleus, which is surrounded by a great deal of cytoplasm that becomes disrupted when the tissue is being processed for microscopic examination so that the nucleus is left sitting in an empty hole in the tissue section.

The identity of the normal cell from which the Reed-Sternberg cell arises has been a source of tremendous controversy; B cells, T cells, follicular dendritic cells, macrophages, and granulocyte/lymphocyte "hybrids" have all been candidates. At present, Reed-Sternberg cells are believed to derive from very severely damaged germinal center B cells that can no longer make immunoglobulin.

Nodular sclerosis classical Hodgkin lymphoma

Nodular sclerosis is the most common subtype of Hodgkin lymphoma, representing well over half of all cases of Hodgkin lymphoma. It is diagnosed most frequently in young adults (with incidence peaking in the twenties). Unlike with the other forms of Hodgkin lymphoma, the incidence of nodular sclerosis has recently been on the rise, particularly in young women. Epidemiological data suggest that nodular sclerosis Hodgkin lymphoma may arise after infection with some common disease-causing organism at a relatively late age, so that someone who gets the infection as a small child is less likely to get nodular sclerosis Hodgkin lymphoma than someone who gets it as an adolescent. The identity of the postulated infection remains unknown.

Nodular sclerosis Hodgkin lymphoma is characterized by the appearance of the lacunar variation of the Reed-Sternberg cell as well as by bands of tissue that resembles scar tissue (the "sclerosis" in the name) that divides up the nodules of lymphoid tissue. Nodular sclerosis Hodgkin lymphoma frequently involves lymph nodes in the neck, above the collarbone, and in the mediastinum. It is most frequently diagnosed at Stage I or II.

Mixed cellularity classical Hodgkin lymphoma

Mixed cellularity is the next most common form of Hodgkin lymphoma, representing a quarter to a third of all cases. The incidence of mixed cellularity

Hodgkin lymphoma increases with age, and it is the most common form of Hodgkin lymphoma diagnosed in people over fifty. (It's also the kind most commonly diagnosed in children.) There is some evidence suggesting that mixed cellularity Hodgkin lymphoma is associated with Epstein-Barr virus infection.

The tumors in mixed cellularity Hodgkin lymphoma consist of diffusely growing cells. In addition to relatively frequent Reed-Sternberg cells, the tumors contain small T cells, plasma cells, eosinophils, neutrophils, and macrophages. As in the other forms of Hodgkin lymphoma, T cells tend to ring the Reed-Sternberg cells. Mixed cellularity is more commonly diagnosed at Stage III or IV than is nodular lymphocyte predominant Hodgkin lymphoma or nodular sclerosis classical Hodgkin lymphoma.

Lymphocyte-depleted classical Hodgkin lymphoma

Lymphocyte-depleted classical Hodgkin lymphoma is a rare form of Hodgkin lymphoma that is decreasing in incidence. Possibly, some of this decrease occurred because some cases of NHL were formerly classified as lymphocyte-depleted Hodgkin lymphoma. It occurs most commonly in people over forty, and the incidence increases with age.

Reed-Sternberg cells are common, sometimes occurring in sheets. Areas of cell death and tissue scarring are also common. Lymphocyte-depleted Hodgkin lymphoma is likely associated with Epstein-Barr virus infection and is found in people with Hodgkin lymphoma who are also infected with HIV. It is more commonly diagnosed at a higher stage and frequently involves lymph nodes in the abdomen.

Lymphocyte-rich classical Hodgkin lymphoma

Lymphocyte-rich classical Hodgkin lymphoma clinically resembles lymphocyte predominant Hodgkin lymphoma, except that it strikes a somewhat older population. It may also resemble lymphocyte predominant histologically (it can grow in either diffuse or nodular patterns). However, the malignant cell is identical to the classical Reed-Sternberg cells found in mixed cellularity classical Hodgkin lymphoma and shows the classical Reed-Sternberg cell immunophenotype.

Stage

The severity of lymphoma, as well as a person's likely response to a given therapy, is determined not only by the specific type of lymphoma (according to the Working Formulation, WHO system, or other classification system) but also by the *stage* of the disease, which defines how extensively the cancer has spread. Whereas the kind of lymphoma is defined by the histological findings and clinical course of the disease, stage is determined by physical findings, certain symptoms, and imaging techniques, like X-rays and CT scans (see Chapter 2).

The stage of the disease is important in choosing the most appropriate therapy for a given individual. For example, some Stage I and Stage II lymphomas are curable with radiation therapy. People whose disease falls into this category may be treated with radiation with the intent to cure their disease. However, people with Stage IV disease are not generally considered curable with this treatment regimen. Therefore, radiation therapy would not generally be used on them as a stand-alone treatment, unless a particular site of disease was causing some problem, in which case radiation might be used to shrink the involved lymph nodes rather than as a cure for the disease.

People diagnosed with different stages of disease may respond differently to various treatment regimens; accurate staging allows oncologists to evaluate how well patients at different stages respond to a particular therapy. This is important when new therapies are tested, so that the effectiveness of different treatment regimens on patients with similar disease characteristics can be compared. Staging is also important in determining how effective a given treatment has been. By evaluating the extent of disease before and after treatment, staging provides an objective measure of the effectiveness of the treatment.

Ann Arbor staging system

The most common system for determining the extent of a patient's lymphoma is called the Ann Arbor staging system. Under this system, the disease is staged at one of four levels. Stage I represents the most restricted and localized disease, and Stage IV represents the most widely disseminated. The defining characteristics of the four stages are as follows:

Stage I   Lymphoma is confined to a single lymph node region such as the neck, armpit, or spleen (see fig. 2.1), or there is localized involvement of a single organ or site outside the lymphatic system. If the involved site is lymphoid (generally inside a lymph node, but also in extranodal lymphoid structures such as the spleen, thymus, appendix, Peyer's patches in the intestine, and the lymphoid region around the mouth and throat containing the tonsils and adenoids called *Waldeyer's ring*), it is simply designated Stage I. If the involved site is nonlymphoid, the disease is given the designation of Stage I E (for *extra*lymphatic).

Stage II   Lymphoma is present in two or more lymph node regions or lymphoid structures (Stage II), or there is localized involvement of a single extralymphatic organ or site as well as one or more lymph node regions or lymphoid structures (Stage II E). However, all involved lymph node regions, lymphoid organs, and extranodal sites are on the same side of the diaphragm, a thin, dome-shaped muscle that separates the upper cavity of the trunk (officially called the thorax and containing the heart, lungs, and thymus) from the lower cavity (officially called the abdomen and containing the stomach, liver, kidneys, pancreas, and intestines).

Someone with Stage II disease could have disease in the lymph nodes in the neck, above the collarbone, and in the armpit—but not *below* the diaphragm. Or a person could have involvement of lymph nodes in the groin and behind the knee—but not *above* the diaphragm. In either case, a single extralymphatic structure on the same side of the diaphragm as the affected lymph nodes could also be involved.

Sometimes, Stage II is further characterized by a subscript denoting how many lymph node regions are involved.

Stage III   Lymphoma is present on both sides of the diaphragm. This may include involvement of lymph node regions or lymphoid structures on both sides of the diaphragm with or without involvement of the spleen, and/or localized involvement of a single, extralymphatic organ or site.

Stage IV   Lymphoma is spread throughout one or more extralymphatic nonlymphoid organs (as opposed to a single, focal site of extranodal involvement), with or without involvement of neighboring or distant lymph nodes. Bone marrow or liver involvement always implies Stage IV disease.

The different sites that may be involved are designated with a letter, as follows:

N = lymph *n*odes
H = liver (for *h*epatic, from the Latin for liver)

           UNDERSTANDING LYMPHOMA

L = *l*ung

M = bone *m*arrow

S = *s*pleen

P = *p*leura (the membranes that surround the lungs)

O = bone (for *o*ssa, from the Latin for bones)

D = skin (*d*ermis)

In addition to the purely anatomic elements of the staging classification, the stage is further designated as "A" or "B" to reflect the presence or absence of certain symptoms. A "B" indicates presence of any of these symptoms.

The "B" symptoms include significant unexplained weight loss, unexplained fevers that last for more than a week, and drenching night sweats (see Chapter 2). Profound, generalized recurrent itching is sometimes included as a "B" symptom, but this is controversial.

The Ann Arbor system was initially devised to stage Hodgkin lymphoma, and it is a reasonably good system for determining the extent of disease in people with Hodgkin lymphoma. In Hodgkin lymphoma, the tumor usually starts out above the diaphragm and spreads from one involved nodal region to adjacent sites. At the time that the Ann Arbor system was initially devised, radiation therapy was the treatment of choice for persons whose disease could be encompassed within a radiation field. The stages defined by the Ann Arbor system are useful in defining the regions to which radiation is delivered in Hodgkin lymphoma (see Chapter 4).

The Ann Arbor system is less useful as a stand-alone measure in evaluating the extent of disease in people with non-Hodgkin lymphoma, in which disease can start anywhere and "jump" from one area of the body to another. In cases in which disease crops up at widely separated sites, the official Ann Arbor designation may only poorly reflect the actual burden of diseased tissue. For example, someone with a single very large tumor might have a more serious illness than someone with two very small tumors: one in the armpit, and one in the groin. Other, more indirect measures of the extent of disease are therefore often used together with the Ann Arbor system to evaluate the severity of NHL (see Chapter 2).

Other staging systems

Non-Hodgkin lymphoma in children, which is typically highly aggressive and often appears extranodally, is frequently staged according to different systems.

The most commonly used staging system for childhood non-Hodgkin lymphoma is the St. Jude system, which is applicable to all the different non-Hodgkin lymphoma types found in children (diffuse large B cell, anaplastic large cell, lymphoblastic, and Burkitt's).

The St. Jude classification system differs from the Ann Arbor system mainly in that extranodal disease in multiple sites is not considered more serious than nodal disease in multiple sites, that disease originating in the abdomen or mediastinum is considered to represent a more advanced stage than disease originating in peripheral lymph nodes, and that involvement of the bone marrow or the central nervous system is explicitly recognized as particularly serious.

St. Jude staging system for childhood NHL

Stage I   A single tumor (extranodal)

or a single anatomic area (nodal), excluding the mediastinum or the abdomen

Stage II   A single tumor (extranodal) with involvement of the regional lymph nodes,

or two or more nodal areas on the same side of the diaphragm,

or two single extranodal tumors with or without regional involvement on the same side of the diaphragm

or a primary gastrointestinal tract tumor, usually in the area around the end of the small intestine and the beginning of the large intestine, with or without involvement of associated nodes only

Stage III   Two single tumors (extranodal) on opposite sides of the diaphragm,

or two or more nodal areas above and below the diaphragm,

or all tumors originating in the thorax (this includes the mediastinum, the lungs, and the thymus)

or all tumors originating in the abdomen that cannot be completely removed by surgery,

or all tumors that impinge upon the spinal cord, regardless of other tumor sites

Stage IV   Any of the above with initial involvement of the CNS and/or the bone marrow

UNDERSTANDING LYMPHOMA

Mycosis fungoides and TNM classification

A specialized staging system has also been developed for mycosis fungoides, since the clinical course of the disease is significantly different from that of most other types of lymphoma and spread to the lymph nodes or the viscera indicates that the disease has become more severe. This staging system is similar to that used for many cancers other than lymphoma, with the classification determined by the size of the primary tumor ("T"), spread of the disease to the lymph nodes ("N"), and metastasis to distant parts of the body ("M"). Such a classification system is inappropriate for most forms of lymphoma, in which the primary tumor often *starts out* in lymph nodes and the implication of metastasis is less clear (since normal lymphocytes circulate through the blood and lymph at certain developmental stages).

In mycosis fungoides, separate designations indicate the spread of lymphoma from the skin to the rest of the body. Specific designations are given to indicate which parts of the body are involved, and these are incorporated into the final stage. The specific designations are "T" for skin involvement, "N" for lymph node involvement, "M" for involvement of the viscera (internal organs), and "B" for the abnormal cells circulating in the blood. Within the "T," "N," and "M" categories, the extent of disease is quantitated with a number. Overall stage is then determined by the extent of disease in these three categories. Skin, nodal, visceral, and blood involvement are rated as follows:

T (skin)

TI   Limited patch or plaque, covering less than 10 percent of the total skin surface

T2   Generalized patches or plaques, covering more than 10 percent of the total skin surface

T3   Tumors

T4   Generalized erythroderma (reddening of the skin covering essentially the entire skin surface)

N (nodes)

N0   Lymph nodes apparently uninvolved

NI   Lymph nodes are enlarged, but a biopsy shows that this is an inflammatory response and not invasion of the lymph nodes with lymphoma

N2   Lymph nodes do not appear diseased, but a lymph node biopsy shows evidence of lymphoma

N3   Lymph nodes are enlarged, and a biopsy demonstrates lymphoma

M (viscera)

MO   No involvement of the viscera

MI   Involvement of the viscera

B (blood)

BO   Fewer than 5 percent of the circulating cells are malignant

BI   More than 5 percent of the circulating cells are malignant

The cumulative T, N, and M rankings are used to determine the clinical stage (blood involvement is not used in determining the clinical stage, although it defines the classification as Sézary syndrome):

Stage IA	TI	N0	M0
Stage IB	T2	N0	M0
Stage IIA	TI–2	NI	M0
Stage IIB	T3	N0–I	M0
Stage IIIA	T4	N0	M0
Stage IIIB	T4	NI	M0
Stage IVA	TI–4	N2–3	M0
Stage IVB	TI–4	N0–3	MI

Staging systems based on the TNM classification system have also been proposed for lymphomas that arise in other extranodal areas, including lymphomas that arise in certain areas of the head, such as the nasal cavities and the sinuses, and lymphomas that arise in the stomach.

SUGGESTIONS FOR FURTHER READING

The medical texts on lymphoma in the reference section for Chapter 1 all have chapters covering lymphoma classification.

Several excellent general review articles worth consulting are:

Aisenberg AC. (1997). "Understanding non-Hodgkin's lymphoma." *Science & Medicine* 4:28–37.

Skarin AT, Dorfman DM. (1997). "Non-Hodgkin's lymphomas: Current classification and management." *CA—A Cancer Journal for Clinicians* 47:351–372.

Urba WJ, Longo DL. (1992). "Hodgkin's disease." *New England Journal of Medicine* 326.678–687.

The following three articles are those that introduced the Working Formulation, the REAL classification, and the WHO classification.

The NHL Pathologic Classification Project. (1982). "National Cancer Institute sponsored study of classifications of non-Hodgkin's lymphoma." *Cancer* 49:2112–2135.

Harris NL et al. (1994). "A revised European-American classification of lymphoid neoplasms: A proposal from the International Lymphoma Study Group." *Blood* 84:1361–1392.

Harris NL et al. (1999). "The World Health Organization classification of neoplastic diseases of the hematopoietic and lymphoid tissues: Report of the Clinical Advisory Committee meeting." *Annals of Oncology* 10:1419–1432.

The final version of the WHO classification was published as:

Jaffe ES, Harris NL., Stein H, Vardiman JW, eds. (2001). *World Health Organization Classification of Tumours: Pathology and Genetics of Tumours of Hematopoietic and Lymphoid Tissues.* Lyon, France: IARC Press.

The following five publications provide information on lymphoma classification and incidence:

Armitage JO, Weisenburger DD. (1998). "New approach to classifying non-Hodgkin's lymphomas: Clinical features of the major histologic subtypes." *Journal of Clinical Oncology* 16:2780–2795.

Fisher RI, Miller TP, Grogan TM. (1998). "New REAL clinical entities." *Cancer Journal from Scientific American* 4 (Suppl 2):S5–12.

Harris NL. (1999). "Hodgkin's lymphomas: classification, diagnosis and grading." *Seminars in Hematology* 36:220–232.

Non-Hodgkin's Lymphoma Classification Project. (1997). "A clinical evaluation of the ILSG classification of non-Hodgkin's lymphoma." *Blood* 89:3909–3918.

Ries LAG et al., eds. (2002). *SEER Cancer Statistics Review, 1973–1997.* Bethesda, Md.: National Cancer Institute.

These two articles introduced the Ann Arbor staging system and its later modification:

Carbone PP, Kaplan HS, Musshoff K, Smithers DW, Tubiana M. (1971). "Report of the Committee on Hodgkin's Disease Staging Classification." *Cancer Research* 31:1860–1861.

Lister TA et al. (1989). "Report of a committee convened to discuss the evaluation and staging of patients with Hodgkin's disease: Cotswolds Meeting." *Journal of Clinical Oncology* 7:1630–1636.

For online resources, see:

The American Society of Hematology image bank, which has pictures of many lymphoid malignancies: www.asimagebank.org/

Dr. David Weissmann's absolutely wonderful hematopathology tutorial: pleiad .umdnj.edu/~dweiss/

Dr. Patrick Treseler's article on the WHO updates: www.pathmax.com/who.html
This article has a great drawing of the different types of lymphoma cells that really gives you a feeling for what histologists mean by "small," "cleaved," "convoluted," and so forth.

SEER online: www.seer.cancer.gov

Steven J. Gould's essay on applying statistics to cancer survival: www.cancerguide .org/median_not_msg.html

CHAPTER 11

Possible Causes of Lymphoma

At some point, many people who are diagnosed with lymphoma become focused on the question "Why did this happen to me?" Wanting to understand what caused a catastrophic illness is natural and may be a universal drive. But for most people with lymphoma this is not yet a question that can be easily answered. We still don't know enough about what causes the disease.

Eventually, for most of us with lymphoma, what caused the illness becomes somewhat immaterial: what really matters is dealing with the disease as best we can. And I think it's important for all of us who have been diagnosed with lymphoma to remember that *we didn't choose to get this disease.* Still, pondering from time to time about what could have caused our illness is inescapable. While a clear-cut cause for most occurrences of lymphoma remains elusive, this chapter explores some of the factors that may be involved in promoting the development, or *pathogenesis,* of lymphoma.

If you have turned to this chapter first, please take a quick look at Chapters 8, 9, and 10 before going any further. You need to understand something about the different types of lymphoma and the nature of cells and the immune system before you can understand how various factors might interact to cause lymphoma.

Environmental factors

The ultimate cause of *all* the different kinds of lymphoma is an alteration in gene expression (see Chapter 8). There may be a mutation in some gene that causes its protein product to be abnormal. Or there may be a mutation that disrupts gene regulation so that more or less of a normal protein is made than appropriate. In many lymphomas, these abnormalities in gene expression result from disruptions of chromosomes, particularly translocations.

In many cases, chromosomal translocations may result from random chance—in other words, plain bad luck, helped along by the DNA shuffling that is a part of the normal process of lymphocyte development. In other cases, they may result from some sort of "environmental insult"—something a person was exposed to increased the probability that chromosomal breakage and inappropriate recombination would occur. In this case, a specific environmental insult may be associated with the disruption of a specific chromosome and hence a specific version of lymphoma.

This chapter is concerned with environmental factors that may cause the sorts of cellular mutations that can lead to a person developing lymphoma. The term *environmental factors* can be used to mean different things. Some people would restrict the term to pollutants or other toxins found in air, food, and water. Others would include substances people might encounter at work or aspects of their lifestyle, such as sunbathing, diet, exercise, or smoking. In this chapter, I use the broadest possible definition of *environmental factors* to include everything a person might be exposed to. The possible role of viruses, diet, environmental toxins, and disruption of the immune system will be explored. Any lymphoma is likely the result of a combination of factors. For example, a weakened immune system might be ineffective at controlling certain viral infections, making it more likely that one could develop a form of lymphoma in which viral infection is involved. And, of course, the converse is also true—certain viruses, like HIV, profoundly suppress the immune system.

In searching for the possible causes of one's own illness (as opposed to general information about factors that tend to enhance the probability of developing the disease), there are many pitfalls for the unwary, and it's important to remember that statistical data apply to large populations of people rather than to individuals. Shortly after I was diagnosed with lymphoma, I read that celiac disease was linked to NHL. Having had a celiaclike syndrome as a baby, I wondered if this was connected to my later development of NHL. I also wondered why none of my doctors inquired about this possible link. It was not until much later that I realized that celiac disease was linked to enteropathy-type intestinal T cell lymphoma—a completely different disease than the mediastinal large B cell lymphoma with which I was diagnosed.

It's painfully easy to jump to this sort of conclusion and to make connections that may be erroneous. Unless you have a form of lymphoma that has been *clearly* linked to a specific cause—such as adult T cell leukemia/lymphoma and infection with HTLV-I—it is unlikely that you will ever be able to determine the exact combination of factors that led to your developing lymphoma. In learning about causes of the disease, I eventually decided that it was best to remove myself from the picture as much as possible.

Using epidemiology to assess the role of environmental factors in causing disease

In assessing the role of environmental factors in causing a relatively rare event, like lymphoma, researchers rely on *epidemiology*, the branch of medicine that studies the occurrence of disease in large groups of people. In the practice of epidemiology, researchers hypothesize that a specific factor increases the chances of developing a certain disease; they gather information about a large number of people; and then they look to see whether people with the disease are more likely to have encountered a potential cause than people who do not have the disease. Epidemiological studies are often useful in suggesting what predisposes people to developing a certain disease. For instance, epidemiological studies have shown that people who got blistering sunburns in childhood are more likely to get a form of skin cancer called melanoma than people who never got a bad sunburn. However, in the world of epidemiology, things are rarely as clear as one might like, and it's unusual to prove a connection beyond reasonable doubt.

There are a number of complicating issues worth keeping in mind when sifting through the evidence on the causes of lymphoma. Many of the epidemiological studies on this topic have shown contradictory results. For instance, some studies suggest that drinking a lot of milk is associated with an increased risk for developing NHL, while others don't. Indeed, one of the latter studies indicated that increased consumption of milk might be associated with a slightly *decreased* risk for developing NHL. Similarly, a number of epidemiological studies have indicated that farmers are at increased risk of developing NHL, while several others haven't.

Why should such disparities exist? First, epidemiological studies rely on statistics to determine the likelihood that there is a *real* association between two things rather than an *apparent* association due to chance. Statistics depend on examining what happens to large groups of people. After gathering information about the incidence of disease, researchers report the likelihood that the association between the disease and a potential cause is real by indicating the *probability* that the number of cases of disease they observed under a certain condition is different from the number of cases they would expect to see by chance.

If the numbers indicate that the likelihood that an apparent association between two things is due to chance is 5 out of 100 or less, the association is statistically significant. It is *likely* to be due to a real relationship. The larger the study, the more likely that any relationships will be statistically significant. With a small population, random chance can play impish tricks on the unwary.

I know five neurobiologists whose last names begin with the letter "A" (including myself). Three of us have been diagnosed with lymphoma. That's an astonishing correlation! Moreover, not one of the many neurobiologists I know whose last name does *not* begin with "A" has developed the disease. But before I start looking for some mechanism by which these two factors could have some sort of lymphomagenic effect (did we sit alphabetically in the front of the class and get spattered with strange toxins by overenthusiastic lecturers?), I'd want to increase the size of my population. Otherwise, it's likely that the same forces that made nine of my twelve mixed-color gladioluses grow red flowers are in play. (On the other hand, if I were Dr. A #4 or #5, I think I'd be scrupulous about getting my annual checkup—just in case.)

Even with a good-sized population and a statistically significant relationship, there's still a chance that the association isn't real. If you investigated the possible role of twenty different factors in causing lymphoma and each of them showed a 95 percent probability of being associated with the disease, there's a good chance that one of those associations would be false. Ideally, you'd like to have a study linking some factor with the pathogenesis of lymphoma that showed a probability of something like 1 in 100,000 of being false. However, because epidemiological studies rely on real people who live complex lives, rather than carefully controlled experimental subjects who differ only in the one factor under investigation, such studies rarely produce information this clear-cut.

Additionally, development of lymphoma is likely to be multifactorial—a number of things may need to go wrong before someone develops the disease. This is analogous to a good driver who got into a car crash only because it was dark, and it was raining, and he swerved to avoid hitting a deer, just as someone passed on the right. For instance, researchers think that developing endemic Burkitt lymphoma may require infection with Epstein-Barr virus at a young age, together with chronic malaria infection, together with eating certain plants. If each of several contributing factors is *necessary* but not *sufficient* for developing the

UNDERSTANDING LYMPHOMA

disease, it may be hard to discern a clear correlation with any one. Similarly, if a multitude of environmental factors each very slightly increases the likelihood of developing lymphoma, it can be excruciatingly difficult to determine the role of each one.

On the other hand, an association between two things doesn't necessarily imply a causal relationship. If both the association between drinking milk and getting lymphoma seen in some studies and the lack of association seen in others is real, one could develop a number of hypotheses to explain these findings. Here are five scenarios.

(1) There could be a lymphomagenic (lymphoma-causing) virus that is transmissible through milk and is killed by heat. The people in the studies that found a correlation lived in regions where most people drink unpasteurized milk, while those in the studies where no association was apparent lived in regions where everyone drank pasteurized milk (heated to kill infectious organisms).

(2) The cows providing the milk in the positive studies ate grass contaminated with carcinogenic compounds; the cows in the negative studies didn't. These compounds showed up in the milk of the contaminated cows.

(3) Drinking milk is innocuous. However, in some cultures, drinking milk is associated with some behavior (eating cookies) that does cause lymphoma.

(4) People in early stages of lymphoma (prior to diagnosis) develop cravings for milk. Whether an association between drinking milk and developing lymphoma shows up in a given study depends on when the dietary analysis was conducted relative to when the participants developed lymphoma.

(5) The people in the studies that showed a positive association varied more widely in their milk-drinking habits (people drank zero to seventy glasses of milk a week) than those in the studies that showed no such association (people drank ten to twenty glasses of milk a week). Thus, a real causal relationship was obscured by the similarity of behavior of the people in the latter studies.

In considering the role of environmental factors in causing lymphoma, it's worth keeping the multiplicity of diseases called *lymphoma* in mind. There is no good reason to assume that they're all "caused" by the same thing. In fact, it's clear that at least some of the different forms of the disease have distinct causes.

Changes in the incidence of the different types of lymphoma suggest that at least some types have different causes. For example, while the overall incidence of NHL has been rising, the overall incidence of Hodgkin lymphoma has declined. Moreover, the increase in incidence for NHL has not been uniform for the different subtypes. According to the SEER data, the incidence of large cell, immunoblastic lymphoma rose nearly twentyfold, from 0.1 cases per 100,000 people per year in the United States in 1978 to 1.9 cases per 100,000 people per year in 1993. Over the same period, the incidence of lymphoblastic lymphoma increased only slightly, from 0.1 cases per 100,000 people in 1978 to 0.2 cases per 100,000 people in 1993. This suggests that whatever factor(s) are involved in the increase in immunoblastic lymphoma do not apply to lymphoblastic lymphoma. In the case of immunoblastic lymphoma, at least some of this increase in incidence was due to the emergence of HIV infection during the 1980s (see below).

The majority of epidemiological studies investigating a role for environmental factors such as diet or exposure to certain chemicals in the pathogenesis of lymphoma have looked either at Hodgkin lymphoma or at NHL but have not subdivided NHL into specific types. If the causes of all the different forms of NHL are similar, this approach would have the advantage of increasing the number of people included in the analysis and therefore the statistical validity of the study. If, however, the different forms of lymphoma have different causes, this approach could obscure the role of a specific environmental factor in causing a specific form of lymphoma.

Such considerations suggest that it might be preferable to look at the epidemiology of the different forms of lymphoma separately. And some studies have investigated causes of the different forms of lymphoma as classified either by the Working Formulation or by groups of Working Formulation subtypes (e.g., "follicular lymphomas"). In such studies, the classifications used must actually represent distinct clinical entities. Moreover, with the rarer forms of lymphoma, it may be difficult for researchers to amass information about enough people to draw statistically valid inferences.

Of course, developing lymphoma, like life itself, is likely to be even more complicated than it first appears. Just as different genetic lesions can lead to apparently identical forms of the disease (e.g., dysregulation of *bcl-2*, *bcl-6*, or *c-myc* can lead to diffuse large cell lymphoma), it's also possible that the same environmental factors could lead to apparently different forms of the disease. With the caveats out of the way, we can now examine some of the environmental factors that may be involved in the pathogenesis of lymphoma.

Viruses and the pathogenesis of lymphoma

Viruses are small infectious organisms that can cause disease in a host organism. Viruses differ from other pathogenic microorganisms (like bacteria and fungi) in several ways. The first is size: viruses were initially defined by their ability to cause disease after being passed through very fine porcelain filters that stop even the smallest bacteria.

Viruses consist of small pieces of DNA or RNA surrounded by a protein coat; they are able to reproduce only inside the cells of a suitable host. The viruses with which we are most familiar take over the genetic machinery of the infected cell and immediately subvert it to their own purposes, using it to churn out many new viruses that can then infect new cells. Usually, the infected cell is destroyed in the process. Sometimes, however, a virus can exist quietly inside the infected cell for extended periods in a latent state. It's the latter sort of infection that has been most frequently associated with virally induced cancers.

At least four (and maybe six) different viruses have been implicated in the pathogenesis of lymphoma. The evidence that infection with certain viruses can lead to lymphoma is strong: there is convincing epidemiological evidence and, in some cases, molecular "footprints" left by the virus as well. This is not to say that these viruses "cause" lymphoma in the same way that influenza viruses cause the flu but, rather, that infection with these viruses increases the chance that an individual will eventually develop lymphoma. Cancers that are caused by a virus, like all forms of cancer, are not transmissible from one person to another, the way an infection might be. You can't "catch" these cancers from another individual (although the underlying viral infection may be transmissible). In all cases, the route from viral infection to development of lymphoma is slow and indirect.

In most of the virus-linked lymphomas, viruses seem to increase the likelihood that a person will develop lymphoma by enhancing proliferation of a population of lymphocytes. They do this by corrupting the cell's control over the manufacture of proteins. They may make the cell synthesize increased amounts of normal cellular proteins that signal the cell to divide or that inhibit apoptosis. Or they may make the cell synthesize a viral protein that is similar enough to a normal cellular protein to inappropriately activate a normal signaling pathway.

Viruses implicated in some forms of cancer make infected cells synthesize proteins that inactivate genes involved in tumor suppression. However, this mechanism hasn't yet been demonstrated for lymphoma. Virally induced expansion of a given population of lymphocytes is abnormal but doesn't, in and of itself, imply malignancy. However, the more frequently a population of cells divides, the greater the likelihood that a mutation may occur. And the more mutations taking place, the greater the likelihood that one will lead to a malignancy.

Herpesvirus-associated lymphomas

The word *herpes* comes from the Greek word *herpein*, "to creep." (This root appears not only in the name of the *herpesvirus* family but also in the term *herpetology* for the study of snakes and other creeping reptiles.) The herpesviruses are characterized by their ability to lie low after the symptoms of the initial infection have passed, hiding quietly inside infected cells until something activates them and they reemerge. The virus genome (DNA) resides in the nucleus of the infected cell, in a latent state.

In the latent state, viral genes may direct the manufacture of viral proteins, but the host cell is not destroyed, no infectious viruses are produced, and there are no overt signs of infection. Most people are familiar with this behavior in connection with the herpes simplex virus, which causes cold sores and may become reactivated by stress, and with the varicella-zoster virus, which initially causes chickenpox but can reemerge years later as shingles (herpes zoster). Two of the viruses associated with lymphoma—one might think of them as dragons rather than serpents—are in this creepy herpesvirus family.

Epstein-Barr virus

Epstein-Barr virus (EBV) is a ubiquitous virus that infects nearly everyone. More than 90 percent of adults throughout the world have been infected with EBV. In developing countries, EBV typically infects young children, whereas in the industrialized world (especially among people of higher socioeconomic status), people are more likely to become infected later in life. When EBV infects young children, it's typically asymptomatic. When EBV infection doesn't occur until late adolescence or early adulthood, it typically causes infectious mononucleosis, the "kissing disease" common among college students, characterized by fever, swollen lymph nodes, and fatigue.

EBV is probably involved in the pathogenesis of several types of lymphoma. Most well established is the link between EBV and endemic Burkitt lymphoma in Africa (see Chapter 10). EBV also seems to be associated with nasal-type NK/T cell lymphoma and several forms of B cell lymphoma found in people who are immunocompromised. It is probably involved in some cases of Hodgkin lymphoma, particularly among young children and the elderly, as well as in some cases of angioimmunoblastic T cell lymphomas, anaplastic large cell lymphomas, and sporadic Burkitt lymphoma. However, the majority of lymphoma types do not appear to be associated with EBV infection.

The precise relationship between EBV infection and any form of lymphoma remains unclear. Indeed, it seems surprising that such a common virus should be implicated in several relatively rare forms of cancer. One factor that does appear to be important is the age of infection—EBV-associated Burkitt lymphoma specifically correlates with infection at an early age.

The exact mechanisms by which EBV leads to lymphoma are uncertain and are probably different for the different forms of EBV-associated lymphoma. EBV infects B cells and induces them to proliferate. These proliferating B cells carry cell surface marker proteins that are characteristic of activated B cells (B cells that have been stimulated to divide in response to antigen). Cytotoxic T cells that recognize EBV antigens then proliferate so they can seek out and destroy the infected B cells, causing the increase in "mononuclear" white cells in infectious mononucleosis.

After the acute infection is over, the general lymphocyte population seems to return to normal. However, while the cytotoxic T cells destroy most of the EBV-infected B cells, a few linger on with the virus in a latent state. In most people, these latently infected B cells never create any problems. Occasionally, however, they lead to EBV-associated lymphomas.

If B cells from a person who has been infected with EBV are placed in a sterile environment with appropriate nutrient medium and no T cells, some of the latently infected B cells will become *immortalized*. Rather than dying out over the course of a few weeks, as would normally happen, the cells keep growing and proliferating indefinitely. They have been transformed into an essentially immortal strain.

These immortalized cells manufacture EBV-associated proteins, which would ordinarily target them for destruction by cytotoxic T cells. The EBV-transformed cells observed in vitro (out of the body, literally "in glass"), in a safe environment where there are no T cells, closely resemble the EBV-containing immunoblastic large cell lymphomas that sometimes occur in immunocompromised people, and it is likely that this capacity of EBV to immortalize cells, together with a loss of ability of cytotoxic T cells to recognize and destroy such immortalized B cells, is involved in the development of EBV-associated lymphomas in these individuals.

The role of EBV in the pathogenesis of endemic Burkitt lymphoma is less clear. One possibility is that infection with EBV somehow leads directly to the translocations of chromosome 8 that cause dysregulation of the *myc* gene. And, in fact, an EBV protein found in Burkitt lymphoma cells enhances the activity of enzymes involved in immunoglobulin gene recombination. In this scenario, increased activity of enzymes involved in *normal* processes of gene rearrangement might increase the chance that an *inappropriate* gene rearrangement could take place.

Alternatively, EBV-induced immortalization of a population of B cells may simply increase the probability that a translocation will occur. In other words, the larger the size of a population of cells, and the more frequently they divide, the greater the likelihood that a mutation will lead to malignancy. In this case, the chromosome 8 translocation might occur by random chance or in response to some other rare instigating event—perhaps related to infection with malaria.

Unlike the transformed B cells seen in EBV-associated lymphomas in immunocompromised people, the EBV-infected malignant lymphocytes found in Burkitt lymphoma do not carry EBV-related antigens recognized by cytotoxic T cells. They are therefore more readily able to escape detection by an intact immune system.

The role of malaria in Burkitt lymphoma remains to be determined. This may involve effects on both T cells and B cells. For instance, suppression of T cells by the malaria parasite, combined with a constant stimulus to EBV-immortalized B cells to divide in response to exposure to malaria antigens, could lead to enhanced proliferation of an abnormal population of B cells. The possible role of additional factors, such as drinking certain plant extracts that promote the immortalization of B cells by EBV, also remains to be elucidated.

Since EBV usually infects B cells, it's surprising that EBV is associated with some NK and T cell lymphomas. It's been suggested that these malignancies may represent abnormal infections of cell types that are not "adapted" to EBV infection.

Human herpesvirus 8

Another virus in the herpes family, called either Kaposi's sarcoma herpesvirus (KSHV) or human herpesvirus 8 (HHV8), is associated with a rare type of lymphoma called primary effusion lymphoma (PEL, formerly known as bodily cavity–associated lymphoma), which usually occurs in people who are also infected with HIV. EBV genetic material is frequently found in PEL cells as well. In addition to PEL, KSHV/HHV8 is also associated with two other forms of cancer. These are Kaposi's sarcoma and multiple myeloma, one of the sister diseases to lymphoma. Kaposi's sarcoma and PEL are both associated with concurrent infection with HIV and KSHV/HHV8.

KSHV/HHV8 may promote the development of these malignancies

through the activity of viral proteins that resemble cellular regulatory proteins. Viral proteins that resemble Bcl-2 (which inhibits apoptosis and is implicated in the pathogenesis of follicular lymphomas), cyclins (proteins involved in regulating the cell cycle, implicated in mantle cell lymphoma), and a growth factor called interleukin-6 (IL-6) are produced by cells infected by KSHV/HHV8. Of these viral impostor proteins, IL-6 is perhaps the most strongly linked to lymphoma.

IL-6 is a growth factor, or cytokine, that stimulates B cell and T cell growth and differentiation. KSHV/HHV8 directs infected cells to manufacture a viral protein that resembles IL-6. While this protein, called vIL-6, is not identical to true IL-6, it is similar enough to fool target cells into thinking they have received a signal to divide. Again, this leads to a scenario in which a population of B cells is aberrantly stimulated to proliferate and is therefore more likely to acquire a deleterious mutation.

Myeloma cells also proliferate in response to IL-6, and KSHV/HHV8 may play a role in the development of multiple myeloma. In this scenario, which has been called "cancer by remote control," supporting cells in the bone marrow are infected with the virus and secrete vIL-6. This vIL-6 acts on neighboring plasma cells, inducing them to proliferate. This is a novel mechanism for viral-induced carcinogenesis, since the malignant cells are not themselves infected with the virus but nearby apparently normal cells are infected. It is possible that such mechanisms are more widespread than is now realized and that other cancers by remote control may be induced in a similar fashion.

Retrovirus-associated lymphomas

Unlike the herpesviruses, which, like humans and other higher organisms, have genomes based on DNA, members of the retrovirus family have genomes based on RNA. Reversing the usual order of things genetic, retroviruses that have infected a target cell use a special enzyme called reverse transcriptase to copy their RNA into DNA. The virally derived DNA is inserted into the chromosomes of the host cell, becoming integrated into the host cell's genome. This means that a given cell will carry a retroviral infection for its entire lifetime.

Moreover, since the entire genome of the cell is copied every time it splits into two daughter cells, all the infected cell's offspring will carry the integrated viral genome. (If infection of additional cells can be prevented, it may be possible to clear the *person* of a retroviral infection by making the population of infected cells die off.) Viral genes that have been incorporated into the host cell genome can direct the manufacture of RNA and protein that are useful for the virus. Two members of the retrovirus family have been associated with lymphomagenesis. These are human T cell lymphotropic virus I (HTLV-I), which was the first human retrovirus to be discovered, and human immunodeficiency virus (HIV), which is more familiar as the cause of AIDS.

Human T cell lymphotropic virus I

Human T cell lymphotropic virus I (HTLV-I, a retrovirus) has been implicated in the development of adult T cell leukemia/lymphoma (ATLL). HTLV-I, and therefore ATLL, are much more prevalent in southern Japan and the Caribbean than in most of the rest of the world. In areas where HTLV-I is endemic, fully 50 percent of adults with lymphoid malignancies have ATLL. (Recall that, in general, all the T cell lymphomas *combined* account for about 15 percent of lymphomas.)

Like KSHV/HHV8, HTLV-I increases the likelihood of someone developing lymphoma by stimulating a population of lymphocytes to divide with a growth factor. HTLV-I causes abnormal proliferation of infected T cells by influencing the production of and sensitivity to a growth factor called interleukin-2 (IL-2).

As with all viruses, HTLV-I co-opts the infected cell's protein synthetic machinery for its own purposes. HTLV-I instructs infected T cells to make a protein called *Tax* that increases the rate at which the cell makes other viral proteins. Tax also forces the cell to make increased levels of certain of its own proteins. Among the proteins whose production is stepped up are the receptor for the growth factor IL-2 and, in early stages of the disease, IL-2 itself.

T cells that have been activated by antigen produce IL-2 as well as increased levels of the cell membrane receptor that allows them to recognize and respond to IL-2. IL-2 signals the T cell to proliferate and differentiate into an armed effector T cell (see Chapter 9). In a parody of the normal process of T cell activation, enhanced production of IL-2 in response to the viral protein Tax, together with the increased sensitivity to IL-2 caused by the rise in the number of IL-2 receptors, leads to abnormal T cell proliferation.

Since only a small percentage of people infected with HTLV-2 develop ATLL, and because progression to lymphoma occurs many years after infection, it is likely that this enhanced proliferation of T cells simply increases the *probability* of a deleterious mutation taking place.

Human immunodeficiency virus

Infection with HIV, the retrovirus that causes AIDS, is associated with several forms of lymphoma. Indeed, NHL in people infected with HIV is considered an AIDS-defining condition. Like Kaposi's sarcoma, *Pneumocystis carinii* pneumonia, or a drop in the number of helper T cells to two hundred cells per microliter of blood or fewer, NHL in people who are HIV positive can define the transition from HIV infection to actual AIDS. NHL is the second most common malignancy associated with AIDS.

It's not clear whether Hodgkin lymphoma is also associated with HIV infection. Some studies indicate that there is an increased incidence of Hodgkin lymphoma in people who have HIV; however, it is possible that this apparent association occurs because HIV infection and Hodgkin lymphoma frequently occur in people in the same age group (twenties and thirties). Since there is considerable evidence that Hodgkin lymphoma occurring in this age group is associated with an infectious agent, the increased levels of Hodgkin lymphoma in persons with HIV may simply reflect concurrent infection with the two pathogens. The increase in incidence of Hodgkin lymphoma in persons with HIV is much less dramatic than the increase in incidence of NHL, and at present, Hodgkin lymphoma is not considered an AIDS-defining condition.

The majority of lymphomas found in conjunction with HIV are small noncleaved cell lymphomas (both Burkitt and Burkitt-like lymphoma) and diffuse large B cell lymphomas. A greater percentage of the diffuse large cell lymphomas have immunoblastic histology than is typical of persons who do not have HIV. These are all aggressive diseases, and lymphoma in people with AIDS tends to be widely disseminated at diagnosis.

Extranodal disease is common in HIV-associated lymphoma. The most common extranodal site for AIDS-related lymphoma is the central nervous system (CNS, the brain and spinal cord). CNS involvement is far more common in AIDS-associated lymphomas than in other cases of lymphoma, occurring in up to two-thirds of patients with AIDS-associated lymphoma. Primary CNS lymphomas, appearing only in the CNS, which account for about 20 percent of AIDS-associated lymphomas, occur at rates several thousand times higher in people with AIDS than in people who are not infected with HIV. Extranodal lymphomas of the gastrointestinal tract also occur in HIV-infected patients, as well as a rare form of lymphoma called primary effusion lymphoma (PEL), which appears as a lymphomatous effusion (fluid filled with lymphoma cells) inside body cavities including the pleural cavity (surrounding the lungs), the pericardial cavity (surrounding the heart), and the peritoneal cavity (inside the abdomen). PEL is always associated with KSHV/HHV8 and often with EBV.

While HIV exerts its effects on the immune system primarily through the infection and destruction of helper T cells, most HIV-associated lymphomas involve B cells and are generally believed to involve indirect mechanisms, rather than direct infection by HIV of the malignant cells. Different factors lead to the development of the different forms of lymphoma found in association with HIV infection, but suppression of the immune response likely plays a role.

Immunosuppression is probably particularly important in HIV-associated lymphomas that have an immunoblastic morphology and those arising in the CNS. Both of these types of lymphoma tend to be diagnosed when the immune system is more profoundly affected than it is when small noncleaved cell lymphomas are diagnosed, and both are usually (always for AIDS-associated primary CNS lymphomas) associated with EBV infection. EBV is associated with primary CNS and immunoblastic lymphomas occurring in people who are immunocompromised for other reasons, and this class of EBV-associated lymphomas likely reflects the inability of their T cells to recognize and destroy cells displaying EBV-associated membrane proteins. Defects in the immune response may also increase the likelihood of other virus-associated lymphomas—such as PEL.

A number of other factors likely contribute to HIV-associated development of NHL, including disruption of the normal balance of cytokines, leading to increased proliferation of nonmalignant B cells and expansion of the B cell population; stimulation of B cell proliferation by continual exposure to HIV-associated antigens; HIV-mediated destruction of follicular dendritic cells (which may expand the B cell population by permitting the survival of B cells that would ordinarily be eliminated in the germinal center); and inappropriate expression of various cellular factors that promote the growth of lymphoma cells. For example, research has indicated that when cells that line bone marrow blood vessels are infected with HIV, the pattern of proteins on the cell surface changes so that they promote the growth of B cell lymphomas.

Hepatitis C virus

Although the link is not as strong as that for the four viruses discussed so far, some evidence suggests that infection with the hepatitis C virus (HCV)—which has long been implicated in liver cancer—may also be involved in the development of certain forms of lymphoma. HCV infects lymphocytes as well as liver cells, and infection with HCV is associated with a B cell disorder called *essential mixed cryoglobulinemia*, which is characterized by the presence of *cryoglobulins*—serum immunoglobulin complexes that become insoluble at low temperatures—and inflammation of the blood vessels.

Recently, an association between HCV infection and certain low-grade B cell lymphomas has been reported, although details of this association are unclear. Some studies suggest a very high correlation between HCV infection and lymphoma, while others don't. Moreover, different studies have suggested that HCV is specifically associated with different forms of lymphoma (lymphoplasmacytic, marginal zone, or follicular). Some of the variation may relate to the prevalence of HCV in the general population in the particular geographical area where the study was conducted, as well as the rarity of lymphoplasmacytic lymphoma in most areas of the world.

HCV seems to be most frequently—but not exclusively—associated with lymphoplasmacytic lymphoma. Since lymphoplasmacytic lymphoma frequently involves cryoglobulin production, it is perhaps not surprising to find a relationship between this disease and essential mixed cryoglobulinemia. In cryoglobulinemia associated with lymphoplasmacytic lymphoma, the cryoglobulins are monoclonal—they represent the same immunoglobulin produced by a clonal population of "identical twin" cells—while in mixed cryoglobulinemia, multiple immunoglobulin species are produced by distinct cell siblings. The exact role of HCV in the pathogenesis of any form of lymphoma has not yet been defined, but it is most likely indirect.

Simian virus 40

In 1960, a virus that was given the name *simian virus 40* (SV40) was discovered in monkeys. Viruses can reproduce only inside living cells, and during the late 1950s and early 1960s, poliovirus used to make vaccines was grown in cultured rhesus monkey kidney cells. Some of these monkey kidney cells turned out to carry SV40 as a passenger. It is estimated that, between 1955 and 1963, millions of people were inoculated with polio vaccine contaminated with live SV40. (Polio vaccine has been free of SV40 since 1963.) Although SV40 is generally innocuous to healthy monkeys, it can cause various kinds of cancer—including lymphoma—in rodents. SV40 DNA has been detected in several forms of human cancer, including lymphoma, but whether SV40 *causes* these cancers is controversial and remains unclear. It's kind of like an eyewitness report stating that a known criminal was seen in the neighborhood where a murder victim has been found. This sort of circumstantial evidence is suggestive, but not the same as a smoking gun.

Viruses: conclusion

Several viruses have been linked to lymphoma. Different viruses are associated with different forms of lymphoma, although they may sometimes work together—for example, EBV-associated lymphomas are often found in people also infected with HIV. Frequently, virally induced lymphomagenesis is associated with increased proliferation of nonmalignant lymphocytes, mediated through viral mimicry of cytokines and other cell-signaling molecules. It seems likely that additional virus links to lymphoma remain to be uncovered. It has long been suspected that forms of Hodgkin lymphoma that are not linked to EBV are related to some infectious agent, most likely a virus. At present, the identity of the elusive "Hodgkin virus" remains unknown.

Carcinogenic compounds

Exposure to carcinogens probably increases the risk of developing lymphoma. Studies suggest that specific occupations are associated with an increased likelihood of developing lymphoma, and, presumably, this reflects occupational or work site exposure to lymphomagenic substances. The incidence of lymphoma appears to be elevated in people who work with wood, in meat packers, in dry cleaners, and in chemists. However, it's maddeningly difficult to pin down any specific substance as a culprit. Correlations between exposure to any given substance and subsequent development of lymphoma tend to be weak and/or inconsistent from study to study.

I first heard of NHL when media attention was given to a report linking it to long-term use of hair dyes. I decided never to dye my hair, even though lymphoma seemed like a terribly obscure disease and the association was particularly strong for black dyes (I was interested in being a redhead). And for a number of years, hair dye was considered to be one of the best established of the environmental factors in the pathogenesis of lymphoma. More recent studies have failed to corroborate this. Years wasted! I considered rectifying the situation with a red wig when I lost my hair to chemotherapy, but I finally opted for a wig that matched my own brown curls.

Various studies have suggested a link between lymphoma and organic solvents, such as benzene. Moreover, the risk of developing lymphoma is elevated in people with occupations likely to involve exposure to organic solvents like benzene, formaldehyde, and carbon tetrachloride (such as chemists and dry cleaners). However, which specific solvents are involved is less certain. While benzene has been linked to leukemia, the association with lymphoma remains controversial.

The evidence linking lymphoma (both NHL and Hodgkin's) to exposure to phenoxy herbicides such as 2,4 D and 2,4,5 T (or to contamination of these herbicides by dioxin) is somewhat more compelling. The combination of these two herbicides made up Agent Orange, known for its use as a defoliant during the Vietnam War. While the link between herbicide exposure and development of lymphoma remains controversial and is far from proven, a committee appointed by the National Academy of Sciences' Institute of Medicine found that there was sufficient evidence to conclude that there was a statistical association between exposure to Agent Orange and the subsequent development of Hodgkin lymphoma and NHL. Therefore, Vietnam veterans who contract lymphoma are presumed to have developed it as a result of exposure to Agent Orange and are entitled to receive compensation for ensuing disabilities.

Another study suggests that the incidence of NHL is higher in women with endometriosis than in women who don't have this condition. Since endometriosis has been linked to dioxin exposure, if the association between NHL and endometriosis is confirmed, it would tend to substantiate a relationship between dioxin and NHL. Contamination of well water with high levels of nitrates in highly agricultural areas with heavy usage of fertilizer also appears to be associated with NHL. Finally, the chemotherapy regimens that cure Hodgkin lymphoma slightly increase the risk of subsequently developing NHL.

Diet

Should you give up those rare hamburgers and milkshakes? Diet has been implicated as a possible factor in the development of several forms of cancer. A diet low in fiber may be associated with colon cancer, while a diet high in certain fruits and vegetables may protect against lung cancer. Diets high in animal fats and red meat may increase the likelihood of developing colon, prostate, and breast cancer. A diet high in pickled food may increase the risk of developing stomach cancer.

The American Cancer Society estimates that the incidence of cancer could be reduced as much as 30 percent if everyone followed certain dietary guidelines.

The society recommends eating a diet high in fruits, vegetables, and whole grains and relatively low in fat and protein (particularly fat and protein derived from animal sources, like milk and red meat). However, except for a possible association between eating foods containing the protein gluten (found in wheat and rye flour) and enteropathy-type intestinal T cell lymphoma in people with celiac disease, the relationship between diet and subsequent development of lymphoma is much less clear.

Several studies have tried to determine whether dietary factors can be linked to lymphoma. Although many of these studies have unearthed a positive or negative link between some aspect of diet and the development of lymphoma, one is left with the overall impression that diet does not play a major role in the pathogenesis of lymphoma. The results of different studies have been contradictory, and the magnitude of the observed effects has not been overwhelming. It's therefore difficult to draw any firm conclusions on the role of dietary factors in the pathogenesis of lymphoma.

Some (but not all) studies suggest a mildly protective effect of a diet high in fruit and/or vegetables. One study from Italy suggests that consuming large amounts of pasta and whole-grain products decreases the risk of developing NHL. I've already mentioned the conflicting results found regarding the relationship between drinking milk and NHL.

A study that was widely reported in the media found about a twofold increase in NHL in women with diets high in animal fat who ate large amounts of red meat—particularly hamburger. This is consistent with a previous epidemiological study, suggesting an increase in the occurrence of both NHL and Hodgkin's with increased consumption of animal protein. Moreover, research has indicated that rats fed a high-protein diet have an increased incidence of lymphomas compared with rats fed a low-protein diet. However, two other epidemiological studies failed to find such a connection.

One of the interesting things about the hamburger study was that the association with NHL was strongest for *rare* hamburger. This could indicate (this is total speculation here) that it's not red meat (or even hamburger per se) that's associated with lymphoma but some pathogen present in the meat (perhaps a virus) that is destroyed with thorough cooking. This is consistent with research suggesting an increased incidence of NHL in meat packers and slaughterhouse workers because they handle raw meat and could inadvertently infect themselves with such a virus by touching their eyes or mouth. Another possibility is that the culprit is some fat-soluble herbicide that gets rendered out during cooking. If the hamburger connection is real and can be verified in future studies, I suspect that trying to associate rare hamburger consumption with specific *types* of NHL may help elucidate these possibilities.

So far, all the links between lymphoma and diet have been inconclusive. It makes sense to eat a diet high in fruits, vegetables, whole grains, and fiber and to avoid consuming excessive fat (particularly saturated fat) and animal protein. And I would feel a bit uneasy about subsisting *solely* on hamburgers and milkshakes. But sometimes cancer simply happens as a result of bad luck.

NHL and dysfunction of the immune system

Some forms of NHL are strongly linked with conditions that lead to dysfunction of the immune system. Given that lymphomas are *cancers* of the immune system, it's perhaps not too surprising that anything that disrupts the harmony of the carefully balanced and orchestrated immune response would enhance the likelihood of lymphomagenesis.

Various conditions that lead to immunodeficiency (suppression of the immune response) all increase the risk of developing NHL. These conditions include inherited immunodeficiency diseases (primary immunodeficiency, obviously not an "environmental factor") and secondary immunodeficient states resulting from infectious diseases like AIDS or from suppressing the immune system with drugs to prevent rejection of transplanted organs.

NHL is the most common malignancy found in people born with immunodeficiencies as well as in persons undergoing immunosuppressive therapy following transplants. Several immunodeficiency states are also associated with an increased incidence of Hodgkin lymphoma, although Hodgkin lymphoma appears to be less globally associated with immunodeficiency than does NHL. As discussed in the section on viruses, the risk of developing NHL, and possibly Hodgkin lymphoma, is increased in persons who become immunodeficient following infection with HIV.

Several factors contribute to the increased likelihood of lymphomagenesis in persons with immunodeficiencies. Lymphoma in immunocompromised people, particularly people who develop lymphomas after undergoing organ transplants, is frequently associated with Epstein-Barr virus. As discussed in the section on HIV and lymphoma, suppression of the immune response and disruption of the normal cytokine balance can result in inability of cytotoxic T cells to control EBV immortalized cells. This, in turn, increases the likelihood of an EBV-linked malignancy.

Genetic lesions that lead to a primary immunodeficient state, such as faulty immunoglobulin or T cell receptor production, can themselves lead to difficulty in containing virally transformed cells. However, as with HIV infection, not all lymphomas occurring in other immunodeficient states are associated with EBV infection. Contributing to the development of these other lymphomas are disrupted cytokine balance as well as enhanced B cell proliferation in response to chronic antigenic stimulation resulting from the inefficient clearance of pathogens from the body.

While being immunocompromised increases the risk, a person doesn't need to be immunosuppressed to get NHL. Indeed, NHL is associated with both immunosuppression *and* overstimulation of the immune response. Gastric lymphoma associated with *Helicobacter pylori* infection may fall into the category of overstimulation and also lymphomas associated with autoimmune diseases and intestinal T cell lymphoma.

This apparent paradox is less surprising when you consider that several of the factors that lead to lymphomas in immunocompromised people are associated with excess stimulation of B cells. In autoimmune diseases, the immune system becomes sensitized to normal constituents of the body. These antigens cannot be cleared from the body, and they continuously stimulate the proliferation of lymphocytes. In distinction from the lymphomas occurring in immunocompromised people, lymphomas associated with autoimmune disorders are frequently low-grade marginal zone (MALT or monocytoid) lymphomas. Autoimmune diseases associated with increased incidence of NHL include rheumatoid arthritis, Hashimoto thyroiditis, lupus, Sjögren syndrome, and mixed cryoglobulinemia.

Since self-reactive T cells and B cells are eliminated during lymphopoiesis, it's difficult to understand how autoimmune diseases can exist. Genetic predisposition is likely involved, and the hormonal status of the affected individual is also significant: many autoimmune diseases are biased toward one gender or the other. Not infrequently, autoimmune diseases appear following infections.

A pathogen may lead to development of an autoimmune disease in several ways. For example, it could damage a cell or tissue so that normally hidden antigens are suddenly exposed. If such a tissue is damaged, it may be scavenged by macrophages that act as professional antigen-presenting cells. Since developing B and T cells never saw these antigens, they will be perceived as foreign and will elicit an immune response. Specific lymphocytes will seek out these antigens and attack them (and the cells carrying them), just as they would a foreign antigen.

Another possibility is "molecular mimicry," in which portions of the pathogen's proteins may resemble normal proteins found in the host. Lymphocytes trained to rout the offending pathogen can become confused and turn on the normal proteins. Finally, certain pathogens may contain polyclonal activators, capable of rousing lymphocytes that have become *anergic* (unresponsive; see Chapter 9) to self-antigens to wake up and ride to battle again.

SUGGESTIONS FOR FURTHER READING

The medical texts on lymphoma in the reference section for Chapter 1 all have information on possible causes of lymphoma. For more information on the causes and epidemiology of lymphoma, see:

Brinton LA, Gridley G, Persson I, Baron J, Bergqvist A. (1997). "Cancer risk after a hospital discharge diagnosis of endometriosis." *American Journal of Obstetrics and Gynecology* 176:572–579.

Butel JS, Lednicky JA. (1999). "Cell and molecular biology of simian virus 40: Implications for human infections and disease." *Journal of the National Cancer Institute* 91:119–134.

Glaser SL, Jarrett RF. (1996). "The epidemiology of Hodgkin's disease." *Bailliere's Clinical Haematology* 9:401–416.

Luppi M, Torelli G. (1996). "The new lymphotropic herpesviruses (HHV-6, HHV-7, HHV-8) and hepatitus C virus (HCV) in human lymphoproliferative diseases: An overview." *Haematologica* 81:265–281.

Lyons SF, Liebowitz DN. (1998). "The roles of human viruses in the pathogenesis of lymphoma." *Seminars in Oncology* 25:461–475.

Shivapurkar N et al. (2002). "Presence of simian virus 40 DNA sequences in human lymphomas." *Lancet* 359:851–852.

Straus DJ. (1997). "HIV-associated lymphomas." *Current Opinions in Oncology* 9:450–454.

Vilchez RA et al. (2002). "Association between simian virus 40 and non-Hodgkin lymphoma." *Lancet* 359:817–823.

Weisenburger DD. (1994). "Epidemiology of non-Hodgkin's lymphoma: Recent findings regarding an emerging epidemic." *Annals of Oncology* 5: (S1):S19–24.

For online resources, see:

Dr. Paul Levine's article on risk factors for Hodgkin lymphoma: www.seer.cancer.gov/publications/raterisk/risks140.html

Dr. Gregory M. Lucas's article on HIV-associated lymphomas: www.hopkins-aids.edu/publications/report/jan01_7.html

Dr. Sheila Zahm's article on risk factors for NHL: www.seer.cancer.gov/publications/raterisk/risks170.html

Afterword

The last time I saw my lymphoma oncologist, she told me that I was almost certainly cured of NHL. And she said "cured," not "durable, long-term remission." It was a bittersweet moment: I was glad to leave my lymphoma behind, but by that time I'd already been diagnosed with a new form of cancer and had moved on to a new oncologist, a new form of chemotherapy, a new course of radiation. The cancer journey continues.

I have met people who told me that they considered a diagnosis of cancer a gift because it made them so much more aware of how precious their life was to them. I admire such people, but I am not one of them. If my cancer was a gift, it's one that I'd have preferred to send back in exchange for something I chose myself. For the most part, my experience of the past few years has been one of loss. Loss of my sense of invulnerability, loss of my energy, loss of my ability to bear children. I ended up leaving academic research for a new career outside the lab. The year after my diagnosis with lymphoma both of my parents collapsed, and the following year my father died. This has been the deepest loss of all, and I have not discovered a way to invoke humor to cope with it.

Still, the experience has not been entirely one of loss. Paul went to medical school; he is now a doctor, devoting himself to helping people whose lives have been touched by illness. I have made wonderful friends through the lymphoma mailing list. I have learned a great deal—always my greatest joy. And, like a metal that has passed through a great fire, I have been annealed. I find that I am more resilient than I used to be and less upset by minor—or relatively minor—problems.

I hope that by sharing what I have learned and what I have experienced with others I will make their own journey with lymphoma a little easier.

I welcome your feedback on this book. If you would like to write, please send your letter to me in care of

The Johns Hopkins University Press
2715 N. Charles Street
Baltimore MD 21218-4363

Acknowledgments

During the course of my battle with lymphoma, I realized how very important it is for someone struggling with a life-threatening illness to have something to live for. I would first like to acknowledge my family—the people whose love and support during this time were essential to my survival. My love for them gave me something very important to live for: my husband, Paul J. Schwartz; my parents, Ruth W. and Edward Adler; and my sister and brother, Stephanie Adler and Peter Adler.

I would like to thank the people who commented on the manuscript and helped me improve it in many ways: Dr. Stephanie Adler; Dr. Marsha Altschuler; Dr. Anne Atkinson; Dr. Wendy Raymond; Dr. Paul J. Schwartz; my editors, Jacqueline Wehmueller, Kim Johnson, and Grace Carino; my artist, Jacqueline Schaeffer; my indexer, Alexa Selph; and, especially, Dr. Michael Bishop for his thoughtful advice and suggestions. Any remaining faults or errors are my own.

I would like to thank Henry Dreher for bringing hope back into my life when I'd lost it and all of my friends on the NHL and SON listserves who have shared this journey with lymphoma. I would like to take the time to remember Sylvia Brown and Deb Larson, two friends who have now completed their journeys with lymphoma.

My Aunt Shirley, who gave me the book of poetry containing "Cancer Garden," has now embarked on her own lymphoma journey. She has been much in my thoughts as I have worked on completing this book, and I wish her a safe return to health.

I would like to thank Dr. Marsha Altschuler and Dr. Elaine Beretz for their help and support during the very difficult time when, still coping with severe debilitation, I returned to teaching.

Finally, I would like to thank Dr. Irene Kuter for saving my life.

Glossary

ABVD (*A*driamycin, *b*leomycin, *v*inblastine, *d*acarbazine). The chemotherapy regimen most commonly used to treat Hodgkin disease.

activated lymphocyte. A lymphocyte that has encountered an antigen it recognizes and has thereby been stimulated to proliferate and differentiate.

active immunization. Exposure to an antigen in order to elicit a specific immune response against that antigen from the cells of the adaptive immune system.

acupuncture. A branch of traditional Chinese medicine in which fine needles are inserted into specific locations of the body for therapeutic purposes; in the related technique of acupressure, these locations are stimulated, but the skin is not actually pierced.

acute graft-versus-host disease. A complication of allogeneic stem cell transplants in which the donor lymphocytes attack the recipient's body.

acyclovir (brand names, Avirax, Zovirax). An antiviral drug.

adaptive immune system. The part of the immune system that involves specific responses to particular antigens and is responsible for the phenomenon of immunological memory; includes T cells and B cells.

adenoids. Lymphoid structures found in the nasal cavity.

Adriamycin (generic names, doxorubicin, hydroxydaunomycin, hydroxydoxorubicin; other brand names, Doxil; Rubex). An antineoplastic drug used in treating lymphoma that is classified as an anthracycline.

adult T cell leukemia/lymphoma (ATLL). A form of lymphoma associated with infection with the retrovirus HTLV-I.

advanced disease. Bulky Stage II, Stage III, or Stage IV lymphoma.

Agent Orange. An herbicide that is suspected of contributing to the pathogenesis of lymphoma.

aggressive disease. Lymphoma that progresses quickly, so that someone who remained untreated would be expected to survive only months to a few years after diagnosis.

AIDS (acquired immune deficiency syndrome). A viral disease that leaves people susceptible to many pathogens and that is a risk factor for developing aggressive forms of non-Hodgkin lymphoma.

alemtuzumab (brand name, Campath). A monoclonal antibody directed against CD52, a protein found on the cell surface of both B cells and T cells.

alendronate (brand name, Fosamax). A drug that inhibits the loss of calcium from the bones.

alkylating agents. A class of antineoplastic drugs.

allogeneic transplant. A stem cell transplant in which the donor is neither the recipient nor the recipient's identical twin.

allopurinol (brand names, Aloprim, Lopurin, Purinol, Zyloprim). A drug used to prevent massive release of uric acid when many tumor cells die at once.

alopecia. Hair loss.

alternative therapies. Nontraditional therapies used instead of conventional medicine.

amino acids. The chemical building blocks that make up proteins.

amphotericin (brand names, Amphocin, Fungizone). An antifungal drug.

amplification. A mutation in which sections of a chromosome are inappropriately repeated many times.

anaplastic large cell lymphoma (ALCL). An aggressive T cell lymphoma.

anemia. Any condition in which there are low levels of hemoglobin, the iron-bearing protein found in red blood cells.

anergic. Refers to lymphocytes that have become unresponsive to the antigen that they recognize.

angiogenesis. Growth of blood vessels.

angioimmunoblastic T cell lymphoma (AIL). An aggressive T cell lymphoma.

Ann Arbor "B" symptoms. Fever, weight loss, and night sweats, used as part of lymphoma staging.

Ann Arbor staging system. The most common system for defining how far lymphoma has spread through your body.

anthracyclines. A class of antineoplastic drugs.

antiangiogenesis. A therapeutic approach aimed at inhibiting the growth of new blood vessels to tumors.

antibody. A secreted protein that specifically recognizes and binds to an antigen.

antibody-dependent cellular cytotoxicity. A mechanism in which natural killer cells are recruited to cells that antibodies have bound to so that the antibody-coated cells can be destroyed.

antigen. A substance capable of eliciting a specific immune response.

antigenic determinant. The part of an antigen that a particular antibody recognizes.

antimetabolites. A class of antineoplastic drugs.

antimitotics. A class of antineoplastic drugs.

antineoplastic agents. Drugs used to treat cancer; chemotherapy drugs.

antioxidant. A substance that prevents oxidation, which can therefore protect cells from oxidative damage caused by highly reactive substances called free radicals.

antisense gene therapy. A therapeutic approach in which a sequence of nucleotides complementary to a particular stretch of messenger RNA is given to someone to inhibit production of the protein encoded by that messenger RNA.

apheresis. A procedure in which whole blood is withdrawn, some component of the blood removed, and the rest returned to the body.

apoptosis. A process of programmed cell death whereby unnecessary or nonfunctional cells can be eliminated.

appendix. A lymphoid structure that projects from the gut.

aspergillus. A fungal pathogen.

autoimmune disease. A disease in which the immune system attacks the body's own tissues.

autologous transplant. A stem cell transplant in which the donor and the recipient are the same person.

autonomic nervous system. The part of the nervous system involved in regulating involuntary aspects of bodily function such as blood pressure and heart rate.

band cells. Neutrophils in the next-to-last stage of maturation.

barium. A substance that is opaque to X-rays, which therefore may be given to improve visualization in some radiographic procedures.

basophils. A class of white blood cells.

B cells. See *B lymphocytes.*

B cell chronic lymphocytic leukemia. A form of leukemia that is equivalent to small lymphocytic lymphoma.

B cell mitogen. A substance that stimulates B cells to divide.

bcl-2. A gene that is abnormally expressed in follicular lymphomas; its protein product inhibits apoptosis.

BCNU (bischloroethylnitrosourea; also called carmustine). An antineoplastic drug that is classified as an alkylating agent; used to treat lymphoma.

benign. Not cancerous.

Bexxar (^{131}I-tositumomab). A radiolabeled monoclonal antibody directed against the B cell protein CD20.

B immunopoiesis. The stage of B cell development that takes place after a B cell has encountered an antigen it recognizes.

biological therapies. Therapies that use living cells to create an anticancer response.

biopsy. A procedure in which a small piece of tissue is removed from the body so that it can be examined for evidence of disease.

bleomycin (brand name, Blenoxane). An antineoplastic drug that is similar to the anthracyclines.

B lymphocytes (also called B cells). The class of cells responsible for the humoral limb of the adaptive immune response.

bone marrow. The spongy tissue in the center of our bones where the progenitor cells that give rise to the different types of blood cells live.

bone marrow suppression. A condition in which the numbers and/or activity of the progenitor cells that reside in the bone marrow are limited so that fewer blood cells are formed; a common side effect of certain types of chemotherapy.

bone marrow transplant. A form of stem cell transplant in which the stem cells are obtained directly from the donor's bone marrow.

"B" symptoms. See *Ann Arbor "B" symptoms.*

bulky disease. Generally defined as a tumor that is greater than 10 cm in maximal diameter or, for mediastinal disease, one-third or more of the width of the chest cavity.

Burkitt lymphoma (formerly called Burkitt's lymphoma). A very aggressive form of lymphoma.

Campath. See *alemtuzumab.*

cancer. A disease characterized by the existence of a population of abnormal cells that accumulate without the normal restraints governing cell growth and that can invade normal tissue.

cancer cachexia. A syndrome of weight loss, muscle wasting, and malnutrition that sometimes occurs in people with cancer.

cancer vaccines. Various therapeutic strategies designed to elicit an active immunological response against tumor-associated proteins.

Candida. A pathogenic fungus.

capillaries. The smallest type of blood vessels.

carbohydrates. A class of chemical compounds consisting of both sugars and larger molecules made from sugar polymers.

carcinogens. Environmental agents that increase the likelihood that one will develop cancer.

carmustine. See *BCNU.*

catheter. A flexible tube that can be inserted into the body.

CAT scan. Computerized *axial tomography*; see *CT scan.*

CBC. See *complete blood count.*

CD4. A protein found on helper, inflammatory, and regulatory T cells.

CD8. A protein found on cytotoxic T cells.

CD20. A protein found on normal B lymphocytes as well as in some forms of lymphoma.

celiac disease. An intestinal disease characterized by inability to tolerate gluten.

cell. The fundamental unit of living organisms.

cell cycle. The sequence of events involved in duplicating a cell that spans the time between one cell division and the next.

cell membrane. The substance that surrounds an individual cell and separates the cell interior from the extracellular environment; the cellular equivalent of the skin.

central line. An intravenous tube that has been placed so as to give semipermanent access to the large veins near the heart.

central lymphoid organs. The bone marrow and the thymus.

central nervous system (CNS). The brain and spinal cord.

centroblast. B cells at a developmental stage following exposure to antigen in which they rapidly proliferate within the germinal center.

centrocytes. B cells at the next developmental stage after centroblast.

cerebrospinal fluid. The clear fluid that bathes the brain and spinal cord.

chemoreceptor trigger zone. A specialized region of the brain that detects noxious substances circulating in the bloodstream.

chemotherapy. The use of drugs to treat disease, particularly cancer.

chlorambucil (brand name, Leukeran). An antineoplastic drug used in treating lymphoma that is classified as an alkylating agent.

CHOP (*cyclophosphamide, hydroxydaunomycin, Oncovin, prednisone*). A chemotherapy regimen commonly used to treat aggressive forms of non-Hodgkin lymphoma.

chromosomes. Long, double-stranded lengths of DNA found in the cell nucleus that contain many individual genes linked together.

chronic lymphocytic leukemia (CLL). A form of leukemia that is equivalent to small lymphocytic lymphoma.

circulatory system. The system of interconnected vesicles that carry blood throughout the body.

cisplatin (brand name, Platinol). An antineoplastic drug used in treating lymphoma with a mechanism of action similar to that of an alkylating agent.

cladribine (2-chlorodeoxyadenosine; brand name, Leustatin). An antineoplastic drug used in treating lymphoma that is classified as an antimetabolite.

classical Hodgkin lymphoma (formerly called classical Hodgkin's disease). The four types of Hodgkin lymphoma that are characterized by the appearance of Hodgkin cells and multinucleated Reed-Sternberg cells (rather than the L&H, or popcorn, Reed-Sternberg cell variant seen in nodular lymphocyte predominant Hodgkin lymphoma).

classical Hodgkin's disease. See *classical Hodgkin lymphoma.*

clinical entity. A specific disease that can be differentiated from other diseases.

clonal. Refers to a group of cells that are descended from a single cell.

CNS. See *central nervous system.*

coding sequence. The order of nucleotides in a strand of DNA or RNA that specifies the amino acid composition of a particular protein.

colony-stimulating factors (CSFs). Hematopoietic growth factors; chemical messengers that promote the differentiation and proliferation of particular classes of blood cells.

combination chemotherapy. Chemotherapy in which several different drugs—typically drugs with differing mechanisms of action—are administered together.

combined modality therapy. Combining chemotherapy with radiation therapy, chemotherapy with monoclonal-antibody therapy, or radiation therapy with monoclonal-antibody therapy or combining all three forms of treatment.

complement. A group of plasma proteins that can be recruited by antibodies to kill antibody-coated cells; used by the immune system to kill pathogens.

complementary therapies. Nontraditional therapies meant to be used together with conventional medicine.

complete blood count (CBC). The total number of red cells, white cells, and platelets present in a microliter (µl) of blood.

complete molecular remission. A remission in which not only are there no clinical signs of disease but no evidence of abnormal DNA can be detected.

complete remission. A remission in which no clinical evidence of disease can be detected by CT scan or physical examination.

computerized axial tomography (CAT scan). See *CT scan.*

conditioning. High-dose chemotherapy intended to eliminate all cancer cells; given in preparation for a stem cell transplant.

consolidation phase. In a leukemia-type chemotherapy regimen that involves multiple phases, the consolidation phase is given after a complete remission has been attained during the induction phase.

constant region. The portion of an antibody that is common to all antibodies of that class.

contiguous. Touching.

controlled clinical trial. A clinical trial in which one randomly assigned group of individuals is given the investigational therapy and another randomly assigned group is given the therapy that is the current standard of care and the efficacy of the two treatments is directly compared.

cord blood. Blood obtained from the umbilical cords of newborns, used as a source of stem cells.

corticosteroids. Anti-inflammatory compounds produced by the adrenal cortex and the family of drugs related to them; some corticosteroids are used in chemotherapy, and some are used to prevent nausea.

cryoglobulins. Serum immunoglobulin complexes that become insoluble at low temperatures.

cryoprotectant. A substance that protects against damage caused by freezing.

CSFs. See *colony-stimulating factors.*

CT scan (also called CAT scan). An X-ray-based technique for obtaining a detailed three-dimensional picture of internal structures.

cutaneous T cell lymphoma. A form of non-Hodgkin lymphoma that involves the skin.

cyclophosphamide (brand name, Cytoxan). An antineoplastic drug used in treating lymphoma that is classified as an alkylating agent.

cyclosporine (brand names, Neoral, Sandimmune, SangCya). An immunosuppressive drug.

cytarabine (cytosine arabinoside, ara-C; brand name, Cytosar-U). An antineoplastic drug used in treating lymphoma that is classified as an antimetabolite.

cytokines. The chemical messengers by which one cell type conveys information to another.

cytomegalovirus. A virus that sometimes infects people who are immunosuppressed following a stem cell transplant.

cytometer. A cell counter.

cytoplasm. The jellylike substance with which cells are filled.

cytosine arabinoside. See *cytarabine.*

cytotoxic T cells. The class of T cells whose job it is to kill virally infected cells.

dacarbazine (brand name, DTIC-Dome). An antineoplastic drug used in treating lymphoma that is classified as an alkylating agent.

daunorubicin (brand names, Cerubidine, DaunoXome [liposomal daunorubicin]). An antineoplastic drug used in treating lymphoma that is classified as an anthracycline.

deletion. A mutation in which one or more nucleotides are omitted.

dendritic cells. The class of professional antigen-presenting cells that are the most powerful stimulators of T cell responses.

dendritic cell vaccine. A therapeutic approach in which dendritic cells are grown outside the body in the presence of tumor-associated antigen and then reintroduced into the body with the hope that they will stimulate an antitumor T cell response.

denileukin diftitox (brand name, Ontak). A drug in which the cytokine interleukin-2, which binds to T cells, is fused to a portion of the toxin produced by the bacterium that causes diphtheria.

dexamethasone (brand names, Decadron, Dexameth, Dexone, Hexadrol). A corticosteroid.

differential. A complete blood count in which the different types of white blood cells are identified and counted.

differentiated properties. The specific properties characteristic of a mature cell that distinguish it from other cell types and allow it to carry out its particular function.

diffuse follicle center lymphoma. A form of non-Hodgkin lymphoma.

diffuse large B cell lymphoma (DLBCL). The most common form of aggressive non-Hodgkin lymphoma (defined according to the REAL and WHO classification systems).

diffuse large cell lymphoma. The most common form of aggressive non-Hodgkin lymphoma (defined according to the Working Formulation).

diffuse mixed small and large cell lymphoma. A form of non-Hodgkin lymphoma that is defined as intermediate grade in the Working Formulation and that usually involves malignant T cells.

dioxin. A contaminant of the herbicides used in making Agent Orange, which is suspected of contributing to the pathogenesis of lymphoma.

directed therapies. Highly selective treatments designed to target some specific property that is characteristic of cancer cells but is not shared by most normal cells.

DNA (deoxyribonucleic acid). A large molecule found in the cell nucleus that comprises the genetic material that acts as blueprint to specify how to construct and maintain a living being.

dopamine. A neurotransmitter.

dose-limiting toxicity. A drug side effect that becomes critical at a certain drug dose so that the drug cannot be safely administered at higher doses.

doxorubicin. See *Adriamycin.*

drenching. When referring to night sweats, "drenching" means so heavy that you need to change your sheets; drenching night sweats are one of the Ann Arbor "B" symptoms.

duplication. A chromosomal abnormality in which there is an extra copy of a particular chromosome.

EBV. See *Epstein-Barr virus.*

effector (or armed effector). When referring to lymphocytes, an effector cell is one that is ready to fulfill its immunological functions without undergoing further differentiation.

electrolytes. Dissolved salts (used to refer to salts dissolved in bodily fluids).

engraftment. The process whereby transplanted stem cells find their way to the appropriate sites inside bone and start generating new hematopoietic cells.

enteropathy-type T cell lymphoma (also called intestinal T cell lymphoma). A form of non-Hodgkin lymphoma that is associated with gluten intolerance.

enzyme. A protein that catalyzes some chemical reaction.

eosinopenia. Having too few eosinophils.

eosinophil. A type of white blood cell.

eosinophilia. Having too many eosinophils.

epidemiology. The study of the causes and distribution of disease in general populations.

Epstein-Barr virus (EBV). A herpes-family virus implicated in the pathogenesis of certain forms of lymphoma.

erythrocyte. A red blood cell.

erythrocyte sedimentation rate (ESR). A blood test that measures the speed with which red cells settle out of a sample of blood in a tube. The sedimentation rate can be elevated in a variety of inflammatory conditions.

erythropoietin. A growth factor produced by the kidneys that stimulates the production of red blood cells.

escape mutation. A mutation that allows a pathogen or a cancer cell to survive a therapy directed against some component that is lost or changed.

esophagus. The tube that carries food from the mouth to the stomach.

ESR. See *erythrocyte sedimentation rate.*

etoposide (also called VP-16; brand name, VePesid). An antineoplastic drug used in treating lymphoma that acts through a mechanism similar to an anthracycline.

evidence-based medicine. Choosing therapeutic approaches based on the results of controlled clinical trials.

excisional biopsy. A surgical procedure in which a suspicious lymph node (or lump or other suspicious area) is removed from the body so that it can be examined for evidence of disease.

extended field radiation. Radiation therapy in which the treatment area includes not only the sites of known disease but also adjacent lymph node chains.

external beam therapy. Radiation therapy in which the radiation is applied from outside the body.

external tunneled catheter. A semipermanent central line in which a flexible tube is placed into a central vein and tunnels a short distance under your skin before emerging from your body.

extracellular fluid. The fluid that bathes and surrounds cells.

extracellular matrix. The solid parts of a tissue that exist outside cells.

extracorporeal photopheresis. A procedure in which a sample of blood is removed from the body, treated with psoralens, and exposed to light before being returned to the body.

extranodal. Refers to disease that is found outside lymph nodes.

extranodal marginal zone B cell lymphoma of mucosal-associated lymphoid tissue (MALT lymphoma). An indolent form of non-Hodgkin lymphoma that involves mucosal-associated lymphoid tissue.

extranodal NK/T cell lymphoma, nasal type. A form of non-Hodgkin lymphoma that involves the nose and pharynx and is associated with Epstein-Barr virus infection.

fatigue. A state of exhaustion in which your ability to function normally is impaired by your lack of energy.

fine needle biopsy. A procedure in which a small sample of tissue is removed from a suspicious lymph node (or lump or other suspicious area) through the bore of a needle so that it can be examined for evidence of disease.

fixed. Tissue that has been treated so that all the small structures that make up the cells remain in place during treatment and can be visualized under a microscope in permanent sections.

flow cytometry. A diagnostic procedure in which fluorescently labeled antibodies are used to determine the presence or absence of specific marker proteins.

fluconazole (brand name, Diflucan). An antifungal drug.

fludarabine (brand name, Fludara). An antineoplastic drug used in treating lymphoma that is classified as an antimetabolite.

fluorescence. The property of glowing when exposed to light.

folic acid. A B vitamin required by rapidly dividing cells.

follicular. Having to do with follicles, regions of lymph nodes or other lymphoid tissues that are rich in B cells.

follicular dendritic cell. A type of cell found in lymphoid follicles.

follicular lymphoma (FL). The most common form of indolent non-Hodgkin lymphoma (grade 3 as defined by the WHO system may be considered aggressive disease). The malignant cells in follicular lymphoma resemble centrocytes and centroblasts and commonly grow in patterns that resemble lymphoid follicles. In the variant known as "diffuse follicle center lymphoma," cells do not grow in the follicle-like pattern.

fractionated doses. Radiation applied as a series of treatments, rather than all at one time.

free radicals. Highly reactive substances that can damage cells.

frozen sections. A way of preparing tissue from a biopsy so that it can be visualized immediately (i.e., while the person is still on the operating table)

gallium. A substance used for imaging lymphoma cells.

ganciclovir (brand name, Cytovene). An antiviral drug.

gastrointestinal tract. The stomach, intestines, and associated structures.

G-CSF. See *granulocyte colony-stimulating factor.*

gemcitabine (brand name, Gemzar). An antineoplastic drug used in treating lymphoma that is classified as an antimetabolite.

gene. A sequence of DNA found at a particular spot on a chromosome that specifies how to construct a particular protein (or protein chain).

genome. All the genetic material for a given organism.

germinal center. The site in a lymphoid follicle in which activated B cells are rapidly proliferating.

glucocorticoids. The class of corticosteroids that influence carbohydrate, protein, and fat metabolism.

gluten. A protein found in wheat.

GM-CSF. See *granulocyte/macrophage colony-stimulating factor.*

gout. A condition in which uric acid crystallizes from the blood.

graft failure. In a stem cell transplant, graft failure occurs when the donor stem cells are unable to take hold in the recipient.

graft-versus-host disease. A condition in which donated stem cells in an allogeneic transplant attack the recipient's body.

graft-versus-lymphoma effect. A condition in which donated stem cells in an allogeneic transplant attack and help eliminate any residual lymphoma cells.

graft-versus-tumor effect. See *graft-versus-lymphoma effect.*

granulocyte. A member of the class of white blood cells that includes neutrophils, eosinophils, and basophils.

granulocyte colony-stimulating factor (G-CSF; also known as filgrastim [brand name: Neupogen] and pegfilgrastim [brand name: Neulasta], which is a long-acting form). A growth factor.

granulocyte/macrophage colony-stimulating factor (GM-CSF; also known as sargramostrim [brand name: Leukine]). A growth factor.

growth factors. Chemical messengers that stimulate cells to grow, differentiate, or reproduce (or some combination thereof).

hairy cell leukemia. An indolent lymphoid malignancy.

half-life. The amount of time it takes a given radioisotope to decay by half.

Hashimoto thyroiditis. An autoimmune disease.

Helicobacter pylori. A kind of bacteria that live in the stomach, which are associated with the development of ulcers as well as of gastric mucosal-associated lymphoid tissue (MALT) lymphomas and other stomach cancers.

helper T cell. A class of T lymphocytes.

hematologist. A physician who specializes in diseases of the blood.

hematopoiesis. The process of making blood cells.

hemoglobin. The red iron-bearing pigment that carries oxygen through blood.

hemolytic anemia. A form of anemia associated with the destruction of red blood cells.

hepatitis C virus. A virus that may be associated with the pathogenesis of some forms of lymphoma.

herpesviruses. A class of viruses, some members of which are associated with the pathogenesis of some types of lymphoma.

herpes zoster. Shingles, a blistering rash caused by the same virus that causes chickenpox; may occur in people who are immunosuppressed.

HHV8. See *human herpes virus 8.*

high-grade. Refers to rapidly progressing forms of lymphoma.

histology. The microscopic appearance of a tissue.

HIV. See *human immunodeficiency virus.*

HLA. See *human leukocyte antigens.*

Hodgkin's disease. See *Hodgkin lymphoma.*

Hodgkin lymphoma (also called Hodgkin's disease or Hodgkin's lymphoma). Those forms of lymphoma that are characterized by the appearance of Reed-Sternberg cells in a background of nonmalignant inflammatory cells.

home. When referring to lymphocytes, the tendency to return to a particular tissue.

HTLV-I. See *human T cell lymphotropic virus 1.*

human herpes virus 8 (HHV8). A virus that is associated with a rare form of lymphoma called primary effusion lymphoma.

human immunodeficiency virus (HIV). The retrovirus that causes AIDS, an immunodeficiency disease that is associated with an increased likelihood of developing various aggressive B cell lymphomas.

human leukocyte antigens (HLAs). The human cell surface proteins that allow T cells to recognize other cells as "self" or "not-self"; see *major histocompatibility complex.*

human T cell lymphotropic virus I (HTLV-I). A retrovirus that is associated with the development of adult T cell leukemia/lymphoma.

humoral immune system. The branch of the immune system in which immunity can be transferred from one individual to another through antibodies in the serum.

hydroxydaunomycin. See *Adriamycin.*

hypercalcemia. A condition in which the blood calcium level is elevated.

hyperpigmentation. An abnormal increase in skin coloring.

hypogammaglobulinemia. Having reduced levels of circulating antibodies.

hypothalamus. The region of the brain that controls the autonomic nervous system.

hypothyroid. Having suboptimal levels of thyroid hormone.

idarubicin (brand name, Idamycin). An antineoplastic drug used in treating lymphoma that is classified as an anthracycline.

ifosfamide (brand name, IFEX). An antineoplastic drug used in treating lymphoma that is classified as an alkylating agent.

IL-2. See *interleukin-2*.

immune surveillance hypothesis of cancer. The idea that cancers frequently arise spontaneously but are kept in check through the normal functioning of the immune system.

immune system. The tissues, cells, and molecules whose function it is to protect against disease.

immunocompromised. A condition in which the function of the immune system is weakened, so that an individual is at increased risk of disease.

immunofluorescence. A histological technique in which proteins are identified by means of specific antibodies to which a glowing molecule has been attached.

immunoglobulin. A member of the class of proteins that can function as antibodies in the immune response.

immunohistochemistry. A histological technique in which proteins are identified by means of specific antibodies labeled with a colored molecule.

immunological therapies. See *immunotherapies*.

immunophenotype. The repertoire of proteins displayed on a cell's surface, as determined by the particular set of monoclonal antibodies that bind to that cell.

immunopoiesis. The stage of B cell development that takes place after a mature B cell encounters antigen.

immunotherapies. Approaches to treating disease that involve using elements of the immune system (such as antibodies) and/or recruiting an immune response.

indolent. Indolent lymphomas are the low-grade slowly progressing diseases in which even someone who remained untreated would be expected to survive for years after diagnosis.

induction phase. With therapies that involve the sequential administration of distinct chemotherapy regimens, the induction phase is the first and is given with the aim of achieving a complete remission.

inflammatory T cells. The class of helper T cells whose job it is to activate macrophages.

innate immune responses. The nonspecific defenses that we are born with; white cells that participate in the innate immune response include granulocytes, macrophages, and natural killer cells, whereas B cells and T cells are involved in the adaptive immune response.

interferons. A class of antiviral cytokines, Interferon alpha promotes increased expression of MHC I proteins (see *major histocompatibility complex*).

interleukins. The class of cytokines produced by white blood cells.

interleukin-2 (IL-2). T cell growth factor, a cytokine that is produced by T cells and also stimulates T cells to proliferate.

intermediate-grade lymphoma. Lymphoma that progresses relatively quickly, so that someone who remained untreated would be expected to survive only months to a few years after diagnosis.

interstitial fluid. The fluid that surrounds your cells.

intestinal T cell lymphoma. See *enteropathy-type T cell lymphoma*.

intrathecal chemotherapy. Delivery of antineoplastic drugs into the cerebrospinal fluid, which bathes the brain and spinal cord.

intravenous. Refers to delivery of a substance into a vein.

in vitro. Outside the body, literally, "in glass."

involuntary. Refers to those aspects of bodily function over which we lack conscious control, such as blood pressure or digestion.

involved field radiation. External beam radiation delivered to known sites of disease.

isotopes. Alternate forms of an element in which the atoms differ slightly in weight.

jaundice. Yellowing of the skin and the whites of the eyes caused by liver malfunction.

Kaposi sarcoma herpes virus (KSHV). See *human herpes virus 8.*

L&H cell (lymphocytic and histiocytic cell; informally called a popcorn cell). The malignant cell in the nodular lymphocyte predominant form of Hodgkin lymphoma.

laparoscopy. A minimally invasive surgical procedure performed through very small abdominal incisions that involves the insertion of a laparascope, a very thin lighted tube with a camera to allow visualization.

laparotomy. A surgical procedure that involves making an incision in the abdominal wall.

large cell, immunoblastic. A high-grade form of non-Hodgkin lymphoma (as defined by the Working Formulation; some would dispute the distinction from diffuse large cell lymphoma, which the Working Formulation defines as intermediate grade).

large, granular lymphocytes. Natural killer cells.

LDH (lactate dehydrogenase or lactic dehydrogenase). An enzyme normally found inside cells that is released into the blood when cells are damaged; note that LDH has nothing to do with LDL, which refers to a form in which cholesterol is carried through the blood.

leukemia. Forms of cancer of the white blood cells or their precursors that involve cells found in the bone marrow and circulating in the blood in preference to cells found in lymph nodes; there is considerable overlap between lymphoma and the lymphoid leukemias.

leukocytes. White blood cells.

Lhermitte syndrome. An unusual complication of radiation therapy in which you develop a tingling or "electric" sensation in your legs and feet after bending your neck.

ligand. A molecule that binds specifically to another (usually larger) molecule such as a receptor.

lipids. Substances like fats and oils.

localized disease. Lymphoma that is localized to a particular region rather than spread throughout the body.

lomustine (brand name, CeeNU). An antineoplastic drug used to treat lymphoma that is classified as an alkylating agent.

low-grade. See *indolent.*

lumbar puncture. Spinal tap, insertion of a needle into the cerebrospinal fluid in the lumbar region of the lower back.

lymph. The clear fluid that is reclaimed from the extracellular (or interstitial) fluid and returned to the circulatory system by way of the vesicles of the lymphatic system.

lymphadenopathy. Enlarged lymph nodes.

lymphangiogram. A technique in which the lower portions of the lymphatic system are visualized by means of a dye.

lymphatic system. The system of interconnected vesicles that return interstitial fluid to the blood, together with the lymph nodes and associated lymphoid tissues, such as Peyer's patches in the gut, the tonsils, and the thymus.

lymph nodes. Small bean-shaped organs found at junctions in the lymphatic system; one of the peripheral lymphoid structures where lymphocytes are activated.

lymphoblastic lymphoma. A very aggressive form of non-Hodgkin lymphoma in which the malignant cells resemble the large, rapidly dividing precursor lymphocytes found at an early stage of development.

lymphoblasts. Large rapidly dividing precursor lymphocytes from an early stage of development.

lymphocyte. A class of white blood cells of which the T cells and the B cells are specialized to recognize and respond to antigen in the adaptive immune response; lymphocytes circulate through the blood and lymphatic system and are also found throughout bodily tissues.

lymphocyte-depleted. A form of classical Hodgkin lymphoma.

lymphocyte-rich. A form of classical Hodgkin lymphoma.

lymphocytopenia. Abnormally low levels of circulating lymphocytes.

lymphocytosis. Abnormally high levels of circulating lymphocytes.

lymphoid. Pertaining to lymphocytes, lymph, or lymphatic tissues.

lymphoid follicle. Clusters of B cells found within a lymph node or the spleen.

lymphoplasmacytic lymphoma (LPL). An indolent form of lymphoma in which the malignant cells correspond to B cells at a late state of development.

macrobiotic diet. A diet that emphasizes whole grains, beans, and certain vegetables.

macrophages. The "big eaters," a class of cells involved in the innate immune response.

magic bullet therapies. Highly directed therapies that take aim at the peculiarities of diseased cells and leave healthy cells intact.

magnetic resonance imaging (MRI; also known as nuclear magnetic resonance [NMR]). A noninvasive procedure by which internal structures can be visualized.

maintenance phase. With therapies that involve the sequential administration of distinct chemotherapy regimens, the maintenance phase is the last and is given to prevent recurrence of the disease.

major histocompatibility complex (MHC). A group of proteins found on the cell surface that are used to present antigen to T cells; it is the MHC proteins that constitute the human leukocyte antigens that must be matched in an allogeneic stem cell transplant.

malignant. Cancerous.

MALT. See *mucosal-associated lymphoid tissue.*

MALT lymphoma. See *extranodal marginal zone B cell lymphoma of mucosal-associated lymphoid tissue.*

mantle cell lymphoma (MCL). A form of non-Hodgkin lymphoma in which the malignant cells resemble the cells found in the mantle zone of lymphoid follicles; it has some features of indolent disease and some features of aggressive disease.

mantle field. Radiation field that encompasses all the major lymph node regions found above the diaphragm.

mantle zone. The region that rings a lymphoid follicle; the cells in the mantle zone are B cells, which, at this stage in development, are called mantle cells.

MAO. See *monoamine oxidase.*

marginal zone. The area surrounding the mantle zones in spleen and mucosal-associated lymphoid tissues. Marginal zone–type cells are also found in the mantle zones of lymph nodes, but in lymph nodes the marginal zone doesn't constitute a distinct region surrounding the follicle.

marginal zone lymphoma (MZL). Indolent forms of non-Hodgkin lymphoma in which the malignant cells resemble marginal zone cells.

mast cell. A cell type related to the basophil that is found throughout the body.

matched, unrelated donor (MUD) transplant. An allogeneic transplant in which the donor is unrelated to the recipient but has human leukocyte antigens that are compatible with those of the recipient.

MCH. See *mean corpuscular hemoglobin.*

MCV. See *mean corpuscular volume.*

mean corpuscular hemoglobin (MCH). The average amount of hemoglobin in each red cell.

mean corpuscular volume (MCV). The average size of each red cell.

mechlorethamine (brand name, Mustargen). An antineoplastic drug used in treating lymphoma that is classified as an alkylating agent.

mediastinal large B cell lymphoma (also known as primary mediastinal large B cell lymphoma). A type of diffuse large cell lymphoma in which the disease arises in the anterior mediastinum, likely from a rare type of B cell found in the thymus.

mediastinum. The region in the center of the chest behind the breastbone and between the lungs.

medullary cord. Lymphoid tissue found in the central region of a lymph node.

megakaryocytes. The cells that give rise to platelets.

melphalan (brand name, Alkeran). An antineoplastic drug used in treating lymphoma that is classified as an alkylating agent.

memory cells. The population of lymphocytes that persist following exposure to a particular antigen so that the immune response is faster and more effective the next time that antigen is encountered.

mesna (sodium 2-mercaptoethane sulfonate; brand names, Mesnex, Uromitexan). A drug that binds to the toxic by-products of cyclophosphamide and ifosfamide metabolism and prevents them from injuring the bladder wall.

messenger RNA (mRNA). RNA that specifies the amino acid sequence for a particular protein.

methotrexate. An antineoplastic drug used in treating lymphoma that is classified as an antimetabolite.

methylprednisolone. A glucocorticoid.

MHC. See *major histocompatibility complex.*

β_2**-microglobulin.** A protein associated with the major compatibility complex that is elevated in most forms of lymphoma and can therefore serve as a marker for the extent of disease.

mineralocorticoid. A corticosteroid that regulates the handling of substances like sodium, potassium, and water.

minimal residual disease. The presence of abnormal DNA in someone in a complete clinical remission.

mini transplant. An informal name for a non-myeloablative or reduced-intensity stem cell transplant.

mitosis. The phase during the cell cycle when a cell divides.

mitotic spindles. Subcellular structures that pull the chromosomes apart during mitosis.

mitoxantrone (brand name, Novantrone). An antineoplastic drug used in treating lymphoma that is classified as an anthracycline.

mixed cellularity. A form of classical Hodgkin lymphoma.

monoamine oxidase (MAO). An enzyme that breaks down a class of compounds called monoamines.

monoclonal antibodies. Antibodies produced by a single clone of B lymphocytes that are therefore directed against one particular antigenic determinant.

monoclonal spike. Greatly increased levels of the particular immunoglobulin made by a given B cell (or plasma cell) clone.

monocytes. A class of white blood cells.

monocytoid B cell lymphoma. An indolent form of non-Hodgkin lymphoma (may be used to refer to the nodal form of marginal zone lymphoma).

monocytosis. A condition in which there are excess circulating monocytes.

morphology. The structure of an organism, a tissue, or a cell.

MRI. See *magnetic resonance imaging.*

mucosal-associated lymphoid tissue (MALT). Lymphoid tissue associated with the mucous membranes that line such organs as the gut and the lungs.

MUD transplant. See *matched, unrelated donor transplant.*

multiple myeloma. Cancer in which the malignant cell resembles a plasma cell.

mutation. A change in the genome, which can lead to a change in the protein that the improperly copied gene codes for.

mycosis fungoides/Sézary syndrome. A form of T cell lymphoma that affects the skin (Sézary syndrome refers to mycosis fungoides in which abnormal cells are found circulating in the blood).

myelodysplastic syndrome. A condition of ineffectual bone marrow that sometimes occurs in people who have undergone an autologous stem cell transplant.

myeloid. Refers to those white cells that are not lymphocytes.

nadir. The lowest white cell count that occurs after receiving chemotherapy.

naive cell. A lymphocyte that has not yet encountered its specific antigen.

natural killer cells (NK cells) A class of lymphocytes that are neither T cells nor B cells and that participate in the innate immune response.

negative selection. (1) The process during lymphocyte maturation by which lymphocytes that recognize normal self-antigen are eliminated; (2) the use of monoclonal antibodies that recognize antigens found on lymphoma cells to destroy those cells in stem cells harvested for an autologous transplant.

nervous system. The brain, spinal cord, peripheral nerves, and ganglia.

neurotransmitters. Chemical messengers that transmit information between nerve cells.

neutropenia. A condition in which there are too few circulating neutrophils.

neutrophil. A type of white blood cell.

neutrophilia. A condition in which there are excess circulating neutrophils.

NHL. See *non-Hodgkin lymphoma.*

night sweats. When drenching, one of the Ann Arbor "B" symptoms.

nitrogen mustards. A group of alkylating agents that include cyclophosphamide, ifosfamide, mechlorethamine, and chlorambucil.

NMR (nuclear magnetic resonance). See *MRI.*

nodal. Pertaining to a lymph node or nodes.

nodal marginal zone B cell lymphoma. An indolent form of non-Hodgkin lymphoma closely related to mucosal-associated lymphoid tissue (MALT) lymphomas but found in lymph nodes; sometimes called monocytoid B cell lymphoma.

nodular lymphocyte predominant. The form of Hodgkin lymphoma that is not classical Hodgkin lymphoma; it is characterized by the appearance of L&H, or popcorn, cells, rather than by classic Reed-Sternberg cells. Many oncologists think that it may actually be a form of non-Hodgkin lymphoma.

nodular sclerosis. A form of classical Hodgkin lymphoma.

nodule. Another name for a follicle.

moncontiguous. Not touching.

non-Hodgkin lymphoma (NHL). Those forms of lymphoma that are not classified as Hodgkin lymphoma.

non-myeloablative transplant. A form of stem cell transplant in which the recipient's bone marrow is not first destroyed.

nuclear medicine. The branch of medicine that involves the use of radioisotopes for diagnostic or therapeutic purposes.

nucleic acids. DNA and RNA.

nucleotides. The individual units that make up the DNA and RNA polymers; many antimetabolite drugs consist of abnormal nucleotides.

nucleus. The large organelle that contains the genome.

Ommaya reservoir. An implantable device used to deliver medication into the cerebrospinal fluid.

oncologist. A physician who specializes in treating people with cancer.

oophoropexy. A surgical procedure in which the ovaries are moved closer to the uterus.

organelles. Cellular "organs," subcellular structures that are specialized to carry out a particular function.

osteoblasts. The cells that make bone.

osteoclasts. The cells that resorb bone (osteoclasts are a type of macrophage).

p53. A protein that acts as a tumor suppressor whose loss or mutation is associated with many forms of cancer.

palliative. Treatment that is meant to alleviate the symptoms of a disease but not to cure it.

partial remission. A remission in which the symptoms of lymphoma recede but some clinical evidence of disease remains.

passive immunization. Injection of antibody into someone to elicit an immune response that does not depend on lymphocyte proliferation and therefore does not lead to the generation of memory cells.

pathogen. An organism that causes disease, such as a bacterium, virus, or fungus.

pathogenic. Causing disease.

pathognomonic. Something that is so decisively characteristic of a particular disease that its presence is diagnostic for that disease.

pathologist. Physician who specializes in identifying disease on the basis of the appearance and molecular characteristics of cells and tissues viewed under a microscope.

PCR. See *polymerase chain reaction.*

pentamidine (brand names, Pentam 300, NebuPent [inhaled pentamidine]). An antibiotic used to treat various protozoal and fungal infections including *pneumocystis carinii.*

peripheral blood stem cell harvest. A procedure in which stem cells for a stem cell transplant are isolated from those circulating in the blood.

peripheral neuropathy. Damage to nerve cells found outside the central nervous system.

permanent section. Tissue prepared for microscopic examination in such a way that it will last indefinitely; permanent sections provide better preservation of cellular structures than do frozen sections (which are more rapidly prepared).

PET scan. See *positron emission tomography.*

petechiae. Tiny purple spots that may appear on the skin of people who have low levels of platelets.

Peyer's patches. Areas of lymphoid tissue found in the small intestine.

phagocytes. Eater cells.

plasma. The fluid portion of blood that is left after the cells have been removed.

plasma cells. The fully differentiated mature form of B cells, whose job it is to secrete antibody.

platelets (also called thrombocytes). Cellular structures found in blood that are involved in clotting.

pluripotent stem cell. A precursor cell that can differentiate in one of many possible directions.

pneumocystis carinii. A protozoal or fungal infection commonly found in people who are immunosuppressed.

polyclonal activator. A substance that can activate many lymphocytes and stimulate them to divide, not just those that specifically recognize it.

polyclonal mitogen. A substance that can activate many lymphocytes and stimulate them to divide, not just those that specifically recognize it.

polymer. A long molecule that consists of many repeating subunits (monomers) strung together.

polymerase chain reaction (PCR). A technique whereby tiny amounts of DNA or RNA can be specifically identified.

polymorphs (or polymorphonuclear leukocytes). The class of white blood cells that includes neutrophils, eosinophils, and basophils.

popcorn cell. See *L&H cell.*

port. (1) An implanted device through which blood can be withdrawn or medications administered; (2) the exact region on the skin where the radiation beam touches the body.

positron emission tomography (PET scan). A method for imaging internal structures or tissues on the basis of their metabolic activity.

precursor B lymphoblastic leukemia/lymphoma. A very aggressive form of non-Hodgkin lymphoma.

precursor T lymphoblastic leukemia/lymphoma. A very aggressive form of non-Hodgkin lymphoma.

prednisone. A corticosteroid with anti-inflammatory properties used in various regimens to treat lymphoma.

primary effusion lymphoma (PEL). A rare form of non-Hodgkin lymphoma associated with human herpes virus 8 infection and usually HIV and Epstein-Barr virus infection as well.

primary lymphoid follicle. A follicle in which the B cells are naive.

primary lymphoid organs. The bone marrow and thymus—the sites in which lymphocytes develop.

primary mediastinal large B cell lymphoma. See *mediastinal large B cell lymphoma.*

procarbazine (brand name, Matulane). An antineoplastic drug used in treating lymphoma that is classified as an alkylating agent.

progenitor cells. "Ancestor" cells that give rise to more specialized cell types.

promoter. A substance that increases the rate of cell division and therefore the likelihood that cancer will develop in a tissue that has been exposed to a carcinogen.

prophylactic. Preventative.

protein. One of the classes of large molecules of which living things are composed.

pruritis. Severe, intense itching.

psoralens plus ultraviolet A. See *PUVA.*

purge. To treat stem cells harvested for an autologous transplant so as to rid them of even minimal residual disease.

purines. One of the two classes of nitrogenous bases used in making nucleic acids.

PUVA (psoralens plus ultraviolet A). A treatment combining substances that make cells sensitive to light with treatment with long-wavelength ultraviolet light.

pyrimidines. One of the two classes of nitrogenous bases used in making nucleic acids.

radiation field. The area of the body that is exposed to the radiation beam.

radiation port. The exact region on the skin where the radiation beam touches the body.

radiation therapy. The use of high-energy radiation, such as X-rays or gamma rays, to treat disease.

radioactive decay. The process in which a radioisotope becomes a different substance by giving off radiation.

radioisotope. An unstable isotope that gives off radiation as it undergoes radioactive decay to become another substance.

R-CHOP (*Rituxan plus cyclophosphamide, hydroxydaunomycin, Oncovin, prednisone*). The combination of CHOP chemotherapy with the monoclonal antibody rituximab, now the most common initial treatment for aggressive B cell lymphoma.

REAL (*Revised European-American Lymphoma*) classification. System for classifying lymphoma and related diseases.

receptor. A protein on a cell surface that is specifically recognized and bound by another substance; binding of a ligand to its receptor generally triggers some sort of response in the recipient cell.

Reed-Sternberg cells. The malignant cells that characterize classical Hodgkin lymphoma.

regulatory region. The part of the gene that does not encode a protein but instead controls how much and under what circumstances that protein is made.

regulatory T cells. The class of T lymphocytes that inhibit the activity of other cells in the immune system.

relapse. The recurrence of disease in someone who has experienced a remission.

remission. A condition in which the physical evidence of disease goes away.

retrovirus. A class of viruses in which the genetic material consists of RNA and the enzyme reverse transcriptase is used to transcribe viral RNA into DNA in the infected cell.

ribonucleic acid. See *RNA.*

Richter syndrome. A condition in which small lymphocytic lymphoma (SLL), an indolent disease, changes into an aggressive large cell form of non-Hodgkin lymphoma.

rituximab (brand name, Rituxan). A monoclonal antibody directed against the B cell protein CD20; often used as solo therapy against indolent B cell lymphomas or combined with chemotherapy to treat aggressive B cell lymphomas.

RNA (ribonucleic acid). A nucleic acid.

RNA polymerase. The enzyme that transcribes DNA into RNA.

salvage therapies. Therapies aimed at saving someone who has not been cured by his or her initial treatment.

secondary lymphoid follicle. The specialized region of a lymph node where activated B cells proliferate.

secondary (or peripheral) lymphoid organs. Structures such as lymph nodes, Peyer's patches, and the spleen in which lymphocytes encounter antigen and become activated to generate an immune response.

self-antigen. A substance that is capable of eliciting an immune response if it is injected into another organism but that does not elicit an immune response from its own parent organism.

sense strand. The DNA strand that corresponds to the messenger RNA that encodes a protein.

serotonin. A neurotransmitter.

serum protein electrophoresis (SPEP). A blood test that can uncover the existence of abnormal production of immunoglobulins.

simian virus 40 (SV40). A virus that may be associated with some forms of non-Hodgkin lymphoma.

6-mercaptopurine (brand name, Purinethol). An antineoplastic drug used in treating lymphoma that is classified as an antimetabolite.

Sjögren syndrome. An autoimmune disease.

SLL. See *small lymphocytic lymphoma.*

small cleaved cells. Cells that resemble centrocytes, which are a class of B cells found in the germinal center; follicular lymphomas are graded by the relative number of small cleaved cells versus large cells.

small lymphocytic lymphoma (SLL). An indolent form of non-Hodgkin lymphoma closely related (some would say identical) to chronic lymphocytic leukemia.

smudge cell. Fragile malignant cells found in small lymphocytic lymphoma (SLL) and chronic lymphocytic leukemia (CLL) that break down during preparation of a microscope slide to view the blood cells.

spade field. The radiation field that includes the spleen and the paraaortic lymph nodes.

SPEP. See *serum protein electrophoresis.*

spleen. An organ that participates in both the cardiovascular and lymphatic systems, the spleen gets rid of red blood cells that are no longer functional and contains lymphoid tissue (white pulp) that responds to bloodborne antigens.

splenectomy. A surgical procedure in which the spleen is removed; formerly performed frequently as part of the staging of Hodgkin lymphoma but now performed only rarely.

splenic marginal zone lymphoma. An indolent form of non-Hodgkin lymphoma.

spontaneous remission. A remission that takes place for no known reason.

Stage I. Lymphoma that is confined to a single lymphatic region.

Stage II. Lymphoma that is found in two or more lymphatic regions that are both on the same side of the diaphragm.

Stage III. Lymphoma that is found on both sides of the diaphragm.

Stage IV. Lymphoma that is spread throughout one or more extralymphatic organs.

staging. The process of determining how far lymphoma has spread throughout your body.

stem cell transplant. A procedure in which either the patient's or a donor's stem cell transplants are harvested so that they can be replaced after exposure to high-dosage therapy has destroyed the bone marrow (except see *non-myeloablative transplant*).

subtotal nodal irradiation. Radiation delivered to the mantle field and the spade field.

sulfamethoxazole-trimethoprim. An antibiotic combination.

superior vena cava. The large blood vessel that returns blood from the head, neck, arms, and upper chest to the heart.

supportive therapy. Treatments that are not meant to directly attack the cancer but to help someone tolerate the side effects of antineoplastic therapy.

SV40. See *simian virus 40.*

sympathetic nervous system. The part of the nervous system that mediates the fight or flight response.

syngeneic transplant. A form of stem cell transplant in which the donor is the recipient's twin.

systemic. Affecting the whole body; systemic symptoms are those, like fever or weight loss, that are not confined to a particular organ or region of the body; systemic therapies, like chemotherapy, are treatments that affect the whole body rather than being delivered locally.

tacrolimus (brand name, Prograf). An immunosuppressive drug.

TBI. See *total body irradiation.*

T cells. See *T lymphocytes.*

T-cell/histiocyte-rich B cell lymphoma. A variant form of diffuse large cell lymphoma.

T cell receptor. The cell surface proteins that allow T cells to recognize antigen or to identify other cells as "self" or "foreign."

template strand. The strand of DNA that is copied during transcription.

thrombocytes. See *platelets.*

thrombocytopenia. A condition in which there are too few platelets.

thymocytes. Young T cells during the stage that they are being educated in the thymus.

thymus. A lymphoid organ in the upper central portion of the chest in which T cell development takes place.

thymus-independent antigens. Antigens that can activate B cells to produce antibody even in the absence of T cells.

thyroxine. A hormone produced by the thyroid.

tingible body macrophages. Macrophages found in the germinal center that have eaten B lymphocytes that committed suicide.

tissue-typed. Tested for which of the human leukocyte antigens are present so that a suitable match for allogeneic stem cell transplant can be identified (refers to both potential donors and potential recipients).

T lymphoblastic lymphoma. A very aggressive form of non-Hodgkin lymphoma.

T lymphocytes (also called T cells). The class of cells that develop in the thymus and are responsible for the cellular (as opposed to humoral) limb of the adaptive immune response.

tonsils. Lymphoid structures found on either side of the throat.

topoisomerase II. An enzyme involved in DNA replication and RNA transcription.

total body irradiation (TBI). Radiation therapy delivered to the entire body.

total nodal irradiation. Radiation delivered to the mantle field, the spade field, and lymph nodes in the groin and pelvis.

transcription. The process of copying DNA into RNA.

transcription factors. Proteins that bind to DNA and help regulate transcription.

translation. The process of making a protein based on a messenger RNA sequence.

translocation. A mutation in which parts of two chromosomes become switched with each other.

trisomy. A chromosomal abnormality in which there are three copies of any given chromosome rather than the normal two copies.

tubulin. A protein that makes up microtubules, subcellular structures that play a role both in cell division and in ferrying substances down the length of nerve cells.

tumor lysis syndrome. A condition in which massive death of cancer cells leads to excess levels of uric acid in the blood.

tumor suppressor genes. Genes such as *p53* whose protein products keep damaged, potentially malignant, cells from progressing through the cell cycle.

tumors. Lumps.

2-chlorodeoxyadenosine (also known as cladribine; brand name, Leustatin). An antineoplastic drug used in treating lymphoma that is classified as an antimetabolite.

umbilical cord blood transplants. Stem cell transplants in which the source of the stem cell is blood from the umbilical cords of newborns.

unconventional therapies. Therapies that are outside the mainstream of conventional medical care.

vaccination. Exposure to a nondangerous form of an antigen associated with a particular pathogen or tumor cell with the intention of eliciting an immune response against that antigen and thereby protecting the individual from the illness caused by that pathogen or tumor cell.

vaccines. Preparations of antigen (or dead or weakened pathogens) used to elicit a protective immune response.

valacyclovir (brand name, Valtrex). An antiviral drug.

variable region. The portion of an antibody that recognizes its particular antigen.

veno-occlusive disease. A possible complication of a stem cell transplant in which blood flow out of the liver is impeded.

ventricles. The fluid-filled cavities found inside the brain.

very aggressive disease. Rapidly progressing but curable forms of lymphoma in which someone who remained untreated would be expected to survive for weeks or months after diagnosis.

vinblastine (brand name, Velban). An antineoplastic drug used to treat lymphoma that is classified as an antimitotic.

vinca alkaloids. Vincristine and vinblastine; antineoplastic drugs isolated from the Madagascar periwinkle.

vincristine (brand name, Oncovin). An antineoplastic drug used to treat lymphoma that is classified as an antimitotic.

viscera. Internal organs.

Waldenström's macroglobulinemia. A condition in which excess secretion of immunoglobulin leads to thickening of the blood.

Waldeyer's ring. The lymphoid tissues around the back of the mouth and the throat.

WHO classification system. World Health Organization classification of tumors of hematopoietic and lymphoid tissues; currently accepted system for classifying lymphoma, as well as other lymphoid and myeloid neoplasms.

Working Formulation classification system. A lymphoma classification system originally designed to "translate" between several different classification systems then in use; it categorizes lymphoma on the basis of histological appearance into ten main groups, which are classified as indolent, aggressive, or very aggressive disease.

X-rays. A form of electromagnetic radiation that can pass through materials opaque to visible light.

Zevalin (generic name, ibritumomab tiuxetan). A radiolabeled monoclonal antibody used to treat B cell lymphoma.

Zinecard (generic name, dexrazoxane). A drug that can protect against the cardiotoxic effects of Adriamycin; it is sometimes used when it is necessary to give Adriamycin-containing therapies repeatedly so that the cumulative dose exceeds that to which people are generally exposed.

Index

abdominal pain, 18

ABVD (combination chemotherapy), 95, 109, 116

Achong, Bert, 310

active immunization, 163

acupressure, 86, 228

acupuncture, 86, 228

acute lymphoblastic leukemia, 107, 315

acyclovir, 192

adenine, 237, 239

adenoids, 256

adenosine, 112

Adriamycin ("Big Red," doxorubicin, hydroxy-daunomycin), 55, 70, 95, 96, 103, 117

  heart damage associated with, 54, 90, 201

  for lymphoblastic lymphoma, 107

  side effects of, 109–11

adult T cell leukemia/lymphoma (ATLL), 36, 104, 246, 315

  AZT for, 109

  and HTLV-I, 109, 162, 315, 316, 344

Agent Orange, 349

AIDS, lymphomas associated with, 109, 309, 311, 345–46

alcohol

  in mouthwashes, 136

  and nausea associated with chemotherapy, 86

  and procarbazine, 122

alemtuzumab. *See* CAMPATHIH

alendronate (Fosamax), 121

alkaline phosphatase, 53, 54

alkylating agents, 68, 69, 90

alkylation, 69

allopurinol, 43, 109, 153, 155, 156

alopecia. *See* hair loss

alternative therapies, 199

amino acid, 237

amphotericin, 191, 192

amplification (in DNA replication), 245

anaplastic large cell lymphoma (ALCL), 102, 316–17, 341

anemia, 36–37, 160

  and chemotherapy, 80

  fatigue associated with, 87–88

  hemolytic, 37

  iron deficiency, 37, 208

  and lymphoplasmacytic lymphoma, 298

  megaloblastic, 210

  microcytic hypochromic, 37

  following stem cell transplant, 185

  as symptom of lymphoma, 3–8, 20–21, 298

  symptoms of, 38

angiocentric lymphoma, 319

angiodysplasia, 6

angiogenesis, 168

central lines, 93

central nervous system (CNS), 27–28, 116

central nervous system (CNS) lymphoma, 94, 116, 120, 144, 315, 345, 346

centroblasts, 270–71, 272

centrocytes, 271, 272

cerebrospinal fluid, 28, 108

chemo brain, 89

chemotherapy

administering of, 91–94

for aggressive lymphomas, 103–25

and anemia, 37

birth control during, 82

blood cell levels during, 76–78

and "B" symptoms, 19

for Burkitt lymphoma, 108, 114

and the cell cycle, 243–44

combination, 91, 94–96, 100–102, 103–10

in combination with rituximab, 154–57

in combination with radiation therapy, 128, 129, 142–44

diet during, 78, 204

for Hodgkin lymphoma, 94–96

how it works, 67–68

for indolent lymphomas, 96–102, 104

by intravenous injection, 91–92

intrathecal, 94, 108, 116

and liver function, 42

for lymphoblastic lymphoma, 107–8, 119

and lymphocytopenia, 36

and MUGA scans, 54

neutropenia during, 78, 80, 122, 125

and neutrophils, 33, 77, 78, 108, 253

palliative, 67

phases of, 107

during pregnancy, 81–82

and reproductive organs, 81–82, 114

risk of infection during, 78–79

risk of leukemia with, 95, 113, 117

secondary malignancy associated with, 90

side effects of, 71–73; anemia, 80; bladder damage, 115; bone marrow suppression, 76–80, 109, 111, 112–13, 114, 115–16, 117, 118, 120, 122, 259; cognitive problems, 89; diarrhea, 76; fatigue, 86–88; fever, 111, 112; gastrointestinal problems, 120; hair loss,

73–74, 109–10, 111, 114, 118, 124; heart damage, 54–55, 110–11, 115; infertility, 81–82, 114, 118; joint pain, 122; kidney damage, 114, 120; liver damage, 120; long-term, 89–90; lung damage, 111, 112, 115, 117; mood changes, 122; mouth sores, 74–76, 109, 116, 120, 122, 125; nail ridges, 74; nausea and vomiting, 82–86, 109, 111, 114, 116, 117, 118, 122; nerve damage, 124; skin changes, 74, 111–12, 114, 122; weight gain associated with prednisone-containing regimens, 120–21

and stem cell transplants, 171–72, 183–84

chicken pox, 192

chimeric antibodies, 152

Chinese medicine, traditional, 227–28

chlorambucil, 69, 113

chlorpromazine, 84

CHOP (combination chemotherapy), 101, 103–6, 114, 121, 212

effectiveness of, 198

with radiation therapy, 143–44

See also R-CHOP

chromosomes, 238–39, 266. See also DNA

chronic lymphocytic leukemia (CLL), 294–96

cisplatin, 83, 90, 107, 113–14

cladribine (Leustatin, 2-CDA, 2-chlorodeoxy-adenosine), 36, 68, 100, 112–13

classical Hodgkin lymphoma, 322–24

cleaved cells, 286

clonal cell lines, 151–52. See also monoclonal antibodies

C-MOPP (combination chemotherapy), 100

CNS lymphoma. See central nervous system lymphoma

coding sequence, 238

cognitive problems, 89

cold sores, 192

colonoscopy, 6

colony-stimulating factors (CSFs), 79–80, 160–61, 184, 192, 259

combined modality treatment, 128, 142–44

compared with chemotherapy alone, 143–44

See also chemotherapy; radiation therapy

COMP, 114

complement, 149

complementary therapies, 196–97, 199–200

diet: as cancer preventative, 202–7; vitamin and mineral supplements, 205, 207–11

exercise, 201–2

lifestyle-oriented, 200–219

herbal medicine, 219–21; dosages of, 226–27; effectiveness of, 221–23; and the immune system, 223–26

physician consultation regarding, 200, 220–21, 229

psychosocial interventions, 213–19

scientific study of, 197–98

traditional Chinese medicine, 227–28

complete blood count, 31–39

computerized axial tomography scan. *See* CT scans

conditioning regimen (for stem cell transplants), 173, 183–84, 194

consolidation phase, 107

constipation, 124–25

cord blood stem cell transplants, 181

corticosteroids, 68, 71, 84, 108, 116, 188

cortisone cream, 102

cryoglobulins, 347

cryoprotectant, 179

CSFs. *See* colony-stimulating factors

CT scans, 22–23

abdominopelvic, 44–45

as diagnostic tool, 44–47, 55

and kidney function, 43

Curie, Marie, 48

Curie, Pierre, 48

cutaneous B cell lymphoma, 102

cutaneous follicle center lymphoma, 300

cutaneous T cell lymphoma, 18

CVP (combination chemotherapy), 100, 114

cyclophosphamide (Cytoxan), 69, 100, 103, 107

for Burkitt lymphoma, 108

side effects of, 114–15

cyclosporine, 188, 190, 192, 194

cystitis, 115

cytarabine (cytosine arabinoside), 68, 107, 108, 115–16, 120, 243

cytidine, 243

cytokines, 19, 20, 21, 71, 79, 254

and Ann Arbor "B" symptoms, 161

and graft-versus lymphoma effect, 190

and neutropenia, 33

and stem cells, 257–60

and T cells, 275

as used in lymphoma treatment, 160–63

cytomegalovirus infections, 192

cytometer, 26

cytoplasm, 235

cytosine, 237, 239, 243

cytosine arabinoside. *See* cytarabine

cytotoxic T cells, 255

Cytoxan. *See* cyclophosphamide

dacarbazine, 69, 95, 116

daunorubicin, 70, 107

deletion (chromosomal), 245, 265, 296

dendritic cells, 164–65, 276

dendritic cell vaccine, 164–65

denileukin diftitox (Ontak), 162

dental care. *See* oral hygiene

deoxyribonucleic acid. *See* DNA

dexamethasone, 71, 84, 100, 107, 116

Dexedrine, 88

dexrazoxane, 55

DHAP (combination chemotherapy), 107

diabetes, 121

diagnosis, lymphoma

biopsies, 22–25

blood work, 31–43

bone marrow biopsy, 26–27

goals of, 21–22

imaging techniques, 43–57

immunophenotyping, 25–26

lumbar puncture, 27–28

medical history, 28–29

physical examination, 29–31

diarrhea, 76, 137

diet

as cancer preventative, 202–7, 349–50

high-fiber, 203

macrobiotic, 206

while neutropenic, 78

as possible causative factor, 349–51

follicular mixed small and large cell lymphoma, 97, 299

follicular small cleaved cell lymphoma, 97, 299

formaldehyde, 24, 349

Fosamax. *See* alendronate

fractionated doses (of radiation), 132, 137

free radicals, 70, 111

frozen eggs, 81

frozen embryos, 81

frozen section, 24

frozen sperm, 81

fungal infections, 191

gallium, 50

gallium scans, 50–52

gamma globulin, 185

gamma rays (γ rays), 128, 159

ganciclovir, 192

gap phase, 242, 243

gastric lymphomas, 101, 352

gastroendoscopy, 6

gastrointestinal problems
    associated with chemotherapy, 120
    associated with radiation therapy, 137, 139

gastrointestinal tract
    bleeding from, 5–6
    and graft-versus-host disease, 187
    and the immune system, 251–52
    lymphoma in, 18, 302

gemcitabine (Gemzar, $2',2'$-difluorodeoxycytide), 117–18

Gemzar. *See* gemcitabine

Genasense, 167

gene expression, 165–66, 238, 333–34

genes, 238–39. *See also* DNA; mutations

genome, 236, 237

germinal center, 270

ginger tea, 220

ginseng, 228

globulins, 39–41

glucocorticoids, 33, 36, 71, 120, 216, 218

gluten enteropathy, 326

graft-versus-host disease, 174, 178, 181, 185, 194
    acute, 187, 274
    chronic, 187–88, 193

graft-versus-lymphoma effect, 174, 175, 190

granisetron, 84

granulocyte colony-stimulating factor (G-CSF), 80, 160, 259

granulocyte/macrophage colony-stimulating factor (GM-CSF), 80, 160

granulocytes, 252–54. *See also* basophils; eosinophils; neutrophils

Groshong catheter, 93

G3139, 167

guaiac test, 5

guanine, 237, 239

Haddow, Alexander, 310

hair loss
    as side effect of chemotherapy, 73–74, 109–10, 111, 114, 118, 124
    as side effect of radiation therapy, 136, 139

hairy cell leukemia, 36, 159

half-life, 48

Hashimoto thyroiditis, 302

heartburn, 139

heart damage
    as side effect of chemotherapy, 95, 110–11, 115, 201
    associated with radiation therapy, 54, 95, 111, 139–40, 201

Helicobacter pylori, 101, 161, 303, 352

helper T cells, 255, 267–69, 275

hematocrit, 6, 7, 36–38

hematopoiesis, 257–60

hematopoietic stem cells, 172, 257–60

hemoglobin, 7, 36, 37, 38, 208

heparin, 94

hepatitis C virus, 298, 346–47

herbal medicine, 219–21
    dosages of, 226–27
    effectiveness of, 221–23
    and the immune system, 223–26

herpes simplex, 192, 340

herpesviruses, 340–43

herpes zoster, 192, 340

hiccups, 136

Hickman catheter, 93

high blood pressure, 123

histiocytes, 255

histology, 24

HIV. *See* human immunodeficiency virus

HLAs. *See* human leukocyte antigens

Hodgkin lymphoma, 10, 18, 161, 273, 301
   and alcohol, 20
   classical, 322–24
   chemotherapy for, 94–96
   combined modality treatment for, 143
   as distinguished from non-Hodgkin lym-
      phoma, 320–21
   incidence of, 11
   nodular lymphocyte predominant, 322
   radiation treatment for, 129–31
   and Reed-Sternberg cells, 25, 322–23, 324
   resemblance of to other lymphomas, 308,
      317
   and small lymphocytic lymphoma, 296
   and T cell function, 21
   treatment of, 94–96
   types of, 321–22
   See also lymphoma

Hodgkin, Thomas, 203, 283–84

Hooke, Robert, 235

hormone-replacement therapy, 122

Hoxsey, Harry, 219

Hoxsey herbal therapy, 219, 225

HTLV-I, 109, 162, 315, 316, 344

human herpesvirus 8, 342–43

human immunodeficiency virus (HIV), 345–46

human leukocyte antigens (HLAs), 175–76,
   177, 179, 190, 274

human T cell lymphotropic virus I. *See*
   HTLV-I

humoral immune system, 148, 271

hydrocortisone, 120

hydroxydaunomycin. *See* Adriamycin

hydroxyurea, 107

hypercalcemia, 41–42

hyperfractionated doses (of radiation), 132

hyperpigmentation, 74

hypogammaglobulinemia, 41

hypothalamus, 215–16

hypothyroidism, 139

ibritumomab tiuxetan (Zevalin), 158

idarubicin, 70

ifosfamide, 69, 107, 115

imaging techniques. *See* bone scans; CT scans;
   gallium scans; MRI; MUGA scans;
   PET scans; radioisotopic scans; thallium
   scans; X-rays

immune responses, 252, 261, 346
   adaptive, 252, 255, 271, 279
   innate, 252, 279
   See also antibodies; immunoglobulin

immune surveillance hypothesis of cancer, 251

immune system, 250–51, 279–81
   deficiencies in, 334, 351–53
   and glucocorticoids, 71
   hematopoiesis, 257–60
   and herbal medicines, 223–26
   humoral, 148, 271
   and the lymphatic system, 256–57
   lymphocytes' role in, 255–56; B cells, 255,
     256, 260–71, 277, 278–79; natural killer
     (NK) cells, 255, 259, 279; T cells, 255,
     256, 271–77, 278, 279
   and lymphoma, 10, 21, 351–53
   overview of, 251–56

immunization. *See* vaccines

immunoblastic lymphomas, 104, 306, 346

immunofluorescence, 25, 26

immunoglobulin D, 266

immunoglobulin M, 266

immunoglobulins, 39–40, 150, 163–65, 260–61,
   266, 270
   and B cells, 261, 262–71
   constant region, 262
   in follicular lymphomas, 166
   following stem cell transplants, 185
   structure of, 265
   variable region, 262–63

immunohistochemistry, 25, 26, 288

immunological memory, 252

immunology, 148

immunophenotype, 25, 150, 288, 308

immunotherapies, 148. *See also* cytokines; monoclonal antibodies; vaccines

implanted ports, 93–94

induction phase, 107

infection
   chronic, 302

MCV (mean corpuscular volume), 38
mechlorethamine, 69, 95–96, 102, 118
mediastinal large B cell lymphoma, 307. *See also* primary mediastinal large B cell lymphoma
mediastinal masses, 17–18
meditation, 216, 217
medullary cord, 271
megakaryocytes, 80
megaloblastic anemia, 210
melanoma, 12
memory B cells, 157, 166, 271
memory T cells, 277
menopause, early, 121–22
mesna (2-mercaptoethanesulfonate sodium), 107
Metchnikoff, Elie, 255
methionine, 237
methotrexate, 68, 107, 188, 243
    for Burkitt lymphoma, 108
    for lymphoblastic lymphoma, 107, 108
    side effects of, 119–20
methylprednisolone, 71, 120
metoclopramide (Reglan), 85
MHC molecules, 161, 273–75, 279
microglia, 255
β$_2$ microglobulin, 41
microtubules, 70, 71, 72
Milstein, Cesar, 151, 152
MIME (combination chemotherapy), 107
mind-body interactions, 215–19
MINE (combination chemotherapy), 107
mineralocorticoids, 71
mini-transplants. *See* nonmyeloablative transplants
mitochondria, 235
mitosis, 70, 242–43, 267
mitotic spindles, 70, 71, 72, 242, 243
mitoxantrone, 70, 100, 107
mixed cellularity classical Hodgkin lymphoma, 323–24
monoamine oxidase (MAO), 122–23
monoclonal antibodies, 101, 103, 151–60
    with chemotherapy, 154–57
    effectiveness of, 152–53
    and purging of stem cells, 182–83

radioactively tagged, 158–60
    side effects of, 153, 157, 158–59
monoclonal spike, 40
monocytes, 32, 34, 35, 252, 254
monocytoid B cell lymphomas, 301, 352
monocytopenia, 35
monocytosis, 35
monomer, 237
mood changes with chemotherapy, 122
MOPP (combination chemotherapy), 95–96
MOPP-ABV (combination chemotherapy), 96
mouth sores, 74–76, 109, 116, 120, 122, 125
moxibustion, 228
MRI, 55–56
mucosal-associated lymphoid tissue (MALT), 101–2, 256, 301–3, 319
mucous membranes, 251–52, 256
MUD transplants. *See* matched, unrelated donor (MUD) transplants
MUGA scans, 54–55
multiple-gated cardiac blood pool (MUGA) scans, 54–55
multiple myeloma, 11, 343
mustard gas, 69
mutations, 226, 244–45; as factor in cancer, 234–35, 245–49
myc gene, 246–47, 306
mycosis fungoides, 36, 97, 153, 278, 312–14
    radiation therapy for, 131, 140–41
    staging system for, 329–30
    topical agents for, 102
myelodysplastic syndrome, 193
myelogenous leukemia, 193
myeloid progenitor cells, 260

nadir, 77
nail ridges, 74
naive B cells, 267, 280
National Marrow Donor Program, 176, 178
natural killer cell–derived lymphomas, 311–12, 315
natural killer (NK) cells, 255, 259, 277, 279
nausea and vomiting
    alternative therapies for, 85–86
    causes of during chemotherapy, 83
    drugs to combat, 82–83, 84–85

nausea and vomiting (*continued*)
  prevention of, 85–86
    as side effect of chemotherapy, 82–86, 109, 111, 114, 116, 117, 118, 122
    as side effect of radiation therapy, 133
    and stem cell transplants, 183–84
nerve damage, 124. *See also* peripheral neuropathy
Neulasta. *See* granulocyte colony-stimulating factor (G-CSF), 80
Neumega. *See* interleukin-11
Neupogen. *See* granulocyte colony-stimulating factor (G-CSF)
neurotoxicity, 122, 124
neurotransmitters, 83
neutropenia, 33, 35, 78, 80, 122, 125
neutrophilia, 33
neutrophils, 32, 33, 34, 117, 252–53
  during chemotherapy, 33, 77, 78, 108, 253, 259
  following stem cell transplants, 185–86, 191
NHL. *See* non-Hodgkin lymphomas
night sweats, 19–20
nitrogen mustards, 69
nitrosureas, 111
nodal marginal zone lymphomas (NMZL), 301, 302
nodular lymphocyte predominant Hodgkin lymphoma, 322
nodular sclerosis classical Hodgkin lymphoma, 323
nodules, 322
noncleaved cells, 286
non-Hodgkin lymphomas (NHL), 10, 18
  aggressive: chemotherapy for, 103–9; types of, 303–12, 314–20
  and B cell function, 21
  chemotherapy for, 103–25
  childhood, 328
  combined modality therapy for, 143
  as distinguished from Hodgkin lymphoma, 320–21
  and immunodeficiency, 351–53
  increase in incidence of, 11, 12, 337–38
  indolent, 16, 96–98; antibiotics for gastric, 101–2; chemotherapy for, 98–102; relapsed, 101; types of, 293–303, 312

prevalence of, 11–12
  See also lymphoma
nonlymphocytic leukemia, 90
nonmyeloablative stem cell transplants, 194–95
note taking, importance of, xxi
nuclear medicine, 48–49
nucleic acids, 235
nucleotides, sequences of, 237–38
nucleus, 236
nutrition during chemotherapy and radiation treatment, 203–5

oblimersen, 167
Ommaya reservoir, 94, 108
Oncovin. *See* vincristine
ondansetron, 84
Ontak. *See* denileukin diftitox
oophoropexy, 137
oprelvekin. *See* interleukin-11
oral hygiene
  during chemotherapy, 75
  during radiation therapy, 136
organ damage
  following stem cell transplant, 192
  See also bladder damage; heart damage; kidney damage; liver damage; lung damage
organelles, 235–36
osteoblasts, 42
osteoclasts, 42, 255
osteoporosis, 121–22, 193

paclitaxel, 70–71, 225
passive immunization, 163
pathogenic organisms, 251, 280
pathologist, 24
PBSCH. *See* peripheral blood stem cell harvest
PCR (polymerase chain reaction), 182
pegfilgrastim. *See* granulocyte colony-stimulating factor (G-CSF), 80
pelvic field, 130, 131
pentamidine, 191
pentostatin, 68
peripheral blood stem cell harvest (PBSCH), 178, 179–80, 181, 187

peripheral neuropathy, 117, 124

peripheral T cell lymphomas, 318

permanent section, 24

permanent venous access device, 93

perphenazine, 84

PET scans, 52–53

petechiae, 80

Peyer's patches, 256

p53 gene, 248, 311

phagocytes, 252, 254

photopheresis, 188

photosensitizers, 141

physical examination, 29–31

physician, patient's approach to, xx–xxiii

pilocarpine (Salagen), 136

plasma cells, 151–52, 255, 259, 280

plasma, 31, 261

plasmablasts, 271

platelets, 32

    during chemotherapy, 77

    following stem cell transplants, 185

pleural reaction, 8

pluripotent stem cells, 257–60

Pneumocystis carinii, 191, 345

podophyllin, 116

podophyllotoxin, 116–17

poke, 225

polyclonal activator, 225

polyclonal mitogen, 267

polymerase chain reaction (PCR), 182

polymorphonuclear leukocytes, 252–53

polymorphs, 252–53

popcorn cell, 322

Port-a-Cath, 93–94

ports. *See* implanted ports

positron emission tomography (PET) scans,
    52–53

post-thymic T cell lymphomas, 318–20

precursor B lymphoblastic leukemia/lym-
    phoblastic lymphoma, 304, 315

precursor T cell lymphoblastic leukemia/
    lymphoblastic lymphoma, 314–15

prednisone, 71, 95–96, 100, 103, 107, 116, 188

    for Burkitt lymphoma, 108

    for lymphoblastic lymphoma, 107

    side effects of, 120–22

pregnancy

    and chemotherapy, 81–82

    following radiation therapy, 137

primary effusion lymphoma (PEL), 307, 342,
    345–46

primary mediastinal large B cell lymphoma,
    18, 41, 165, 279, 307

procarbazine, 69, 95–96, 100, 122–23

prochlorperazine, 84, 85

professional antigen-presenting cells, 276

progenitor cell, 260

promoters (of cancerous mutations), 245

prophylactic therapy, 144

proteins, 25, 26, 150–51, 275

    and lymphoma classification, 290–92

    as part of cell structure, 235

    See also monoclonal antibodies

psoralens, 141, 142

psoralens plus ultraviolet A. *See* PUVA radia-
    tion therapy

psoriasis, 141

psychoactive chemicals, 215

psychological support, 213–15

pulmonary symptoms, 8–9

purging (of stem cells), 182–83

purines, 237

PUVA radiation therapy, 141–42, 188

pyrimidines, 237

radiation fields, 129–31, 135

radiation therapy, 36, 95, 96

    blocks used in, 132

    in combination with chemotherapy, 95, 128,
        129, 142–44

    extended field, 129

    and heart damage, 54

    for Hodgkin lymphoma, 129–31

    involved field, 129

    PUVA, 141–42

    secondary malignancy associated with, 140

    side effects of, 133–40; bladder irritation,
        137; bone marrow suppression, 136; de-
        layed, 139–40; esophageal irritation,
        136–37, 138; fatigue, 133; gastrointestinal
        irritation, 137, 139; hair loss, 136, 139;
        hiccups, 136; infertility, 137; nausea, 133;

Epstein-Barr virus, 189, 310, 319, 324, 336, 340–42, 346, 351
  hepatitis C, 298, 346–47
  herpesviruses, 340–43
  human herpesvirus 8, 342–43
  retroviruses, 343–46
  simian virus 40 (SV40), 347–48
visualization, 217
vitamin A, 207
vitamin B$_{12}$, 206
vitamin C, 208
vitamin D, 206, 207
vitamin E, 208
vitamin supplements, 205, 207–11
vitiligo, 141
vomiting. *See* nausea and vomiting

Waldenström's macroglobulinemia, 297
Waldyer's ring, 31
watch-and-wait, 99
Web sites, 13–14, 57, 169–70, 195, 332, 353
weight gain during prednisone-containing chemotherapy, 120–21

weight loss, 20
white blood cells, 252–55. *See also* immune system; neutrophils
white cell differential count, 32–36
  during chemotherapy, 77, 108
  nadir, 77
WHO classification system, 96, 97, 288–92
WHO-modified REAL classification system, 289
Working Formulation classification system, 96, 97, 284–87, 292
World Health Organization. *See* WHO classification system

X-rays, 43–44, 128, 131–32

yeast infections, 6–7
yogurt, 220, 221
yttrium, radioactive, 158, 159

Zevalin (ibritumomab tiuxetan), 158
zidovudine. *See* AZT
Zinecard, 55, 111